*Air*Veda

Ancient & New Medical Wisdom
Digestion & Gas

Volume One

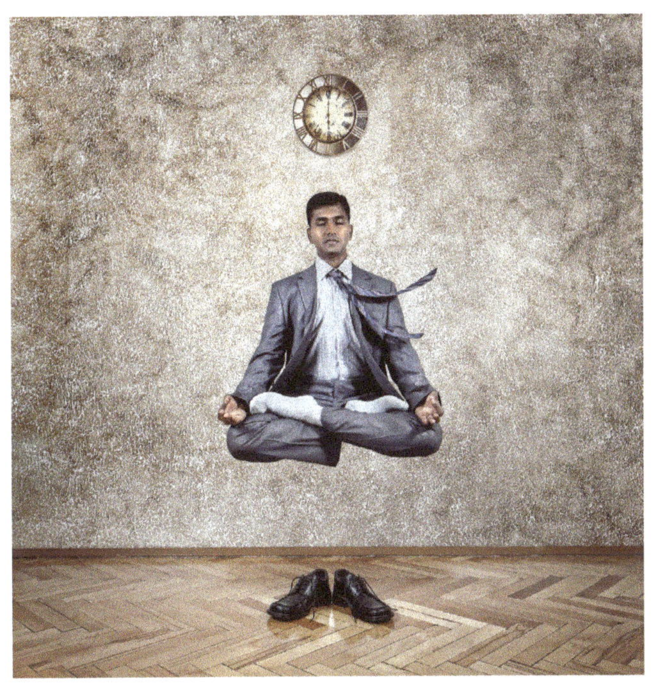

Joseph B. Weiss, MD, FACP, FACG, AGAF
Clinical Professor of Medicine,
Gastroenterology
University of California, San Diego

SmartAsk Books
Rancho Santa Fe, California, USA
www.smartaskbooks.com

ISBN-13: 978-1-943760-18-3 (Color -Volume One)
ISBN-13: 978-1-943760-19-0 (Color - Volume Two)
ISBN-13: 978-1-943760-10-7 (Color – Combined Volumes)

Cover photo: © Byheaven87 | Dreamstime.com license

Last digit is the print number: 9 8 7 6 5 4 3

Dedication

This volume is dedicated to clearing the air of the misperception that intestinal gas is anything other than a normal physiologic process common to all humanity. Nature and natural processes should be universally accepted as one of the cherished principles of fundamental human rights. The pursuit of health and happiness, and the accessible knowledge and resources of how to do so, should be available to all.

I am indebted to my loved ones Nancy, Danielle, Jeremy, Courie, Lizzy, & Indy. They have offered their insights, suggestions, comments, and unwavering support throughout the long process of having this project finally come to pass. You will always be the mighty wind beneath my wings.

Table of Contents – Volume One

Table of Contents – Volume Two

Preface

This is a very unusual book, both in content and intent. Dealing with matters of health and wellness the goal is to be factually correct and accurate, as well as to be informatively entertaining. With time, science and medicine will progress and no doubt a portion of the content will become outdated. In my chosen field of specialization, internal medicine, and especially in my field of sub-specialization gastroenterology, the advances have been dramatic and rapid.

As is to be expected, life, health, wellness, and disease are very complicated and complex subjects. The life sciences such as physiology, genomics, microbiology, etc. are interdependent with the basic sciences of chemistry, biology, physics, mathematics, and others. The applied sciences of engineering, pharmacology, epidemiology, and the myriad others add to the resources for deeper understanding and discovery.

The greatest age of discovery is still ahead of us, and the excitement and challenges in the fields are palpable. The history of medicine and science offer important lessons that are all too often forgotten as time progresses. Some of the most repeated and avoidable errors in health care is that business and profit opportunities from premature marketing of presumed medical and health advances are often later discredited, all too often with serious health consequences and not just financial losses.

This volume, and the others in the series, cover a wealth of topics related to the health and wellness of the digestive process, with an emphasis on intestinal gas and feces as examples of common health concerns that are intimately associated with normal daily health yet are rarely discussed. As a gastroenterologist who has seen tens of thousands of patients from all over the world, and all walks of life, I can unequivocally confirm that they are common concerns across the spectrum of humanity. The humorous references in this volume attempt to be tasteful and light, to compensate for some of the more technical and scientific content provided for those who wish to delve deeper into the subject.

As the book can be read as random short separate entries, or from cover to cover, the reader can choose how they wish to explore the wealth of information contained within these pages. Other volumes in the series provide additional resources for exploring what the author believes to be a fascinating and important subject, although it has been unfortunately suppressed by the embarrassment of cultural and societal norms.

It is ironic and humbling that often times in medicine, it is ancient wisdom that is rediscovered and appreciated anew. As you read these pages the amazing new wisdom and discoveries related to the gut microbiome, genomics, and the brain-gut-microbiome-diet axis were often already reflected in the insights and wisdom of the ancients.

Introduction

Human health and longevity have always been dependent on adequate nutrition, shelter, and avoidance of mortal threats. The average life expectancy was limited to the early reproductive years because of high infant mortality and the lack of effective treatment for most injuries, infections, and illnesses. As communities and social structure evolved, the healing arts developed, often in association with religious beliefs and practices. The oldest known system of the healing arts and medicine was established in Ancient India over five thousand years ago and is known as Ayurveda. The word Ayurveda is derived from the Sanskrit terms Ayu meaning life and Veda meaning knowledge, wisdom, and learning. A major focus of this health system approach, which remains in active practice today, is the vital role of digestion and diet in health and disease.

Ancient Egyptian civilization also developed a system of medicine where digestion and the bowels were a focus of concern and attention. The chief physician of the supreme leader, known as the Pharaoh, was given the honorific title of Keeper of the Royal Rectum. The term physician is a reference back to the priority focus on the digestive organs as the source of health and illness, as the term physic was applied to purgatives and laxatives. A physician was a health professional trained in the use of prescribed physics. Even in more recent Western societies such as the realm of King Henry the Eighth of England the bowel function of the head of state was a closely guarded state secret. The Keeper of the Stool was the given title of the first member of the King's Privy Council, the private closed inner circle of the King's most trusted advisors. The term privy is still in use today as a euphemism for the water closet (WC) or toilet.

Digestive disorders, nutrition, and diet are the most common of health concerns, and justifiably so, since virtually all health matters are ultimately influenced by this basic function and source of vitality. The Greek and Latin term Gastro referring to the stomach, and Entero referring to the intestines, have been added to the suffix -ology meaning knowledge, to arrive at the present name Gastroenterology. Often shortened to the acronym GI for gastrointestinal, it is the name of the internal medicine subspecialty dealing with the digestive organs, health, and disease. Western medicine, most often referred to by the misnomer Allopathic Medicine, tends to focus on disease states and their treatment to allow a return to health. Other healing approaches, especially those taking a more holistic perspective, have gained greater appreciation over recent years. Initially described as Alternative or Complementary Medicine, they are now more often identified as Integrative Medicine. Whatever the name, most practitioners would agree that if the approach provides health and healing benefits, they should be a welcomed addition to the armamentarium of modern medicine.

My own background is based on the Western Allopathic model. My cultural background and early education included Judaic studies of the original ancient Hebrew texts, as well as the original Aramaic texts of the Babylonian Talmud. One of my personal heroes was the compassionate and brilliant Middle Ages Royal Court physician and scholar Maimonides. My interest in medical history has been a lifelong fascination, and I have a profound appreciation for the challenges facing each generation of healers and physicians. It is always the case that we are dealing with a primitive state of medical knowledge, and limited therapeutics, compared to what we know will be the advances to come just over the horizon of time. My cultural and ethnic background exposed me to the common Yiddish exclamation of desperation, Oy Vey! With self-deprecating humor, I would consider the allopathic medicine focus on disease to be a form of OyVeydic Medicine!

Although I pursued a traditional Western medical education in the U.S., I maintained my international and multicultural perspective with postgraduate studies in medicine in Europe, Africa, and Latin America. I completed specialty training in Internal Medicine and Gastroenterology with further interests in tropical medicine, microbiology, nutrition, and metabolism. Maintaining an active clinical practice along with research, teaching, and administrative responsibilities allowed continuous advancement of an extensive experience and education in health matters. Serving in a volunteer capacity for over thirty-five years at the Veterans Administration Medical Center and on the clinical faculty of a major teaching and research university has been extremely rewarding and fulfilling. One of the many significant lessons I learned over and over during my decades of practice in medicine, and being honored with the care entrusted to me by my patients, has been the healing power of empathy and caring. The ability to see the humor that is ever present in the human condition is also a gift worth nurturing. Since I consider myself an amateur humorist, I like to share the philosophy stated in the phrase 'Laughter is the Best Medicine'.

As the culmination of my professional knowledge as a gastroenterologist, my passion for education as a clinical professor at a prestigious university medical school, and my avocation as a humorist and entertainer, I have written a series of books for the lay public. The books are purposefully focused on subjects that are rarely discussed, but that I know from discussions with tens of thousands of patients over the years are of great public interest. Since I have a longstanding interest in medical history, and some knowledge of Ayurveda Medicine, I feel comfortable describing my specialty knowledge (in Sanskrit described as Veda) on digestion and intestinal gas as the founding of the new discipline of AirVeda Medicine.

Since I enjoy sharing what I believe to be valuable and entertaining information, I have published a number of volumes. My books to date include:

AirVeda: Ancient & New Medical Wisdom, Digestion & Gas
The Scoop on Poop! Flush with Knowledge
*You Don't Know Sh*t! Until You Read This Book (same content as Scoop)*
To 'Air' is Human: Everything You Ever Wanted to Know About Intestinal Gas
Artsy Fartsy, Cultural History of the Fart
How Do You Doo? Everybody Pees & Poops!
The Quest for Immortality: Advances in Vitality & Longevity

Now after introducing the reader to my humorous tongue-in-cheek creations of OyVeda and AirVeda, let's return to the original and authentic healing system of Ayurveda. One of the most remarkable aspects of Ayurveda, beyond its ancient history and longevity, is that only recent advances in science and technology have provided a deeper understanding of its properties and benefits. The current research advances in the microbiome, immunology, genomics, epigenetics, diet, nutrition, meditation, herbal remedies, nutraceuticals, and the life sciences in general are opening new appreciation for this ancient and venerable body of knowledge. Ayurveda is the world's oldest health discipline in that it originated in Ancient India over five thousand years ago. It is a holistic approach to body, mind, and spirit which defines disease as the absence of vibrant health. This is a different approach than taken by traditional Western Allopathic Medicine, which typically defines health as the absence of disease. Ayurveda surgical techniques and medical therapies were the basis of many advances adopted by Western medicine. Other aspects are still considered alternative or complimentary medicine, with newer advances in research technology capabilities encouraging their reassessment and adaptation by what we consider Modern Medicine.

In Ayurveda the presence of disease is believed to be attributable to either physical imbalance, emotional turbulence, or spiritual disconnection. Treatment modalities include diet, herbs, massage, meditation, yoga, detoxification, emotional regulation, breath management, and proper sensory input. The balance of Mind, Body, and Spirit are characterized as the three doshas representing various combinations of Akasha (space/potential), Vayu (air/movement), Agni (fire/transformation), Jala (water/protection), and Prithivi (earth/structure). Vata is the combination of space and air, Pitta is the combination of fire and water, and Kapha is the combination of water and earth. Each dosha has a primary site in the body, Kapha is the stomach, chest, and head, Pitta is the small intestine, liver, and blood, and Vata is the colon. Each person has different proportions of each dosha comprising their constitution, and imbalance of the doshas can result in health issues. The Ayurveda approach to treatment is to return the doshas to the proper balance for the individual.

Digestion and nutrition play a vital role in both the Ayurveda and Allopathic Medicine. In Ayurveda health is ascribed to the potency of digestive Agni, defined as the powerful digestive fire. A strong Agni allows the body access to Ojas, the subtle nourishment and nutrition present in food. A weak Agni is unable to properly process and digest intake which allows the accumulation of Ama, the toxic residue and waste of the incomplete digestive and absorptive process. The beneficial Ojas or toxic Ama then enter the Srota, the circulatory channels, and are distributed to the body. The Dhatus are the tissues of the body and are classified as Rasap (plasma), Rakta (blood), Mamsa (muscles), Meda (fat), Asthi (bone), Majja (nerves and bone marrow), and Shukra (reproduction). The waste products are called Mutra (urine), Purisha and Mala (feces), and Sweda (sweat).

The qualities of the Vata Dosha are dry, light, cold, rough, quick, mobile, changeable, irregular, and subtle. Its functions are transportation, movement, and communication. The qualities of the Pitta Dosha are light, hot, sharp, slightly oily, intense, penetrating, acidic, moist, flowing, liquid, and pungent. Its functions are metabolism, digestion, and transformation. The qualities of the Kapha Dosha are oily, heavy, cool, slow, stable, sticky, solid, smooth, steady, enduring, and dull. Its functions are structure, cohesion, and lubrication. In most people, one or two doshas predominate. Although determined at conception and called Prakruti, experience and choice influence an individual's current balance of doshas, called Vikruti.

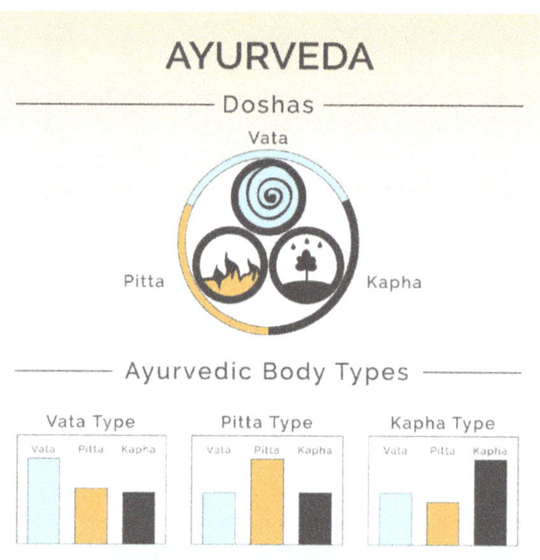

Ayurveda doshas Shutterstock/GL Sonts

Ayurveda describes six tastes: Madhura (sweet), Amla (sour), Lavana (salty), Katu (pungent), Tikta (bitter), and Kashaya astringent. Sweet is considered the taste of energy which builds tissues. Included in this category are grains, pasta, bread, nuts, dairy, oils, sweet fruits, starchy vegetables, animal products, and sugar. The sour taste includes organic acids which promote appetite and digestion. This includes citrus fruits, berries, tomatoes, sour fruits, yogurt, cheese, vinegar, pickles, fermented foods, and alcohol. The taste of salt promotes digestion and includes table salt, fish, meat, seaweed, soy sauce, processed foods, condiments, and sauces. Pungent taste is found in essential oils and is believed to stimulate digestion and assist in detoxification. Examples include pepper, cayenne, ginger, garlic, onions, leeks, chilies, radish, horseradish, salsa, basil, thyme, cloves, and mustard. Bitter taste is considered to be the taste of information and includes anti-inflammatory and detoxifying properties. It is found in green and yellow squash, broccoli, greens, spinach, kale, and Brussels sprouts. The astringent taste is the taste of dryness and lightness and is believed to have healing and compacting properties. It is found in beans, legumes, peas, lentils, tea, cranberries, pomegranate, apples, and dark leafy greens.

In Ayurveda the six stages of disease are Sanchaya (accumulation), Prakopa (aggravation), Prasara (spread), Sthana-samshraya (localization), Vyakti (manifestation), and Bheda (differentiation). The Ayurveda evaluative techniques include Roga Pariksha the examination of the disease and Rogi Pariksha the examination of the patient. Dravya Guna Karma Shastra is the Ayurveda science of pharmacology. The term Dravya describes substances, herbs, and drugs. Guna is the term for their properties and qualities, and Karma is the term for their action and effect. Shastra is the term for science, Veerya means potency, Prabhava is a unique property, and Vipaka is a post-digestive effect. The Ayurveda term Soma is the cooling essence of physiology, Sattva is defined as purity, clarity, and evolution. Additional terms include Rajas meaning dynamism, movement, and energy, and Tamas meaning inertia, darkness, and ignorance.

Pancha Karma is the Ayurveda purification therapy that includes Shodhana and Shamana the terms for detoxification and rejuvenation. The methodology of Pancha Karma detoxification includes Vamana the inducement of vomiting (emesis), especially for the Kapha Dosha. For the Pita Dosha Virechana, the inducement of purgation with laxatives and cathartics, is often prescribed. Nasya, the nasal passage cleansing, using a netti pot and saline solution is often prescribed for the Kapha and Vata Doshas. Basti are colonic enemas that are either Anuvasana (oil based) or Niruha (water based) and often used on the Vata Dosha. Raka Moksha is bloodletting and was used for the Pitta Dosha. Swedena is the use of heat to induce sweating (diaphoresis). Snehana is oleation, the use of oils both internally and externally. Rasayana is the process of rejuvenation utilizing nutrition, rest, exercise, meditation, herbs, and other modalities.

Ayurveda, still predominantly found in India, is taught and practiced around the world. The herb turmeric, often found in curry, is a natural anti-inflammatory product that is just as potent as the strongest prescription pharmaceuticals. Western Allopathic medicine has traditionally taken a reductionist approach, looking for a single key feature or chemical which offers a specific mechanism of action. A limited number of diseases are fully explained and successfully approached with this methodology. Ayurveda takes a more holistic systems biology approach, where multiple compounds in a natural product may require synergy to provide a full benefit. The life sciences are providing more evidence that the systems biology approach is necessary for the vast majority of illnesses and therapeutics. The nearly infinite variability of the human genome, combined with the complexity and interaction of human microbiome diversity, emphasizes the importance of the systems biology approach.

Air is critical for life, and has played a major part in the long history of medicine from the focus on the air nature of the Vata Dosha of Ayurveda to the airborne transmission of communicable diseases and environmental pollutants. The entire specialty of pulmonary medicine deals with the respiratory organs and the absorption and elimination of the various gases that comprise the air we breathe and body metabolism. The gastrointestinal tract also deals with air issues, including the air we swallow, known as aerophagia, the gasses produced by our digestive process, and finally the gasses produced by the microbiome, the community of microbes residing within our body. The purpose of this volume is to offer insight and knowledge about this common concern, which has been all too often been an unnecessary source of confusion and embarrassment.

Many people incorrectly believe the age of discovery and exploration was in the past. The rapid advances in technology over the past century occurred at a dizzying pace. Remarkably the age of flight from the Wright brothers at Kitty Hawk progressed to supersonic jets and man traveling and returning to the moon in less than a hundred years. The first telegraph wire to wireless communication of smart computing phones with video conferencing capabilities to anywhere in the world took place in a blink of evolutionary time. The understanding of a hidden microbial world continues to astound with entirely new life forms identified in only the last few decades. One of these, Archaea, was hiding in plain sight and has the remarkable ability to survive and thrive in places once thought impossible, such as within rocks miles underground, and in extreme temperatures. The recognition that the human microbiome is intimately involved with human health and disease will without doubt revolutionize medicine. Other discoveries of similar or greater magnitude are likely over the years to come, so it remains humbling how little we know.

Air in the gastrointestinal tract is normal. The presence of air, especially if found in excess, can have three or more results. The first is the release of air as an eructation, more commonly known as a burp or belch. The second is distention, also known as bloat. The third result is flatulence, more commonly known as the passage of gas as flatus or as a fart. The word fart is the correct word to use in the English language, and indeed is one of its oldest words. The alternative terms used, such as flatus and flatulence are not original English words as they have been borrowed from the Latin. There is controversy as to the derivation of the word fart. It is thought to have Indo-European roots in the Germanic language word farzen. One thought is that it originated as an onomatopoeia, a word that phonetically imitates the sound of the event it describes. Another thought is that it was related to the term for partridge, as the bird makes a similar sound when it is disturbed in its natural habitat and takes flight.

Farts are ubiquitous, all living creatures generate gas from cellular metabolism and respiration, and humans are no exception. The bacteria of your colonic flora, part of the microbiome of living organisms that lives on and within humans, generate gas which collect in the bowel. They are joined with the air swallowed throughout the day and night, particularly at meals. Aerophagia is universal and we swallow on average three to five cubic centimeters (one teaspoonful) of air with every swallow. Additional gasses are produced during the enzymatic digestive processes as well as the neutralization of gastric hydrochloric acid by pancreatic and duodenal bicarbonate. The result is a significant volume of gasses within and transiting the bowel.

Fortunately, the vast majority of the gasses produced are absorbed by the gut, then into the bloodstream through diffusion and finally exhaled when they each the alveoli of the lungs. The component gasses have very different properties of diffusion through the bowel wall and into the bloodstream. Carbon dioxide readily diffuses and enters solution and is exhaled promptly. Although it is the largest volume of gas generated, and temporarily contributes to distension and postprandial (after meal) discomfort, it is the easiest to eliminate from the bowel and is only a minor contributor to flatulence.

The volume of gasses in the gastrointestinal tract is dependent on the quantity and nature of foods ingested, the body's ability to produce enzymes for the various food types, the microbiome and gut flora, and gastrointestinal transit time. The often quoted figure of twelve farts per day is a reasonable average number of farts passed but there is a very wide range of what is considered normal. The fact is that air is critical for our survival, as well as ubiquitous in nature and in our digestive tract. It is my hope that this book and its companion volumes will serve to inform and entertain the public. The knowledge gained with progress in medicine and the life sciences will hopefully enhance health and vitality as well as extend the human lifespan. Perhaps there is more than a little truth to the phrase Life is a Gas.

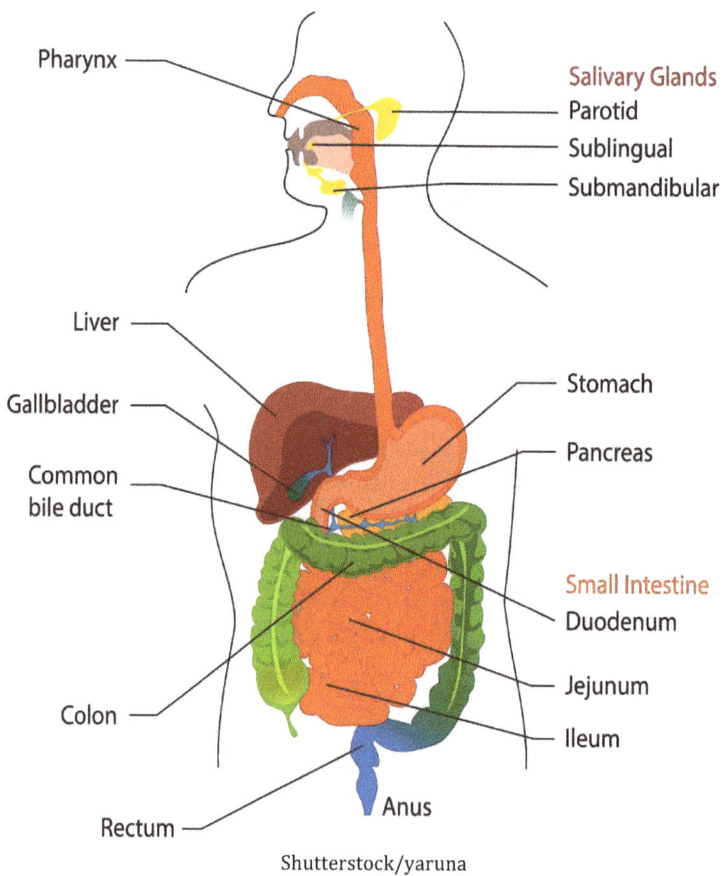

Shutterstock/yaruna

This book is organized in an alphabetical order of subjects, much like an encyclopedia. This allows one the luxury to skip around to read entries of interest, and to spend as little or as much time as one wishes reading at one sitting. The image of the digestive tract on this page is a useful reference to its anatomy and terminology. Reading the entry on digestion is also a very good place to start to give an overview of this fascinating subject vital to good health, as well as understanding the passage of air in the digestive tract.

Activated Charcoal

Commercially available products to trap and contain the dispersion of noxious gasses and toxins have been available for some time. Adapting these properties to address the aroma of a fart have also been marketed with some success. They rely on the adsorptive properties of activated carbon also known as activated charcoal, activated coal, or carbo activatus. Activated charcoal is a form of carbon processed to increase the surface area available for adsorption or chemical reactions.

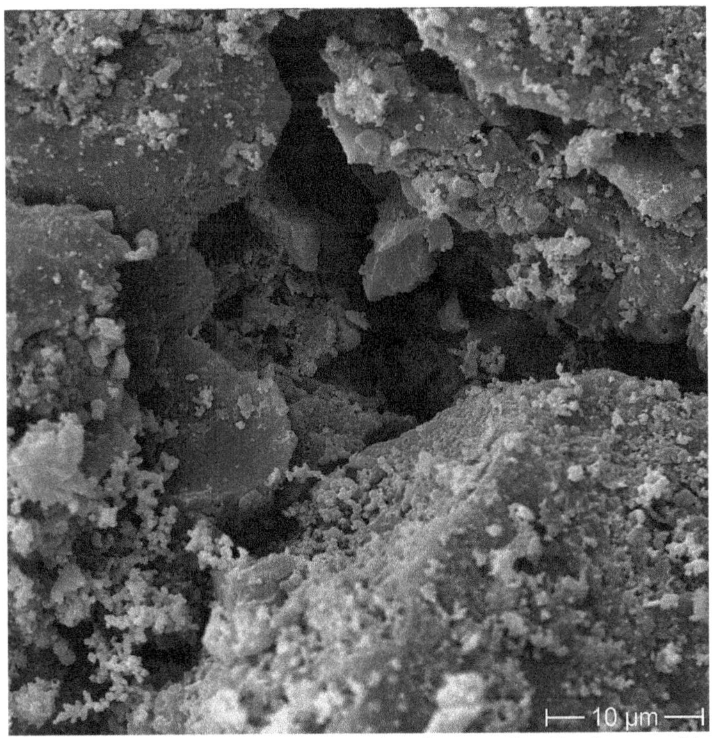

Activated charcoal, microscopic view increased surface area. Creative Commons License

The term adsorption and absorption are frequently confused. Absorption allows another material to be integrated into the volume of the absorptive matter. Adsorption is when the material being incorporated adheres to the surface of the material, and is not absorbed into its interior. An example of the difference between the two terms would be the drinking of water leads to its absorption that is it becomes internalized within your bodily tissues. Water that coats your skin in the shower or after spilling it on yourself is adsorbed, that is it is only on the outer surface of your body, and it is not absorbed.

Its very large surface area is a key concept to understanding the effectiveness of activated charcoal. A single cube of charcoal has a much smaller surface area for adsorption to take place, than an identical volume cube that has been subdivided into many smaller cubes. The following illustration helps to visualize how the surface area can be dramatically increased with the same volume of material.

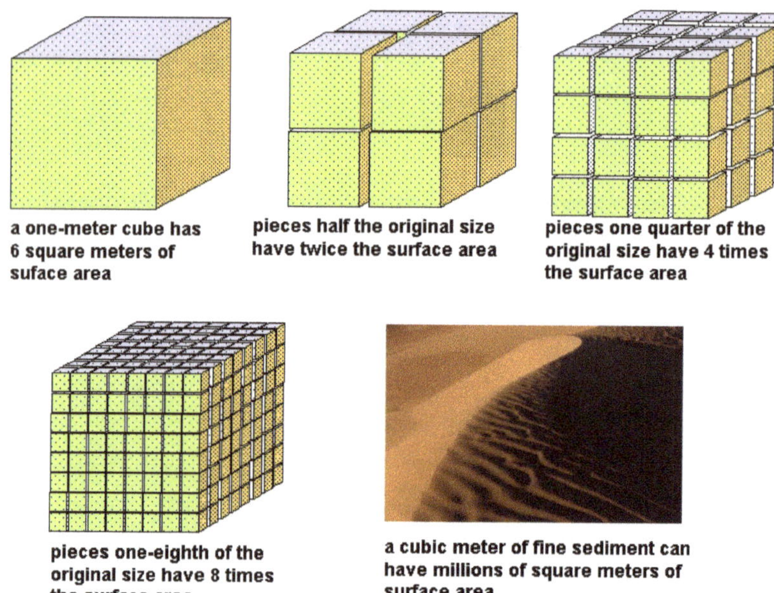

a one-meter cube has 6 square meters of suface area
pieces half the original size have twice the surface area
pieces one quarter of the original size have 4 times the surface area
pieces one-eighth of the original size have 8 times the surface area.
a cubic meter of fine sediment can have millions of square meters of surface area

Increase in surface area illustrated. Phil Stoffer, Ph.D. Geology Cafe geologycafe.com Creative Commons License

Activated carbon is used in the purification, decaffeination, metal extraction, water purification, and sewage treatment processes. It is also used in the air filters in masks and respirators, filters in compressed air, and to filter vodka and whiskey to remove impurities that would affect taste. In cases of the ingestion of toxins or poisons it has been used orally to bind to the toxin to prevent its absorption into the victim.

It is also effective in adsorbing offensive smelling gasses in flatus. Due to its porosity a single gram of activated carbon can have a surface area in excess of five hundred meters squared, with one thousand five hundred meters squared being possible with further refining. Its adsorption ability varies amongst gasses and liquids and it is known to be a poor adsorbent of carbon monoxide, which is toxic and odorless. It is particularly effective in adsorbing most of the volatile odoriferous gasses.

The key to the success or failure of the product is the degree to which the fart can escape without having passed through the activated charcoal. The tighter the seal, the less likely for odiferous gasses to escape. The sitting pad was least effective trapping about twenty percent of gasses. Underwear pads ranged from fifty to seventy-five percent effectiveness, while the tight fitting entirely lined with activated charcoal underwear were the most effective, but also the most expensive.

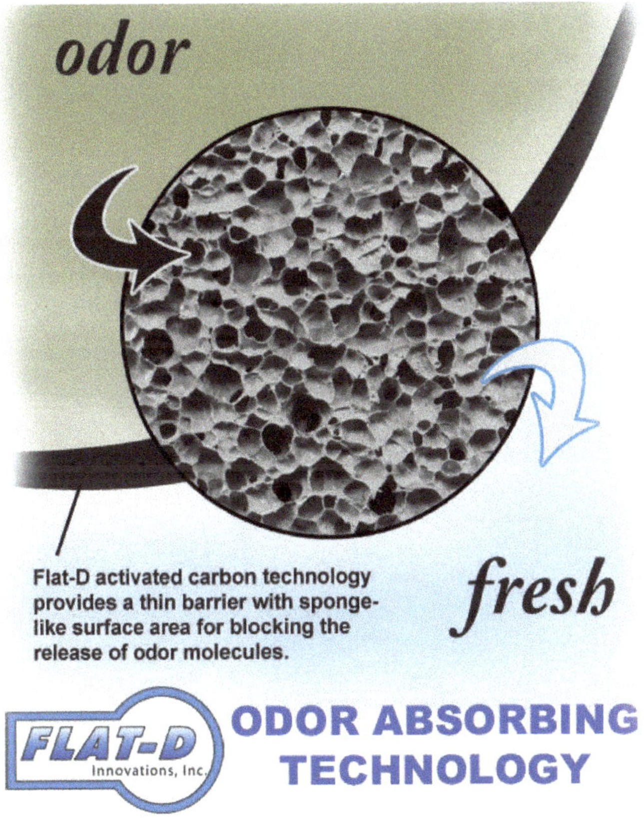
odor
Flat-D activated carbon technology provides a thin barrier with sponge-like surface area for blocking the release of odor molecules.
fresh
FLAT-D
Innovations, Inc.
ODOR ABSORBING TECHNOLOGY

Activated charcoal pad products. Flat-D Innovations, Inc. Used with permission

Activated carbon is used to treat oral poisonings by binding to and preventing the poison from being absorbed by the gastrointestinal tract. The home remedy of eating burnt toast for food poisoning was based on the adsorptive properties of activated charcoal. Charcoal biscuits were marketed in the early 19th century as an antidote to flatulence, and are still sold today for diarrhea, indigestion, flatulence, and as a pet care product. Unfortunately orally ingested charcoal pills are not effective in appreciably reducing intestinal gas. This may be because the adsorptive capacity of the activated charcoal is fully utilized before it finally gets to the colon where its gas adsorbing properties are needed. Fortunately, bismuth products do provide a significant advantage by binding to the sulfur compounds and eliminating them without producing offensive gas.

Aerogel

Aerogel was developed by Samuel Kistler (1900-1975) at the College of the Pacific in Stockton, California in 1931. It was a silica material with a chemical structure similar to glass with gas in its pores rather than liquid. It is an open celled material that is ninety-five percent air, with pores less than one ten-thousandth of the diameter of a human hair. Further refinements allowed the air to be replaced by a vacuum, and the silica to be replaced by other materials. Kistler developed aerogels made of alumina, tungsten oxide, ferric oxide, tin oxide, nickel tartarate, cellulose, cellulose nitrate, gelatin, agar, egg albumen, and rubber. Further advancements and refinements in production have led to greater commercial applications.

The pore diameter being measured in nanometers gives it a nanoporous nature leading to the lowest thermal conductivity of any known solid. It has an extremely high surface area to mass ration with just two grams of aerogel having a surface area of a square kilometer (one thousand meters squared)

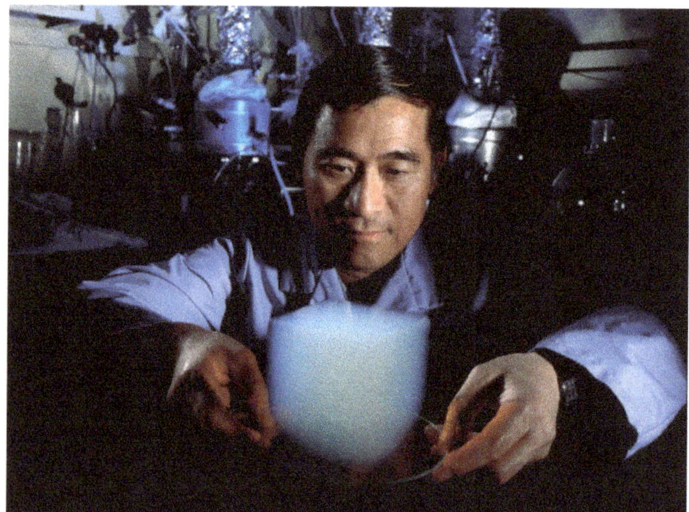

Aerogel. Stardust.jpl.nasa.gov Public Domain

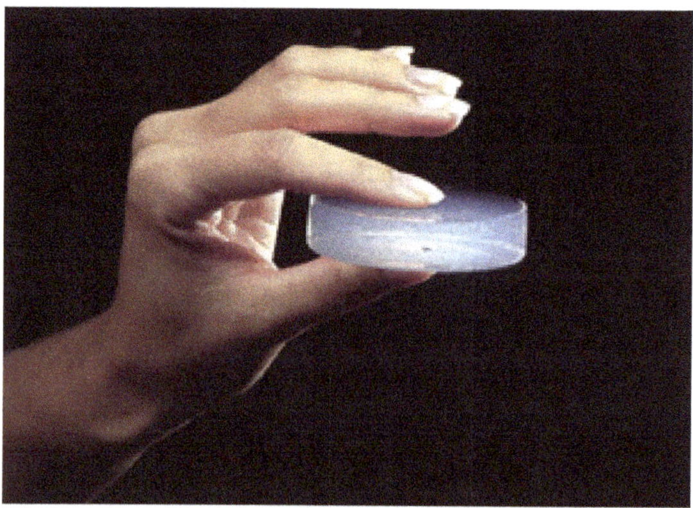

Aerogel is made from a wet gel that is dried. The substance has been described as feeling like volcanic glass pumice; a very fine, dry sponge; and extremely lightweight Styrofoam. NASA Public Domain

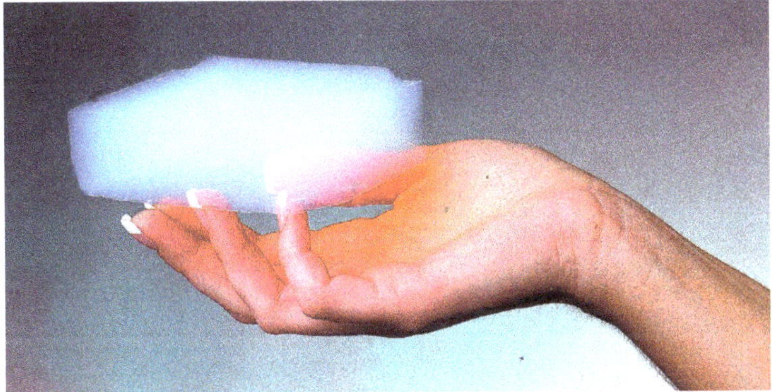

Though with a ghostly appearance like a hologram, aerogel is very solid. It feels like hard Styrofoam to the touch. Aerogel. Stardust.jpl.nasa.gov Public Domain

It is so lightweight that it has unmatched utility as an insulating material and has been utilized by NASA for the space shuttle and space exploration. The development of this product has allowed exploration of extreme environments such as outer space and deep sea exploration, where humans are exposed to the high and low extremes of atmospheric pressure that dramatically effect intestinal gas pressure and volume

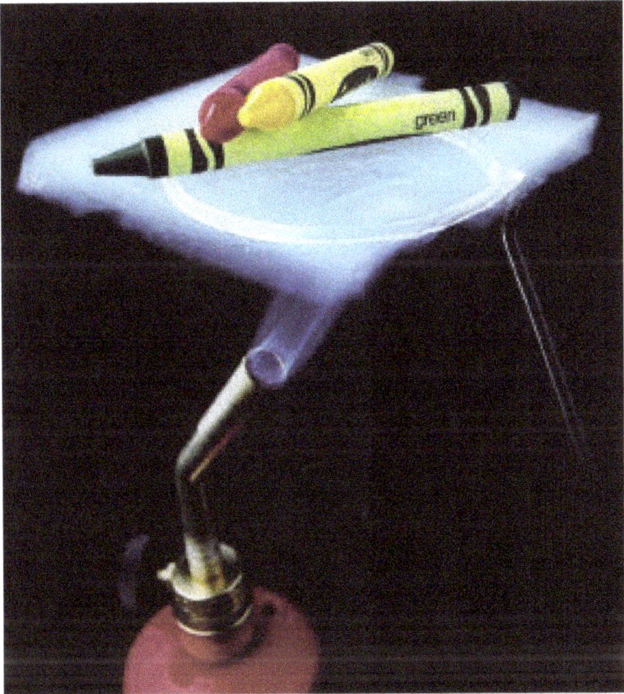

Crayons placed on top of a piece of silica aerogel will not melt from the heat of a flame. Certain types of aerogel provide thirty-nine times more insulation than fiberglass. NASA Public Domain

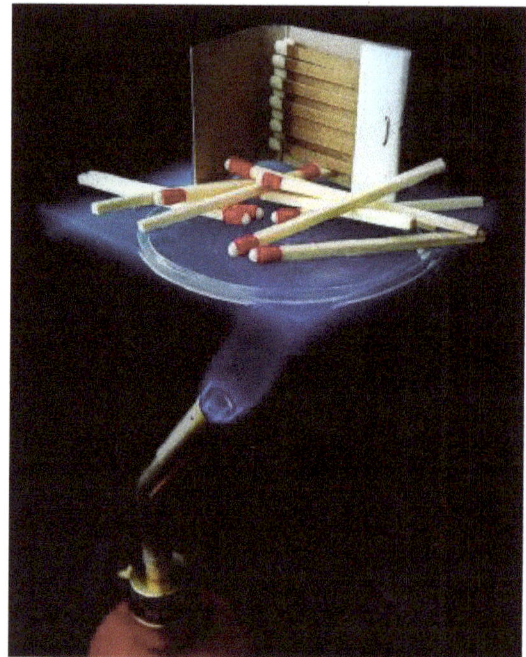

Aerogel. Stardust.jpl.nasa.gov Public Domain

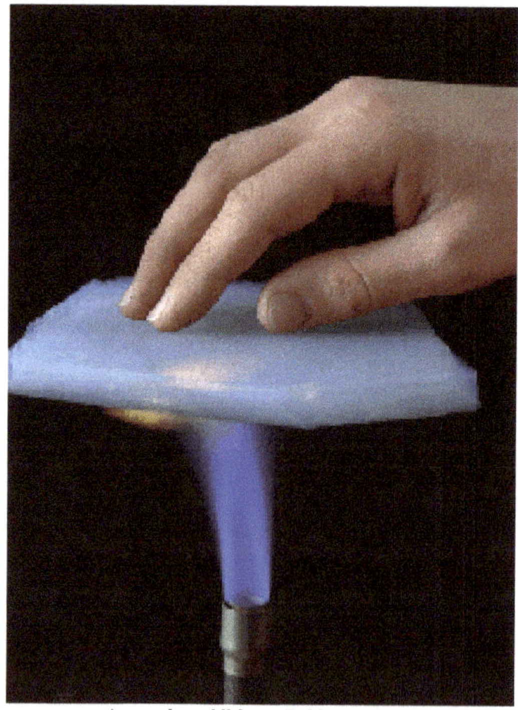

Aerogel eetd.lbl.gov Public Domain

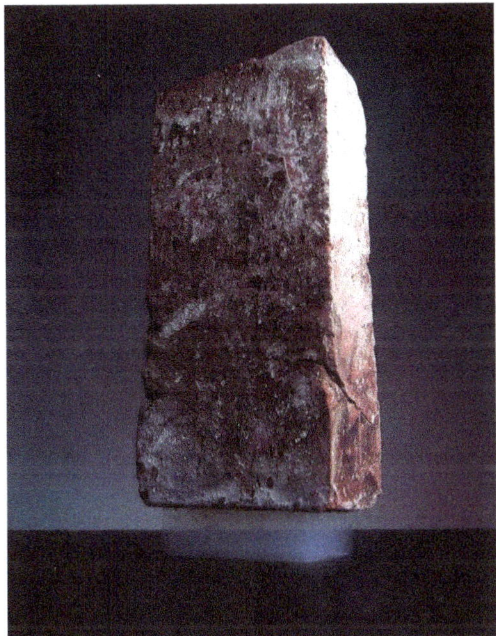

Aerogel. A five-pound (two and one-half kilogram) brick is supported on top of a piece of aerogel weighing only two grams. Stardust.jpl.nasa.gov Public Domain

Aerophagia (Air Swallowing)

Air swallowing is a universal event in humans and is also known as aerophagia. We do it with every one of the on average two thousand swallows we take every day, ingesting approximately five milliliters (one teaspoonful) of air with every swallow. Air is seventy-eight percent nitrogen, which is a poorly absorbed gas. If it is not released in a burp, it will contribute to bloating and distension. The volume of air swallowed is impressive, but is only a small percentage of what the digestive process can generate in terms of gas production.

Aerophagia is the swallowing of air, allowing it to enter the digestive tract, and it occurs naturally and without thinking in every individual. There is a variation of aerophagia in which the behavior becomes a purposeful, and at times obsessive-compulsive, behavior. More often, when excessive spontaneous aerophagia is occurring it is a subconscious or unconscious behavior, much like a nervous tic. The volume of air swallowed in these conditions can be impressive and a plain x-ray of the abdomen may demonstrate that the entire digestive tract is filled with air from esophagus to rectum.

Various studies have estimated the volume of each swallow as approximately twenty milliliters or four teaspoons. Many people swallow larger gulps of food on purpose and some even go to extremes in demonstrating their swallowing abilities. Sword swallowing is just one example where swallowing has been taken to a level of competition or entertainment.

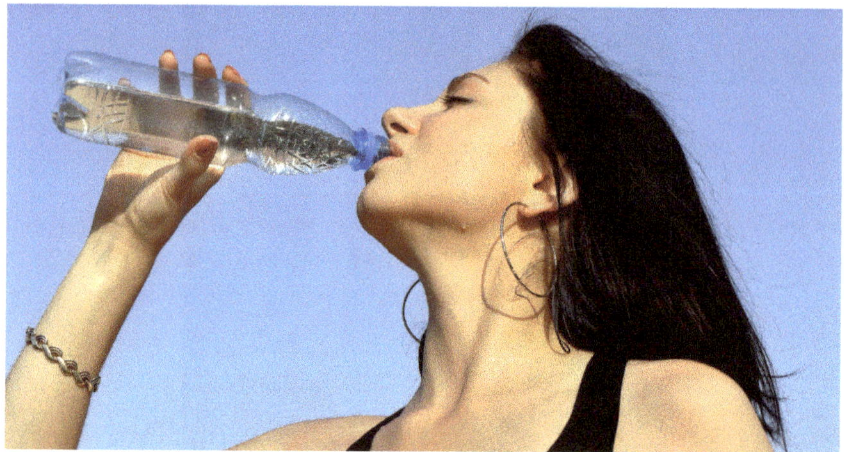

Air swallowing (aerophagia) is universal and occurs with every single swallow including swallows of food, food, saliva, etc. Shutterstock/yuris

At the other extreme, some people take very small swallows and may sip foods at a teaspoon or less per swallow. They may be surprised to learn that sipping smaller volumes may actually increase the total amount of air they swallow. In general, the larger the total number of swallows, the larger the volume of air consumed.

If we took twenty milliliters as the volume of a normal average swallow, and the individual only took in small five milliliters sip of soup, each twenty milliliters swallow would include an additional fifteen milliliters of air. This is why hard candy and chewing gums, which generates small volumes of saliva and frequent swallows that mainly consist of air, lead to excessive aerophagia.

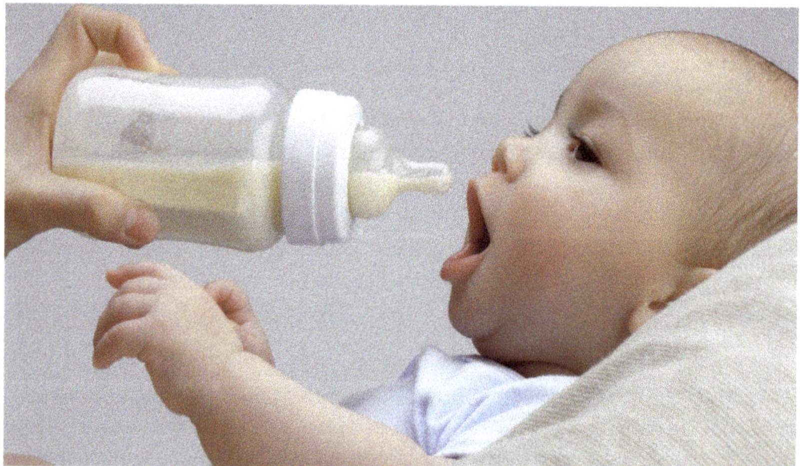

Baby bottles are a common source of aerophagia in infants. If the milk or formula does not completely cover the nipple of the bottle the baby will suck in and swallow air. Shutterstock/Nicolesa

Since the digestive tract of the newborn is sterile, there are no microorganisms generating gas through cellular metabolism. All of the gas the newborn infant begins to pass is swallowed air. If an infant is bottle-fed rather than breast-fed they are much more likely to swallow even more air.

The first exposure to microorganisms that will be swallowed and begin to colonize the infant digestive tract are from the birth mother if the delivery is vaginal. The microorganisms that colonize the infant become its microbiome and play a major role in its ongoing health and wellness. The gut flora is one aspect of the microbiome, with skin, ears, mouth, genitourinary, and every surface of the body exposed to the external environment developing its own unique microbiome. Infants born by Caesarean section have exposure to different organisms, which establish a microbiome that is not believed to be as beneficial as via a natural vaginal delivery.

Baby bottles are a common cause of aerophagia in infants as they suck in and swallow air if the formula does not always cover the nipple. Burping the baby after a feeding is the means of allowing the swallowed air to escape, otherwise it will cause distension and discomfort. Some bottles are designed to use an internal plastic sleeve to prevent air from reaching the nipple, when the formula is depleted the sleeve forms a vacuum so the infant is not sucking in air.

The air swallowed is the same as the air in the atmosphere, about seventy eight percent nitrogen, twenty one percent oxygen, one percent argon, and other gasses. Included in the other gasses that make up one percent of air is argon, comprising the vast majority at zero point nine three percent. In spite of global warming carbon dioxide makes up only a fraction of one percent of air, with the remainder including trace amounts of neon, helium, methane, krypton, and hydrogen. Seventy-eight percent of air is nitrogen and the gastrointestinal tract poorly absorbs this gas compared to oxygen and carbon dioxide.

Once the nitrogen is swallowed it has only two ways to get out of the digestive tract. Coming up as a burp or belch is its closest exit, but it has to overcome the lower esophageal sphincter, the upper esophageal sphincter and the oncoming rush with peristalsis and gravity of more food, fluid, drink, saliva, and yes even more air being swallowed. With every single swallow about five milliliters, or one teaspoonful, of air is swallowed whether you are eating, drinking, or just resting between meals. You swallow approximately every thirty seconds while awake, and about every five minutes while asleep.

The average person swallows about two thousand times a day, but many swallow much more than that. Foods that are extremely hot or cold tend to be swallowed in smaller quantities, resulting in more swallows being necessary to eat or drink the same volume at a moderate temperature. If you chew gum, use a lozenge or sucking candy, or use any product that is a sialagogue, i.e. generates saliva, you will be doing a lot more swallowing. Don't forget that with each swallow you are taking in much more air than saliva.

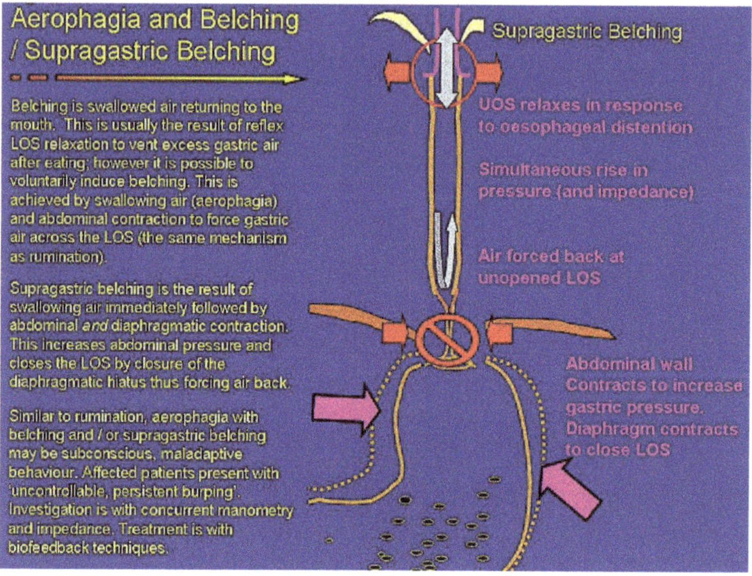

Aerophagia and Belching / Supragastric Belching
Belching is swallowed air returning to the mouth. This is usually the result of reflex LOS relaxation to vent excess gastric air after eating; however it is possible to voluntarily induce belching. This is achieved by swallowing air (aerophagia) and abdominal contraction to force gastric air across the LOS (the same mechanism as rumination).
Supragastric belching is the result of swallowing air immediately followed by abdominal and diaphragmatic contraction. This increases abdominal pressure and closes the LOS by closure of the diaphragmatic hiatus thus forcing air back.
Similar to rumination, aerophagia with belching and / or supragastric belching may be subconscious, maladaptive behaviour. Affected patients present with 'uncontrollable, persistent burping'. Investigation is with concurrent manometry and impedance. Treatment is with biofeedback techniques.
Supragastric Belching
UOS relaxes in response to oesophageal distention
Simultaneous rise in pressure (and impedance)
Air forced back at unopened LOS
Abdominal wall Contracts to increase gastric pressure. Diaphragm contracts to close LOS

www.bmj.com

The same is true of chewing tobacco and even smoking tobacco whether as cigar, pipe, cigarette, or electronic smokeless cigarette. Do you want to hold a conversation while you are eating? Go ahead but it will cause even more air swallowing, as will drinking from a straw or tilting your head back to drink from a bottle or can. Rush through your meals, and you swallow more air than food or drink.

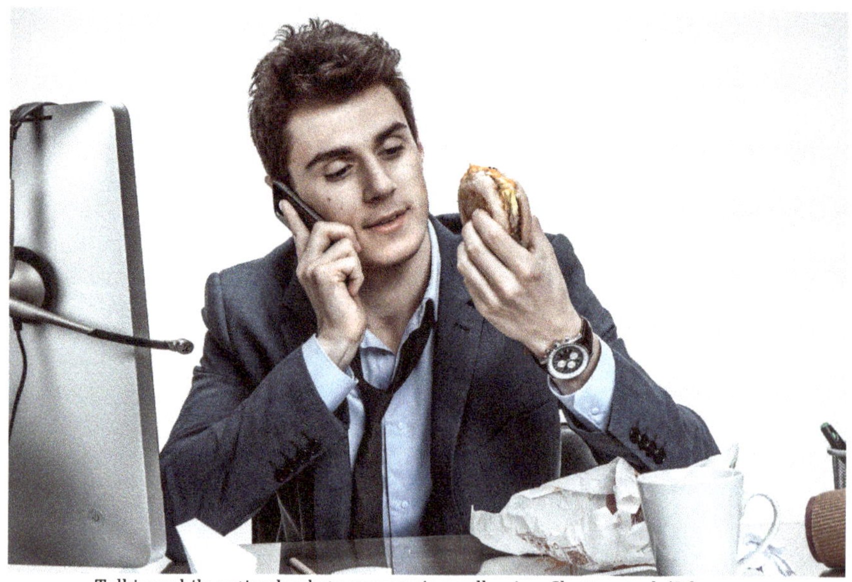
Talking while eating leads to excess air swallowing. Shutterstock/R.legosyn

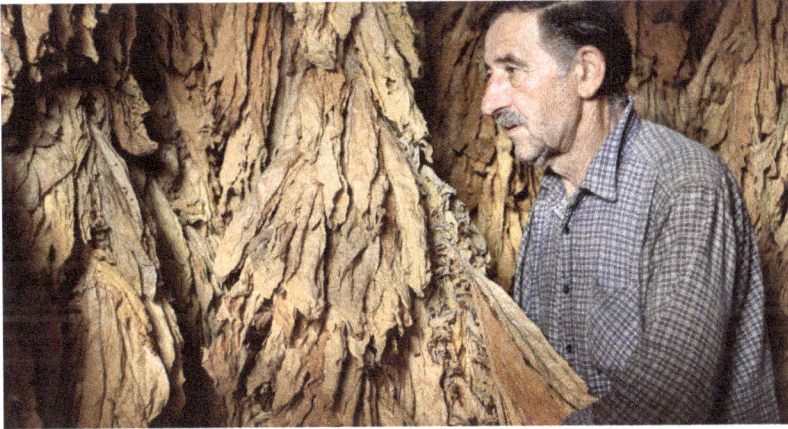

Tobacco smoked as a cigarette, pipe, or cigar, or even chewed contributes to aerophagia Shutterstock/branislavpudar

If you are a baby, just lean back and drink from your baby bottle, even those designed to keep the amount of air swallowed to a minimum. Well, the good news for babies is that most caregivers know how to get them to burp up the air swallowed after a feeding. Then again, the associated spit ups could best be avoided by changing the posture at feeding times to reduce air swallowing.

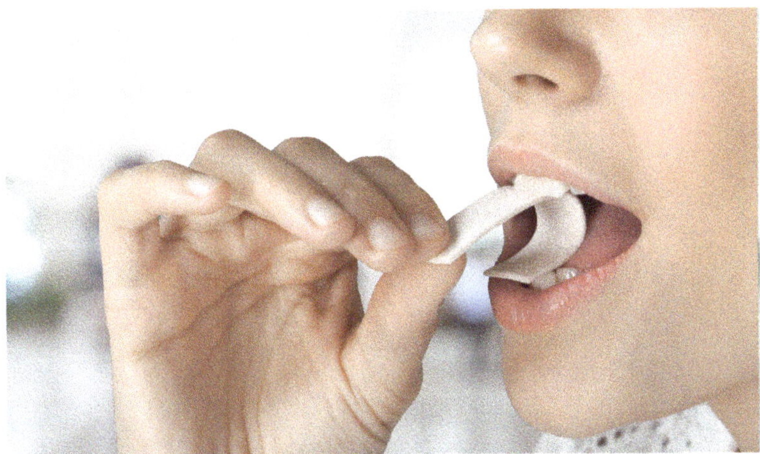

Chewing and bubble gum, as well as use of sucking candy and throat lozenges can lead to excessive air swallowing. Shutterstock/billionphotos

Other conditions recognized to increase air swallowing include poor fitting dentures, not chewing food well, drinking from a straw or bottle, talking while eating, and racing through a meal. In another category is the notorious adolescent male who loves to swallow air on purpose so he can generate belches and burps worthy of a dinosaur. Although he may be proud of his newfound talent, it will take many years to achieve the maturity to recognize the sounds generated are an ineffective mating call to attract the female of the species.

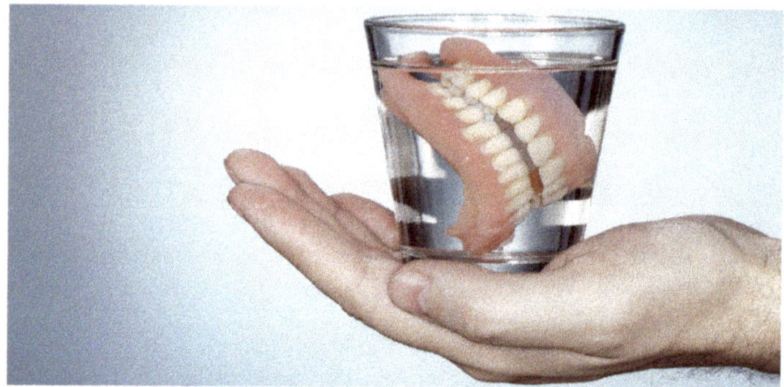

Aerophagia air swallowing is the most common source of excess intestinal gas. Ill-fitting dentures will contribute to more air being swallowed. Shutterstock/stocksnapper

Some individuals also develop a rumination syndrome, where they subconsciously regurgitate and re-swallow food mixed in with even more air. Fortunately, it is unusual to see a different form of purposeful aerophagia since the development of the artificial larynx or voice box. Years ago, individuals who unfortunately developed cancer of the vocal cords or throat and lost their voice box, used to be taught to swallow air and generate esophageal speech. Esophageal speech was primarily air swallowing followed by controlled belching to create a modified vocalization.

Going back to the average of two thousand swallows a day we are talking about ten liters of air swallowed every single day. Even incorrectly assuming that one hundred percent of the oxygen in the swallowed air was absorbed, we are looking at about eight liters of nitrogen that has been taken in and now needs to get out. That is a lot of nitrogen, and the most direct exit, the shortest distance to travel, and the fastest way to get relief, is to burp or belch.

Sometimes the social situation or environment discourages and suppresses the natural inclination to release the swallowed air. Even if you could burp at will that is an awful lot of gas swallowed throughout the day and night. It is much more than the most frequent and dedicated burpers and belchers are able to release through eructation. The retained nitrogen will contribute to bloating and distension, before it eventually makes its way out of the other end of the intestinal tract as flatus, more commonly known as a fart.

Meals with a high fat content trigger the release of hormones that slow down gut motility. As the food spends more time in the digestive tract, continued bacterial fermentation produces increasing quantities of gas. In addition, foods that are extremely hot or cold tend to be swallowed in smaller quantities, resulting in more swallows being necessary to eat or drink the same volume at a moderate temperature. As each swallow contributes an additional quantity of air entering the esophagus and digestive tract, more swallows results in more air ingestion. Foods or snacks that require excess chewing with resultant excess swallowing of saliva, such as chewing or bubble gum, also contribute to excess air ingestion.

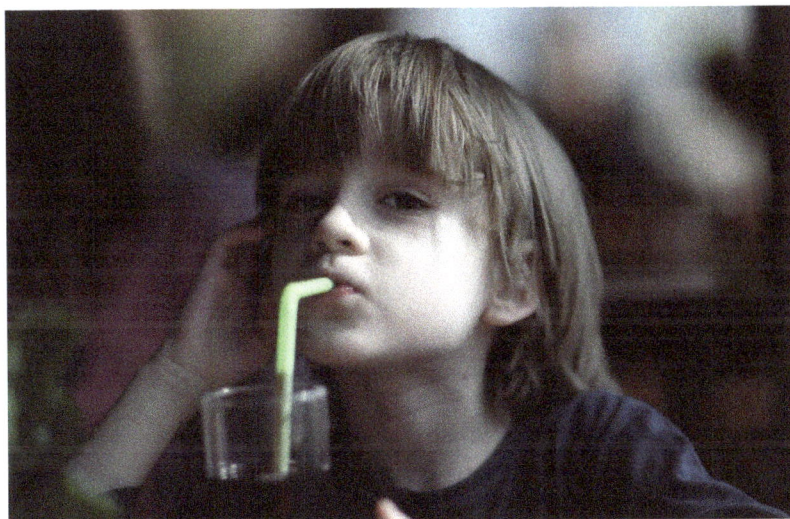

Drinking directly from a bottle or can, or using a straw, can lead to excess aerophagia.
Shutterstock/AnnaJurkovska

A hidden source of swallowed air is the air content present within many foods. Fruits contain a great deal more air than you might have imagined. If you compress an apple and add the volume of the juice and the pressed fruit together you will find that it was only sixty percent of the volume of the original fruit. In other words, of the entire fruit that you swallowed forty percent was air.

We have been in love with ice cream for thousands of years. All ice creams are not prepared in an identical manner. There is another important factor that leads to differences besides the ingredients such as cream or milk fat content, flavorings, sweeteners, stabilizers, emulsifiers, lactose, whey, casein, etcetera. It may be surprising to learn that the two largest ingredients in ice cream by volume are water (between fifty-five percent and sixty-four percent) and air (between three percent and fifty percent).

The other ingredients are measured as a percentage by weight. These include milk fat (minimum ten percent) or in premium ice creams, butter fat (up to nineteen percent). Other ingredients include sweeteners (twelve percent to sixteen percent), milk solids including proteins like casein and whey, and carbohydrates like lactose (between nine percent to twelve percent). Additional ingredients include stabilizers and emulsifiers like agar-agar or carrageenan extracted from seaweed that prevent the fat and water contents from separating (between zero point two percent to zero point five percent). Although air is a large percent by volume, it has virtually zero weight.

The finest ice creams have the lowest percentage of air, but the air is a necessary ingredient to provide a smooth, silky, creamy texture. Without the added air the ice cream would be denser, harder, and feel colder to the tongue. The size of the air bubbles is important as the smallest bubbles provide the smoothest texture. The industry term for air added to foods such as ice cream is 'overrun'. If one liter of ice cream is aerated to double the volume of the mixture to two liters, the overrun is one hundred percent. Most commercial ice creams aim for an overrun of seventy-five percent to one hundred percent, with super-premium ice creams achieving overruns of approximately twenty percent.

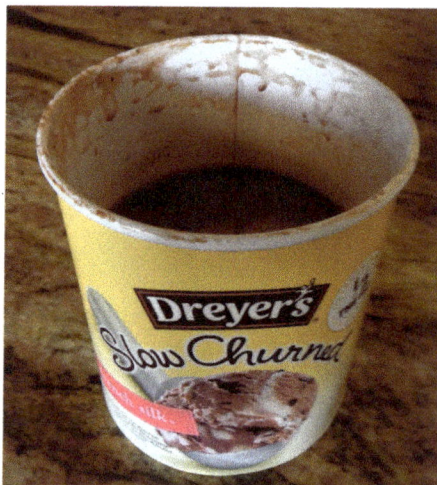

Overrun is the term used to describe air that is added into the finished food product to expand its volume as well as for texture. Air content of ice cream ranges from three percent to fifty percent and has a significant influence on texture, taste, and the value of the product purchased since ice cream is typically sold by volume, not weight. Photo by Lizabeth Weiss.

Have you ever noticed that the volume of ice cream decreases as it melts? If you have accidently left a full container of ice cream out of the freezer and it melted, you would find that it would only be about sixty percent full. You can quickly tell the difference in air content by lifting up equivalent size containers of super-premium ice creams and lower priced competitors. The super-premiums weigh much more, but also contain a lot more content, calories, and fat grams. If half of the volume of ice cream you eat is simply hidden air, you have just been spared half the calories and get the bonus of having swallowed more air to entertain your family and friends.

One of the advantages of a higher overrun, besides higher profits by selling a volume of air at the price of ice cream, is the fact that the air cells as bubbles may prevent ice crystals from forming. If you have ever had ice cream with ice crystals you know that the raspy cutting feeling on the tongue quickly ruins a pleasurable experience. The Food and Drug Administration has standardized the weight of ice cream to not fall below four and one-half pounds to the gallon. This weight standard has limited the amount of air that can be added to the ice cream to approximately fifty percent by volume.

The research team that developed the concept of aeration of ice cream included Baroness Margaret Thatcher, the former Prime Minister of Great Britain and contemporary of US President Ronald Reagan. Perhaps there is a kernel of truth that it was a right-wing conservative conspiracy to allow the addition of air allowing ice cream companies to double their profit by selling half a container of air at the full price of ice cream!

Gelato and ice cream are not identical and have a different composition and nutritional value. In the U.S. ice cream is required to have at least ten percent milkfat, with most medium to high end brands actually containing between fourteen percent to seventeen percent milkfat. Ice cream is churned at a high speed to incorporate air into the mixture to create a smooth and fluffy texture. Ice cream typically contains more than fifty percent air after the churning process both for enhanced mouth feel as well as profitability since it is sold by volume not weight. By contrast, gelato contains between three percent and eight percent milkfat, and twenty -five percent to thirty percent air.

Gelato is denser than ice cream due to its lower air content. A scoop of gelato weighs more than the same size scoop of vanilla ice cream. Since the nutritional comparison is based on ounces of weight and not volume, a scoop of gelato that is the same size as a scoop of ice cream may have more total calories, fat and sugar than ice cream. On average, a three and one-half ounce serving of vanilla gelato contains ninety calories, three grams of fat and ten grams of sugar. A typical three and one-half ounce serving of vanilla ice cream contains one hundred and twenty-five calories, seven grams of fat and fourteen grams of sugar. The fat in content coats the taste buds of the tongue, preventing them from completely experiencing the flavors. Because gelato has a lower fat content the taste buds experience flavors more intensely, and gelato does not need as much added sugar as ice cream for sweetness

The same proposition is true for bread and most baked goods. The baking process often uses baking powder or yeast. When the dough rises you are seeing the additional volume of gasses such as carbon dioxide being produced by the yeast fermentation process. Many foods are whipped with air to increase their volume, which adds to the smoothness and creaminess of the product. It also adds to the bottom line of profitability to the manufacturer, as you are paying for a product typically sold by volume. As long as they don't push it to the detriment of flavor and texture the more air added to a product increases its volume and profitability.

Carbonated beverages are very popular worldwide. In the United States sales of carbonated beverages exceed twenty billion dollars per year, four times the sales volume of dairy products. The majority consumed today already comes carbonated with large amounts of carbon dioxide forced into solution under high pressure. As the pressure seal of the can or bottle is released the carbon dioxide forms bubbles and comes out of the solution, giving a pleasant tickling sensation on the palate, and a full at times bloated feeling in the stomach and gut.

Many soft drinks have high concentrations of simple carbohydrates such as glucose, fructose, and sucrose. Oral bacteria ferment these carbohydrates and produce acidic products, which can erode the tooth enamel beginning the dental decay process. A large number of soft drinks are already acidic and have phosphoric acid added in the manufacturing process bringing their pH level to three or lower. To put this value in perspective, neutral water has a pH of seven and gastric hydrochloric acid has a pH of two. Many dentists advocate avoid the brushing of teeth shortly after an acidic beverage because the tooth enamel is more vulnerable to abrasions after being softened by acid.

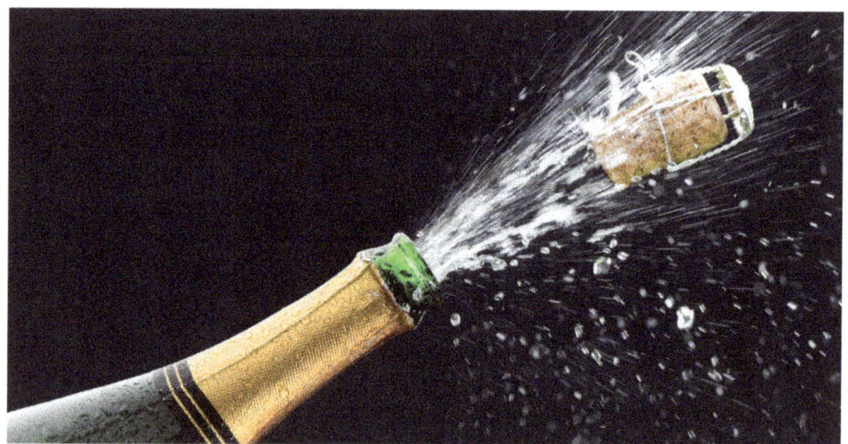

Carbonated champagne uncorking photographed with a high-speed air-gap flash. Shutterstock/lightwork

Mineral water cures were very popular in the middle ages and beyond. Going to the source of mineral springs and the drinking of its contents was referred to as 'taking the waters'. The waters had a variety of mineral content depending on source locale and included various salts and sulfur contents. The sites of such resources became well known as spas, baths, and wells and developed into destinations for the ill and infirm, as well as those who wished to preserve their good health. The term Seltzer water was originally a trademarked name for the German town of Selter that had a famous mineral spring.

The bottling of mineral waters became a profitable enterprise by offering people the opportunity to partake of the presumed beneficial waters in their own locales. An attempt to imitate the effervescent effect of the mineral waters was made by Joseph Priestley in 1767. Some fans of carbonated beverages believe this should be his claim to fame rather than his discovery of oxygen. J. J. Schweppes of Switzerland commercialized the process in 1783, moving his factory and enterprise to England in 1783.

Have you ever wondered how much carbon dioxide gas is released from a soft drink or carbonated beverage. You have already gotten a visual demonstration if the bottle or can was dropped or shaken before being opened. This agitation accelerates the release of the carbon dioxide, and it can form a jet stream of gassy bubbles to be sprayed on everyone within a dozen feet of the demonstration. This social activity is very popular amongst preadolescent boys. The quantification of how much carbon dioxide is in a one liter bottle of a carbonated soft drink is calculated using a formula known as Henry's Law.

The gas content in a one-liter bottle is a surprising two point eight liters. In other words, there is nearly three times the volume of the original container in excess gas under pressure hidden in those tiny bubbles. Do not forget another important law of the physics of gasses, Charles' Law. This law defines the activity of gasses expanding as the temperature increases. If you drink a cold carbonated beverage, and after swallowing it is warmed up to body temperature, it will exhibit another substantial increase in the volume of gasses released. The burping and belching that occurs after drinking a cold carbonated beverage may seem out of proportion to the small amount consumed. Just remember that whatever the volume of liquid carbonated beverage swallowed, there is nearly three times that volume of dissolved gas waiting to be released.

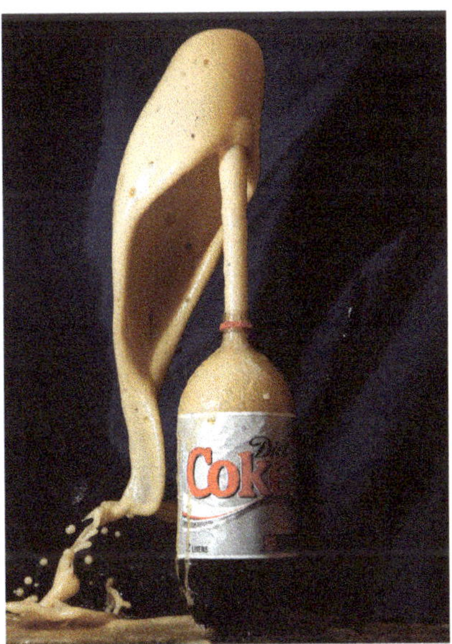

Diet Coke and Mentos Geyser by Michael Murphy Creative Commons License.

If you want further visual proof that Henry's Law is accurate take a look at the photographic evidence of another popular activity. The harmless addition of a Mentos brand mint candy tablet to a liter bottle of a carbonated beverage, such as Diet Coke, sounds like such an innocent activity. This demonstration is repeated in countless elementary school science classes. The *Guinness Book of World Records* described one thousand three hundred and sixty students in the historic university town of Leuven, Belgium creating simultaneous Mentos with Diet Coke geysers. See the entry on carbonation for more details about this process and phenomenon.

In some beverages the carbon dioxide would interfere with the taste and flavor by reacting with the ingredients, giving it an acid taste from carbonic acid. An alternative is to use nitrogen as the gas of choice as it is a neutral gas and would not interact with the beverage. The most popular example is Guinness, which uses nitrogen, or a combination of nitrogen and carbon dioxide, under pressure in kegs.

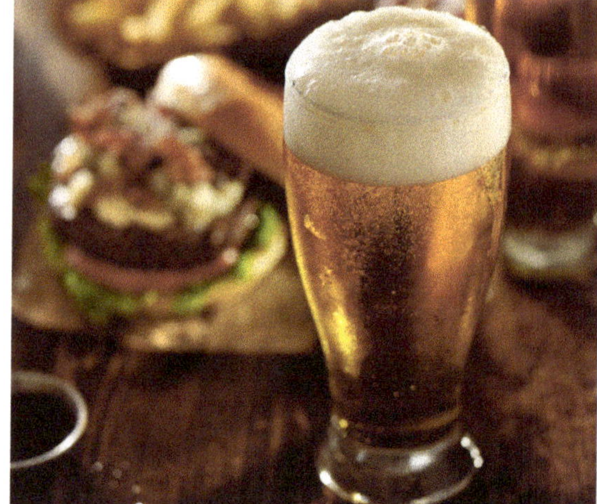

Shutterstock/JoshuaResnick

The nitrogen provides smaller firmer bubbles with a smoother longer lasting head, and other companies have followed their lead. Guinness also pioneered the use of a widget, an irregularity at the base of the container to serve as the nucleation focus for gas bubbles to form at the base of cans and bottles rather than the surface.

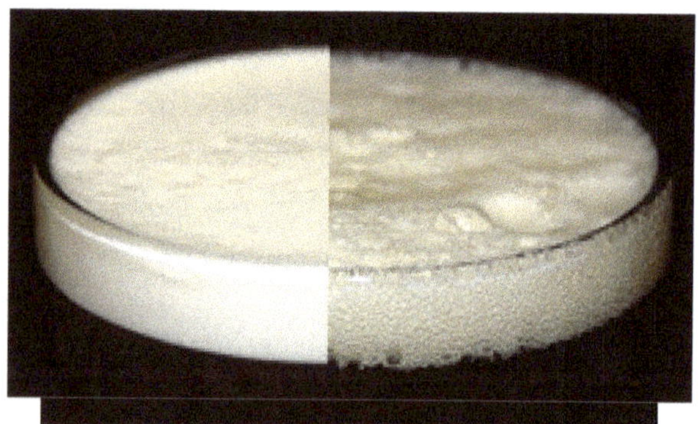

Creative Commons License

Nitrogen is poorly soluble in liquids, and the high density of bubbles contributes to a smooth creamy mouth feel. Most beers are saturated with a combination of thirty percent carbon dioxide and seventy percent nitrogen. The head serves both an aesthetic purpose, as well as accomplishing the dispersal of the beer aroma. You can get an idea of how high the nitrogen content is by looking at the size of the head created. A significant percentage of the volume of your drink is the head, and a friendly bartender will discard some of the head to give you more drink for your money, as well as to encourage a larger gratuity.

Beer drinkers are famous for the burping and belching generated. The added nitrogen gives them an edge up in competitive burping and belching contests since it is not as rapidly absorbed and eliminated via the lungs, as is carbon dioxide. Nitrogen is also used in iced coffee beverages, providing a head of bubbles very similar to that of beer.

Aerospace

Intestinal gas, like gasses everywhere, must comply with the laws of physics and the laws of nature. Boyle's law states that at a constant temperature, the product of the volume and pressure of a gas must remain constant. This requires that they maintain an inverse relationship, if one increases the other has to decrease. As such, an increase in pressure will result in the decrease of the volume of the gas, and vice versa. The atmospheric pressure on earth is defined as a standard of one atmosphere at sea level. As you go deeper down into the earth, such as happens in a mineshaft, or diving deeper into the oceans, the atmospheric pressure increases. As you go higher in elevation, whether climbing flights of stairs, ascending a mountain, or in a hot air balloon, the atmospheric pressure decreases. The atmospheric pressure is also not uniform, constantly changing along with the weather.

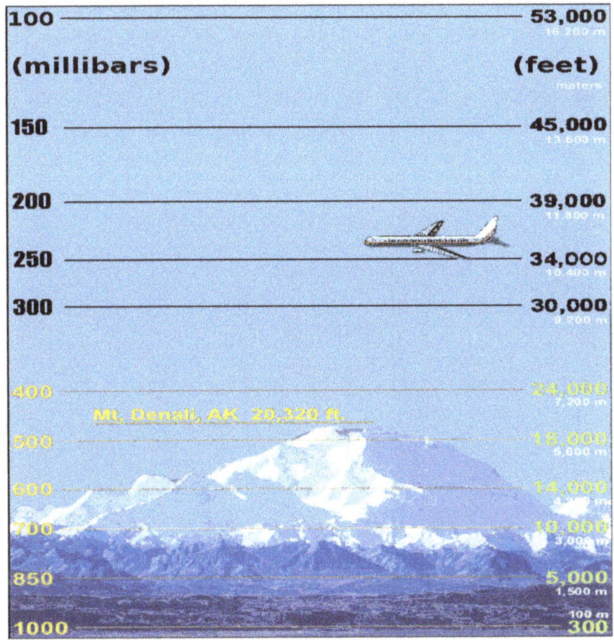

www.wpclipart.com NOAA Public Domain

The changes in atmospheric pressure in aerospace are even more dramatic than in mountain climbers, both in intensity and rapidity. During World War II, flight surgeons found that at altitudes thirty thousand feet or more above sea level, aviators suffered painful abdominal distension. At that altitude, the atmospheric pressure was a fraction of that at sea level, allowing intestinal gas to balloon to nearly four times its original volume. Painful distension of the abdomen was the result of the dramatic volume expansion of trapped intestinal gas. Because the trapped gas was not near the rectum, it could not be readily released as flatus.

Popularly referred to in the military by its abbreviated acronym, High-altitude flatus expulsion (HAFE) is a common gastrointestinal syndrome seen in pilots and passengers of aircraft. It involves the uncontrollable passage of large quantities of intestinal gasses at high altitudes. As the atmospheric pressure decreases with an increase in altitude, the volume of gas in the intestine increases consistent with the principles of physics (Boyle's Law). Military pilots and astronauts have repeatedly verified the existence of HAFE, with its sensation of distension, and the need to expel the expanding intestinal gasses. With commercial aircraft commonly flying at over thirty thousand feet in elevation, the atmospheric pressure outside of the plane is a fraction of atmospheric pressure at sea level. The pressure loss at that altitude would not be tolerable to passengers, so the aircraft is pressurized to simulate what the atmospheric pressure would be at approximately eight thousand feet above sea level.

The retained pockets of air in your gut will expand quickly, and want to be released even if it comes at the expense of your embarrassment. Airlines, pilots, and flight attendants are well aware of this effect, but they rarely offer the passenger any warning or explanation. They assume that you will not comment on the natural discomfort you are experiencing, or the subsequent release of intestinal gas, either your own or of the person sitting directly in front of you. In fact, it is to be expected that there is much more air turbulence inside an aircraft than outside.

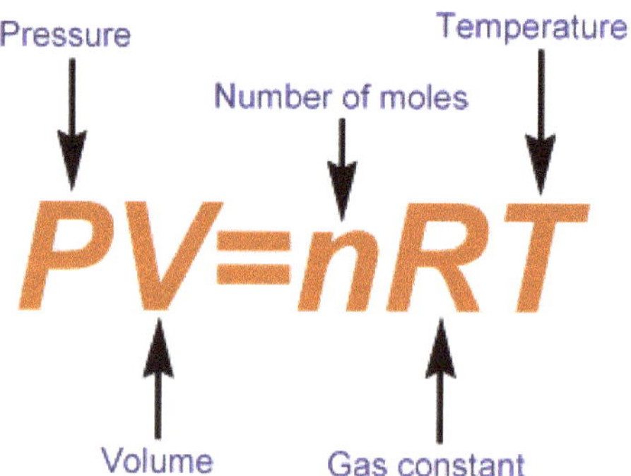

A visual example of the differences in atmospheric pressure between beings on the ground closer to sea level, and at an atmospheric pressure equivalent to an altitude of eight thousand feet is often served to you by a flight attendant. Take a close look at what happens to carbonated beverages served at high altitude. Have you ever noticed that the release of the bubbles of carbon dioxide from a carbonated beverage is much more dramatic when flying? Flight attendants have to spend more time while pouring the carbonated beverages, pausing to let the bubbles release themselves as they fill your glass. If they did not pause to let the gasses be released, you would be handed a container of fizz and foam instead of the beverage you wanted.

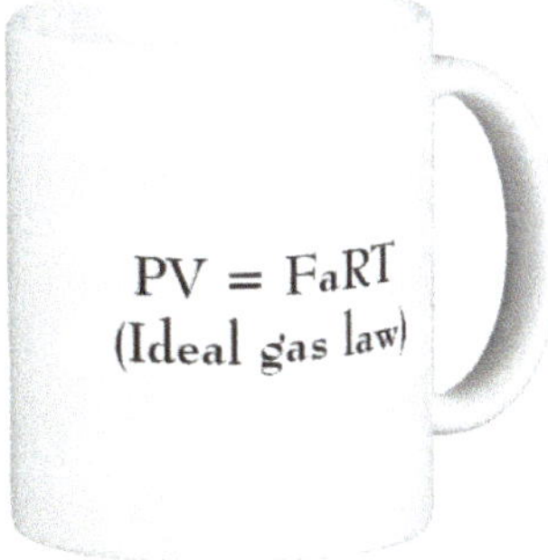

rlv.zcache.com

Aerospace has another concern that increases the volume and frequency of farts within the tight confines of a space capsule or space station. In an environment without gravity, the weightlessness leads to muscle weakness and atrophy. As the abdominal muscles weaken, the intestinal gasses expand further distending the gut and results in an increase in fart volume and frequency. While traveling in space, even in a pressurized space capsule, there is a very significant reduction in pressure, which means that gasses must exhibit a proportional increase in volume.

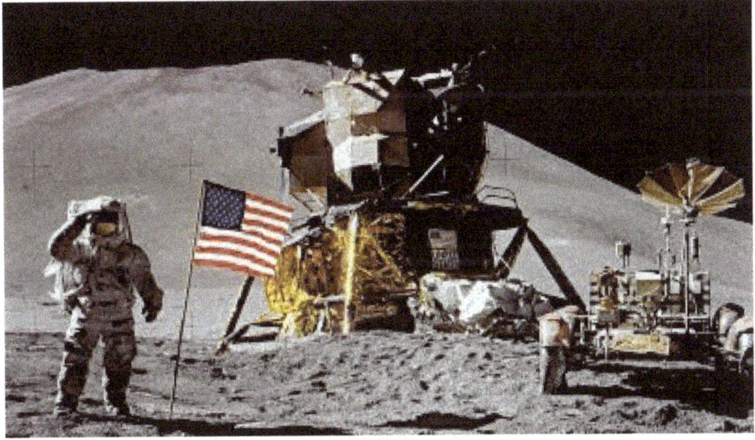
NASA Public Domain

For those involved in space travel, including the growing population of space tourists, the pressure changes are unparalleled. Many people are knowledgeable about the dangers of scuba and deep-sea divers, especially if surfacing from the depths too quickly. The nitrogen gas in the air that is breathed in at higher pressures dissolves in the bloodstream and body fats. When returning to the surface too quickly, the diver is subjected to a rapid drop in atmospheric pressure. The nitrogen gas comes out of solution, and forms bubbles of gas in the circulation. Decompression sickness, caisson disease, or 'the bends' is a risk for the space traveler as well.

The air and space traveler would likewise experience a rapid decrease in atmospheric pressure if not for the ability to pressurize the aircraft or spacecraft. The ambient atmospheric pressure within a spacecraft is typically maintained at fourteen point seven pounds per square inch (psi), or one hundred and one kilopascals (kPa). The most dramatic exposure to a rapid decrease in atmospheric pressure occurs when space travelers leave the pressurized spacecraft for spacewalks, more formally known as extravehicular activity.

Without the pressurized spacesuit, known more formally as extravehicular mobility units, the rapid reduction in atmospheric pressure may be life threatening. The spacesuit is typically pressurized to four point three pounds per square inch (thirty kPa). Without the spacesuit, decompression sickness also known as caisson sickness or the bends can develop in astronauts just as it does in deep-sea divers. As the atmospheric pressure is rapidly reduced the nitrogen gas that was previously in solution forms bubbles. These form in the bloodstream, nerves, joints and can cause pain, as well as circulatory collapse

Because the reductions in atmospheric pressure remain significant and put them at risk of life-threatening decompression sickness, the space travelers are given pure oxygen to breathe for several hours prior to the spacewalk. Breathing pure oxygen for several hours reduces the nitrogen dissolved in their circulation and fat stores, and further reduces the risk of nitrogen bubbles forming in their bloodstream leading to decompression sickness.

The early pioneers of space travel were appropriately heralded as heroes known for 'the right stuff'. They balanced the dangers and unknowns with a mixture of bravado and humor. As space travelers are at the extreme of reduced atmospheric pressure, they have a carte blanche to blame Boyle's Law for any and all gas bubbles they may wish to release. Alan Shepard, Jr. (1923–1998) was an American naval aviator, test pilot, and NASA astronaut. In 1961 Shepard became the first American, and second person after Soviet Cosmonaut Yuri Gargarin, to travel into space. When reporters asked Shepard what he was thinking about as he sat atop the potentially explosive Redstone rocket waiting for liftoff he replied "The fact that every part of this ship was built by the low bidder!" Ten years later, Alan Shepard was at the command of the Apollo 14 mission to the moon. Despite thick gloves and a stiff spacesuit Shepard struck two golf balls on the lunar surface driving the second golf ball "miles and miles and miles."

Benjamin Franklin was quoted as saying "Instead of cursing the darkness, light a candle." Alan Shepard created another memorable quote while waiting for the end of the interminable delays to launch. NASA engineers had delayed his first flight so many times that the Soviets were able to send the first man into orbit. On the day of his successful voyage, Shepard sat on the launch pad, waiting inside his rocket for over four hours while engineers corrected one challenging problem after another. The wait was longer than expected, and Shepard exceeded his bladder capacity. He ended up having to urinate inside his spacesuit. They had to turn off his monitoring equipment so that he did not create a short circuit. When one more problem cropped up, Shepard exclaimed, "Why don't you fix your little problem and light this candle!" The quote became the title of his biography, *Light This Candle.*

The U.S. space program was concerned about intestinal gas during space flight. After liftoff, while experiencing weightlessness, Shepard also experienced this other anticipated consequence of virtually zero atmospheric pressure. His internal gas bubbles expanded with the production of near continuous farting, which he graphically described over the radio communications with mission control. If you listen closely to the recording of the conversations, not all of the background noise was static!

As director of the astronaut program, Shepard received the following memorandum from astronaut John Young. "RE: Safety Issues. No less than six times have I had to listen to Borman complain about his lactose intolerance when someone stole his weird not-milk milk stuff. Additionally, when Borman drinks regular milk, he gets the farts. That's all I'm going to say about that." In the microgravity environment of space, farting results in the body being propelled when the 'digestive gas thruster is fired'. On the U.S.S.R. and Russian space station Mir, restraining devices were installed on the toilet seat, so the user would not be thrust off the seat with a fart.

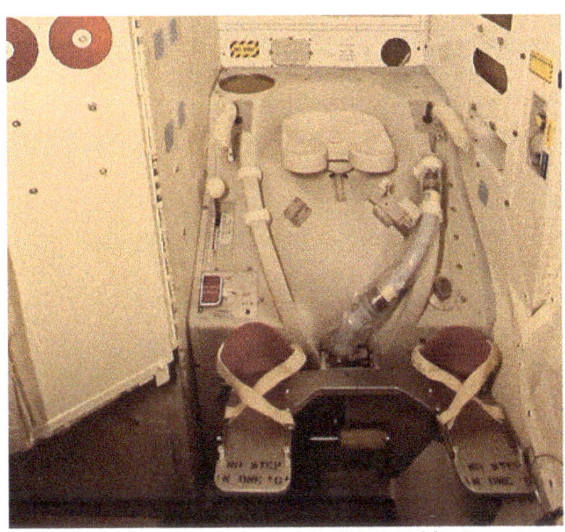

Bathroom on the space shuttle. NASA Public Domain

Gus Grissom was scheduled to go into space two months after Shepard's inaugural flight on Friendship Seven. He insisted that the 'potty' problem had to be solved, and a naval flight surgeon was assigned to the task. He sent one of the nurses into town to buy a women's panty girdle, which was layered with absorbent pads. Grissom was the first astronaut to go into space wearing women's lingerie. Astronauts, cosmonauts, and taikonauts have to deal with bodily functions in space, and modifications have been required. The Hamilton Standard Company was the maker of the U.S. astronaut spacesuits, and male astronauts used a condom catheter under the spacesuits for spacewalks and moonwalks. Ingenuity was required to come up with a comparable solution for female astronauts.

When the Gemini program began, the astronauts graduated to urine and fecal bags and special diapers for spacewalks. Urine waste was disposed of by an overboard dump valve. The solid waste was handled differently with a germicide placed in the storage bag, which was sealed in a locker. Since the lunar model itself was not designed with an overboard dump valve or storage cabinet, astronauts left very personal mementos of their visits behind. More than the national flag of the United States of America was deposited on the moon surface and remains there to this day. At the time the waste was left behind science believed than none of the microbes present in the feces could survive in the hostile environment of outer space or the moon. The remarkable discoveries since then of extremophiles (see Microbiome, Archaea) raises the possibilities that the material left behind still has viable and living microbes that could be the basis of a science fiction thriller with a scatological theme. When the Space Shuttle program was being engineered, a specially designed space toilet called the "Waste Collection Facility" or WCF for short was developed. It was budgeted to cost three million dollars to develop, but with cost over-runs it ended up being the world most expensive toilet by far costing more than thirty million dollars.

For those living in high altitude communities such as Mexico City at over seven thousand feet above sea level, the atmospheric pressure is much lower than at sea level. Commercial aircraft are pressurized to an equivalent of eight thousand feet above sea level. With the atmospheric pressure at just over two-thirds of sea level, the gas volume expands by about forty percent. That is more than enough to cause a person to notice a significant increase in their flatulence, and an increase in the flatulence of everyone else as well.

Air Enema

An air enema is often used during a barium enema study, when the air is inflated into the colon via the enema tube to provide air as a contrast to the barium. This type of barium study is called an air contrast or double-contrast barium enema. Air may also be inflated into the colon as the self-practice of the air enema that is described in the ancient yoga literature. The advanced yogi may develop anal sphincter control, and control of the abdominal muscles to create an abdominal suction effect to vacuum air into the lower intestine.

Shale Basti, also called Vat Basti, Air Basti, is an air enema used as an advanced Hatha yoga technique and is best learned from an expert teacher. There are a number of different approaches and techniques, but mastery of voluntary control of the anal sphincter is a challenging practice. See the entry on yoga for more details, as well as entry on Le Pétomane a stage performer who mastered this technique to great critical acclaim and commercial success.

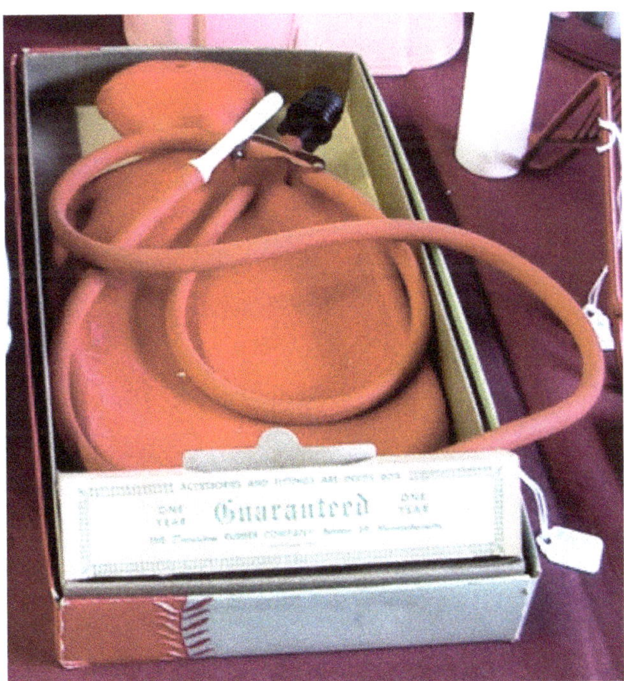

www.flickr.com Creative Commons License

Air Fart

The ability to air fart is the common term for the ability to control the anus and muscles of the abdomen and respiration, including the diaphragm, to cause air to be aspirated into the colon and then released voluntarily as a fart. It is also known colloquially as the ability to butt breathe. The air fart and butt breathe technique is known in more enlightened society as an air enema and has been practiced as a part of yoga colon hygiene for thousands of years. Although usually considered under involuntary control these muscles can be trained, and yogis attain remarkable proficiency. At the turn of the twentieth century, the performer Joseph Pujol, under the stage name Le Pétomane, became an international sensation by demonstrating his prowess at butt breathing. This ability is not limited to trained yogi and stage performers. According to the results of an internet-based survey on farting performed in 2001, with over one thousand three hundred participants, over fifteen percent of respondents were able to accomplish this with the benefit of being able to fart on command.

Fart survey question for men: Can you fart on command also called "Butt Breathe"?

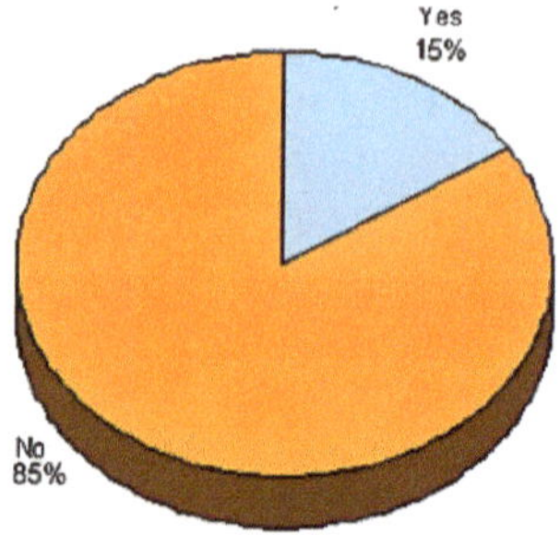

Only fifteen percent of the men surveyed can fart voluntarily by suctioning air into the colon. One-third of all men did not even know that this is possible!

Fart survey question for women: Can you fart on command also called "Butt Breathe"?

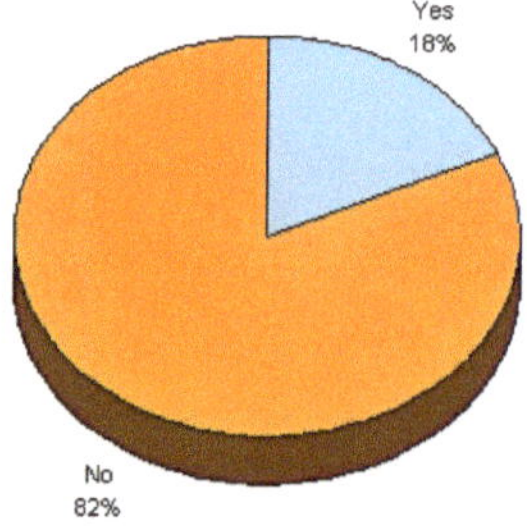

Eighteen percent of the women surveyed can fart voluntarily by suctioning air into the colon. This is either a remarkably high or low number, depending on the perspective.

Air, Gas Composition

If the entire abdomen is distended with air-filled loops of the intestine, a bowel obstruction may be its cause. Marked distension of the stomach can occur with gastroparesis, a neuropathy that delays stomach emptying seen most often in diabetics or when the pyloric channel or upper small bowel is obstructed. Iatrogenic is a fancy way of saying a physician was the cause. Iatrogenic air in the gastrointestinal tract is common after endoscopic procedures such as upper gastrointestinal endoscopy (esophagoscopy, gastroscopy, esophagogastro-duodenoscopy, EGD), endoscopic retrograde cholangiopancreatography (ERCP), or colonoscopy (proctoscopy, sigmoidoscopy, colonoscopy, ileoscopy, enteroscopy). The official name of the endoscopic procedure undertaken is defined by the anatomy of the organs examined.

The coming advances including capsule endoscopy will replace many of these multi-syllable, expensive, and invasive diagnostic tests. Developed initially by Given Imaging, a high-tech company based in Israel, a swallowed capsule travels through the digestive tract like a spying submarine. With remarkable visual clarity, it examines the lining of the bowel for abnormalities. Further development will allow it to obtain tissue samples and even therapeutic lasers bringing the science fiction movie *Fantastic Voyage* one step closer to reality. Other technology companies are pursuing this and other nanotechnology marvels that will travel through the body for diagnostic and therapeutic purposes.

Air is the typical gas inflated, and it may be several hours to up to a day for the excess gas to be eliminated. As described below carbon dioxide is the preferred gas for inflation since it is so readily absorbed and eliminated, but for either ease of access or because of the low cost, air continues to be used by most endoscopists. The radiologist also uses air insufflation with radiographic studies such as the barium enema. When the study is enhanced by air insufflation it is called an air-contrast or double-contrast barium enema.

Barium studies are not performed as often today, but they can provide valuable diagnostic information. A number of years ago I had a patient who was scheduled to have a barium enema to examine the colon, to be followed a few days later by a barium swallow to examine the esophagus. In about twenty percent of patients undergoing barium enema, the contrast material passes through the ileocecal valve and into the small bowel. This can be useful in providing additional diagnostic information about the distal small bowel, such as the presence of inflammatory bowel disease. In this individual, the barium entered the small intestine, but before the radiologist could reduce the pressure of the barium flow it refluxed all the way into his stomach and esophagus and the patient vomited up the barium. With disgust, the patient told the radiologist to cancel the barium swallow. When asked why, the patient told him he would never be able to drink the barium because it tasted like shit!

Iatrogenic (physician caused) distension with gas is routine in the performance of laparoscopy where tube-like visual instruments are used to examine the abdomen and pelvis. The gas used to inflate the abdominal cavity, creating a pneumoperitoneum, is carbon dioxide. The carbon dioxide gas is rapidly absorbed by the body and eliminated via exhalation through the lungs. If air were used the less than one percent component of carbon dioxide would be rapidly absorbed. The twenty-one percent portion of the air comprised of oxygen would be slowly absorbed over a few days. The remaining seventy-eight percent majority consisting of nitrogen is poorly absorbed. The nitrogen gas would remain within the peritoneal cavity for an extended period of time, being slowly absorbed over a period of several days to weeks.

Air, Iatrogenic

Iatrogenic is a fancy way of saying a physician was the cause. Iatrogenic air in the gastrointestinal tract is common after endoscopic procedures such as upper gastrointestinal endoscopy (esophagogastroduodenoscopy, EGD, esophagoscopy, gastroscopy), endoscopic retrograde cholangiopancreatography (ERCP), or colonoscopy (proctoscopy, sigmoidoscopy, colonoscopy, ileoscopy, enteroscopy). The official name of the endoscopic procedure undertaken is defined by the anatomy of the organs examined.

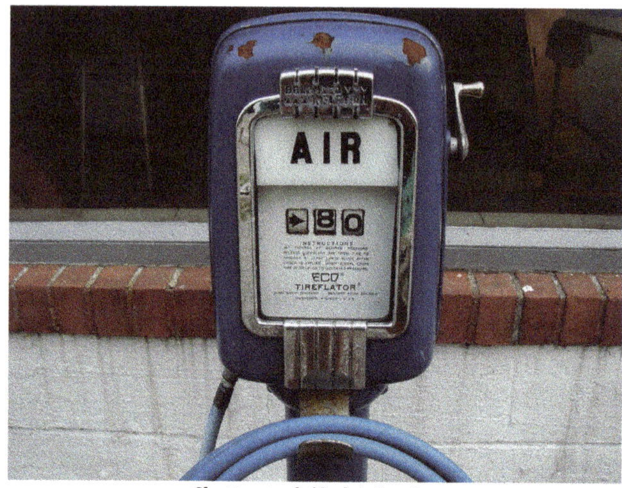

Shutterstock/CedricCrucke

Air is the typical gas inflated, and it may be several hours to up to a day for the excess gas to be eliminated. As described below carbon dioxide is the preferred gas for inflation since it is so readily absorbed and eliminated, but for either ease of access or costs air continues to be used by most endoscopists. The radiologist also uses air insufflation with radiographic studies such as the barium enema. When the study is enhanced by air insufflation it is called an air-contrast or double-contrast barium enema. Iatrogenic (physician caused) distension with gas is routine in the performance of laparoscopy where tube-like visual instruments are used to examine the abdomen and pelvis. The gas used to inflate the abdominal cavity, creating a pneumoperitoneum, is carbon dioxide.

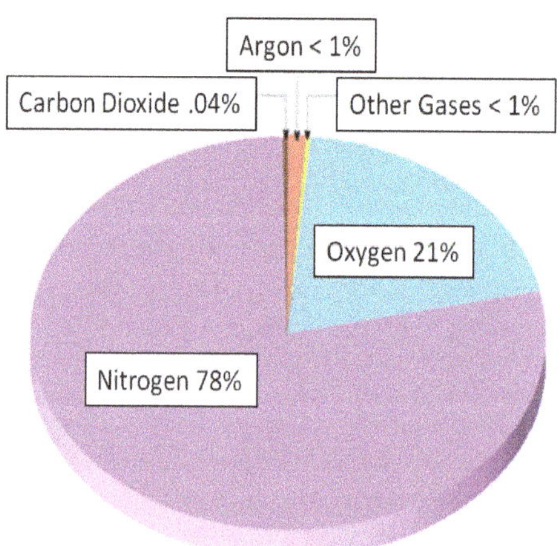

m7science.wikispaces.com Creative Commons License

The carbon dioxide gas is rapidly absorbed by the body and eliminated via exhalation through the lungs. If air were used the less than one percent component of carbon dioxide would be rapidly absorbed. The twenty-one percent portion of the air comprised of oxygen would be slowly absorbed over a few days. The remaining seventy-eight percent majority consisting of nitrogen is poorly absorbed. The nitrogen gas would remain within the peritoneal cavity for an extended period of time, being slowly absorbed over a period of several days to weeks.

Allopathic Medicine (Western Medicine)

Allopathic medicine (Greek ἄλλος, állos, other + πάθος, páthos, suffering) is a description commonly used by homeopaths and advocates of other forms of alternative medicine to refer to mainstream Western or modern medicine. The term was created in 1810 by the founder of homeopathy, Samuel Hahnemann (1755–1843). Allopathic medicine uses pharmacologically active agents or physical interventions to treat the causes and symptoms of diseases or conditions.

Hahnemann used the term allopathic medicine to contrast it from his homeopathic (Greek homeo similar) medicine philosophy of using diluted substances that would cause symptoms similar to the illness being treated. Early in its use, allopathic medicine was considered an offensive term and was not accepted by Western Medicine. Although it is literally incorrect it is now a commonly accepted term to describe Western or modern medicine.

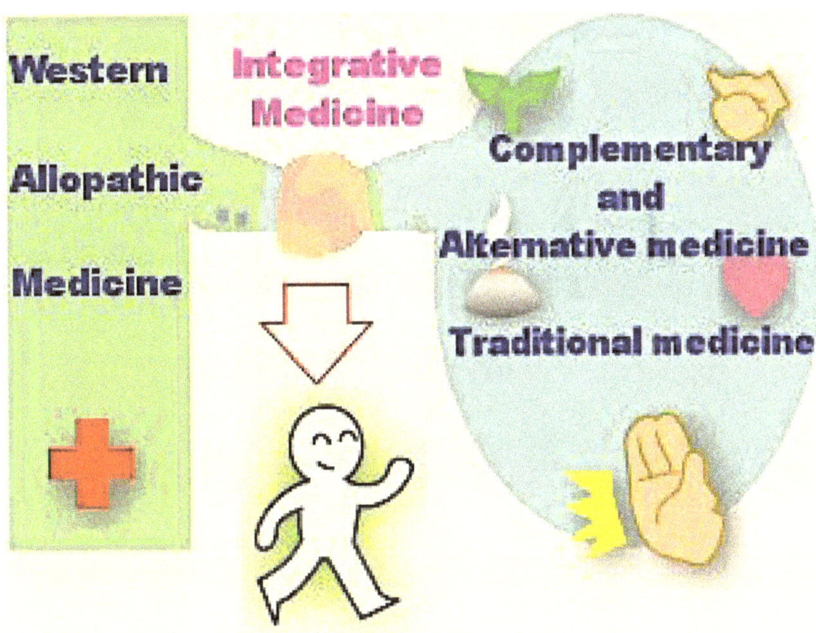

Alpha Galactosidase

Beano, Bean-Zyme, Say Yes To Beans, and competing products are an enzyme-based dietary supplement that is used to reduce the intestinal production of gas from dietary oligosaccharides such as raffinose, stachyose, and verbascose from legumes. Beano contains the enzymes alpha-galactosidase and invertase, which are derived from the fungus *Aspergillus Niger. Aspergillus Niger* and its fermentation products are 'generally recognized as safe' (GRAS) by the United States Food and Drug Administration (FDA). Because pets, such as dogs and cats, also release intestinal gas, the identical product was released to be marketed for pets under the brand name Curtail. Although it may be effective, it reduced the ability of guilty humans to blame a fart on the dog or cat and is no longer on the market as that brand name.

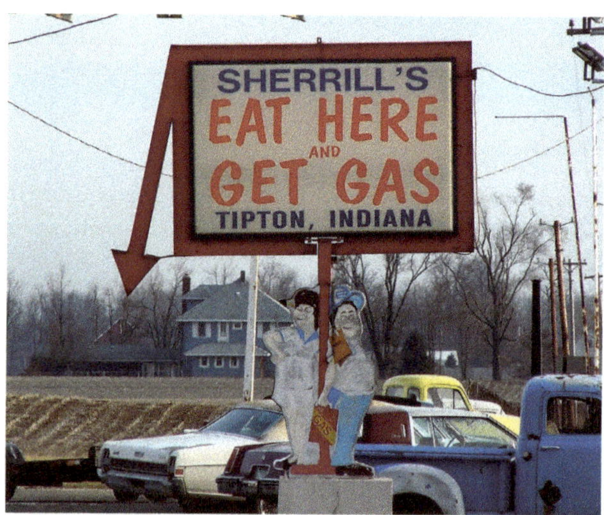

Refueling station and restaurant. Cindy Cornett Seigle www.flickr.com Creative Commons License

The alpha-galactosidase is effective but must be taken with the first bite of food. Because heating inactivates it, it cannot be used in the cooking process, and must be taken when eating the food. It does not have any effect on lactose or other enzyme deficiencies. Additional doses of alpha-galactosidase will be needed if large quantities of legumes are consumed, or a substantial period has passed since the dose was taken.

Another approach is to soak the beans for several hours and discard the fluid, which leaches out some of the complex sugars. Allowing the seeds to germinate allows the bean plant itself to begin to produce alpha-galactosidase. Within twenty-four hours of germination the internally generated enzyme breaks down most of the complex sugars. Using the herb asafetida can also reduce flatulence although the herb itself has an aroma that may be worse than the farts you are trying to prevent. The name of the herb itself may give you a clue as fetida has the same root as the word fetid. These words are derived from the Latin word foetidus and *foetēre* meaning 'to stink'

Certain beans are being developed that have lower concentrations of the challenging complex sugars. The enzyme hydrolyses the polysaccharides and oligosaccharides of the raffinose family including stachyose, verbascose, and galactinol found in foods such as the legumes beans and peanuts, and the cruciferous vegetables cauliflower, broccoli, cabbage, and Brussels sprouts. Beano was marketed by Alan Kligerman of AkPharma, Inc. in 1990. Originally in the dairy farm business, he was the developer of the commercially successful lactase (lactose milk sugar enzyme) supplement Lactaid. Beano received a US patent in 1995, which is estimated to expire in 2015. There are more than fifty competing products on the market. It should be noted that the use of these products enhances the digestibility of certain foods and increases the nutrients and calories absorbed.

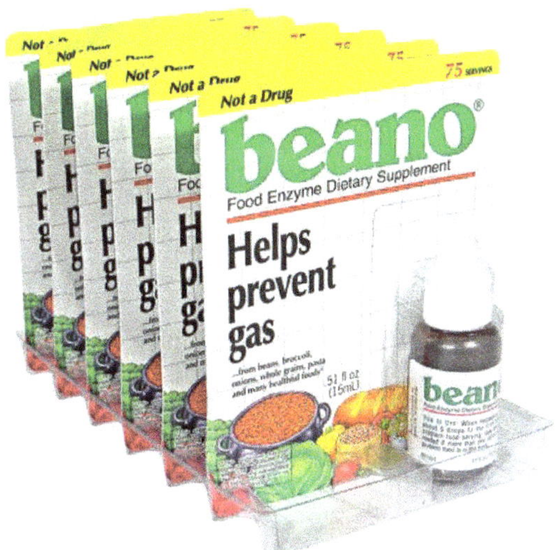

www.flickr.com Creative Commons License

The intellectual concept for a product to reduce or mask the aroma of intestinal gas was proposed in the 1780's by Benjamin Franklin. He submitted an essay "A Letter To A Royal Academy" suggesting that an award be given to the inventor of a food additive that would make the aroma of flatus attractive instead of offensive. Benjamin Franklin was known as for his sense of humor, and although some thought his proposal was serious, it was written tongue in cheek.

Simple sugars are produced in the malting process of barley to brew beer. The complex sugars that are not hydrolyzed or fermented and consumed by the beer drinker may contribute to its well-recognized ability to increase flatulence. Some home brewers have added Beano to the mash in an attempt to reduce this occurrence. The use of the prescription drug Acarbose or Miglitol used in the treatment of diabetes mellitus will cause a dramatic increase in flatulence because of its enzyme inhibitor activity. These drugs are used to treat type 2 diabetes mellitus by inhibiting the glycoside hydrolases, the alpha-galactosidae family of enzymes necessary for the digestion of many starches. It specifically inhibits alpha-glucosidase enzymes in the brush border of the villi of the small intestines, pancreatic alpha-amylase, maltase, isomaltase, glucoamylase, sucrose, and invertase.

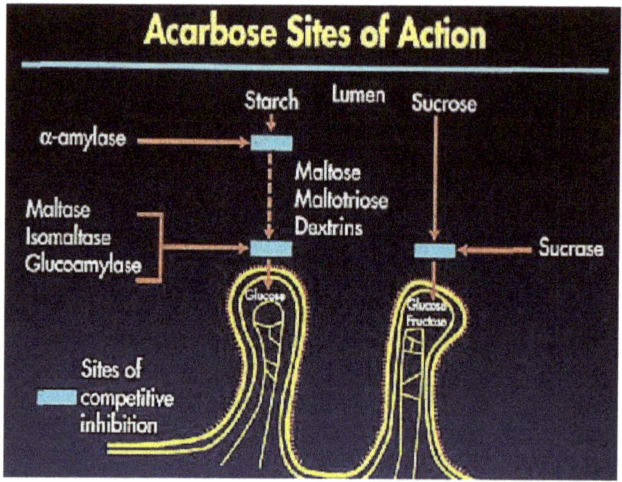

Alpha-glucosidase inhibitors are the competitive, reversible inhibitors of pancreatic alpha amylase and membrane bound intestinal alpha glucosidase hydrolase enzymes. Use of these drugs leads to a blockade of the the enzymatic degradation of complex carbohydrates in the small intestine, decreasing the amount and delaying the absorption of these sugars. Acarbose, which is not absorbed by the body, has the following preferred affinity for blocking the alpha glucosidase enzymes: glycoamylase > sucrase > maltase > dextranase and has no affinity for the alpha glucosidase enzymes, such as lactase. Miglitol is a more potent inhibitor of sucrase and maltase than acarbose and has no effect on alpha amylase.

Pancreatic alpha amylase hydrolyzes complex starches to oligosaccharides in the chyme being digested in the lumen of the small intestine. The intestinal alpha-glycosidase further hydrolyzes oligosaccharides, trisaccharides, and disaccharides to glucose and other monosaccharides at the brush border of the villi in the small intestine. Inhibition of these enzyme systems reduces the rate of digestion of complex carbohydrates and decreases the amount of glucose available for absorption. It should be taken at the start of a meal, and as more complex carbohydrates pass to the colon undigested, increased bacterial fermentation will result. Increased flatulence is reported in the vast majority of patients, and approximately fifteen percent develop diarrhea. The gastrointestinal side effects may diminish with continued use over time. Adverse side effects may also include elevation of liver function tests, which usually resolves with discontinuation of the medicine.

There has been a significant increase in average size and stature of adults in a wide diversity of countries around the world over a span of only one or two generations. The obvious explanation is the improvement in access to not only additional calories but also the critical nutrition role played by vitamins, dietary minerals, and trace elements. The full role of diet, nutrition, hormones, enzymes, the gut flora and microbiome, genetics, epigenetics, and other factors is still in the process of being elucidated.

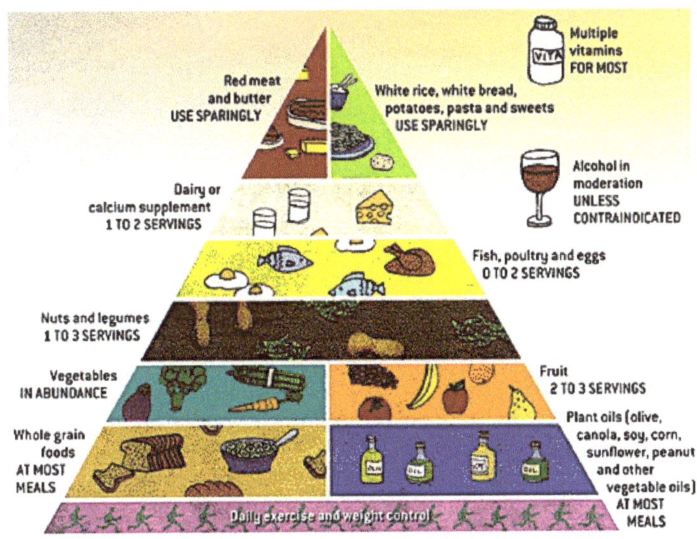

NEW FOOD PYRAMID
outlined by the authors distinguishes between healthy and unhealthy types of fat and carbohydrates. Fruits and vegetables are still recommended, but the consumption of dairy products should be limited.

Public Domain

Certain types of vegetables and fruits contain carbohydrates with substantial quantities of sugars and starches that may be poorly digested by people but happily fermented by bacteria comprising the gut flora. The starches, including potatoes, corn, noodles, and wheat are the source of the majority of gasses generated by the gut microbial flora. Rice is the one starch exception and rarely contributes to intestinal gas production. Wheat has the other 'distinction' of having the protein glutamate, which contains the nitrogen base product that contributes to the generation of ammonia-like aromatic compounds. The most common food intolerance is for the milk sugar, lactose when an individual has decreased quantities and activity of the necessary enzyme for its digestion, lactase.

Amino Acid

Aromatic amino acids are a category of amino acids that include the chemical structure of an aromatic ring. Examples include the essential amino acids phenylalanine, tryptophan, histidine, and the semi-essential amino acid tyrosine. Essential amino acids are those that humans or other animals cannot synthesize for themselves and must be obtained from the diet.

Tyrosine is semi-essential in that it can be synthesized, but only if phenylalanine is ingested. The disorder phenylketonuria occurs when there is an absence of the enzyme phenylalanine hydroxylase, which is required for tyrosine synthesis.

Essential	Conditionally Non-Essential	Non-Essential
Histidine	Arginine	Alanine
Isoleucine	Asparagine	Asparatate
Leucine	Glutamine	Cysteine
Methionine	Glycine	Glutamate
Phenylalanine	Proline	
Threonine	Serine	
Tryptophan	Tyrosine	
Valine		
Lysine		

The twenty standard amino acids, divided into essential, conditionally non-essential and non-essential categories; Non-essential amino acids are synthesized in the body, while essential amino acids must be obtained from food. All plants and microorganisms synthesize their aromatic amino acids, unlike animals, which obtain them through their diet. Animals have lost these energy intensive metabolic pathways, since they obtain aromatic amino acids through their diet. Herbicides and antibiotics inhibiting enzymes involved in aromatic acid synthesis are toxic to plants and microorganisms dependent on this pathway, but not to animals which do not utilize these enzymes.

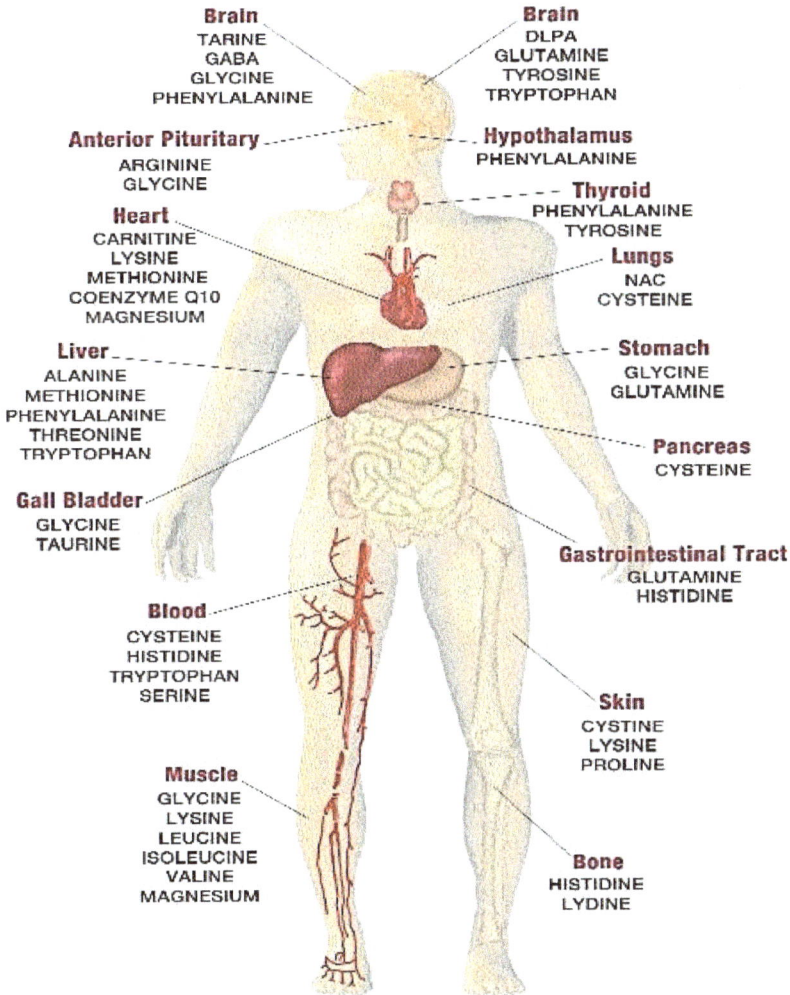

Brain
TARINE
GABA
GLYCINE
PHENYLALANINE

Brain
DLPA
GLUTAMINE
TYROSINE
TRYPTOPHAN

Anterior Pituritary
ARGININE
GLYCINE

Hypothalamus
PHENYLALANINE

Thyroid
PHENYLALANINE
TYROSINE

Heart
CARNITINE
LYSINE
METHIONINE
COENZYME Q10
MAGNESIUM

Lungs
NAC
CYSTEINE

Liver
ALANINE
METHIONINE
PHENYLALANINE
THREONINE
TRYPTOPHAN

Stomach
GLYCINE
GLUTAMINE

Pancreas
CYSTEINE

Gall Bladder
GLYCINE
TAURINE

Gastrointestinal Tract
GLUTAMINE
HISTIDINE

Blood
CYSTEINE
HISTIDINE
TRYPTOPHAN
SERINE

Skin
CYSTINE
LYSINE
PROLINE

Muscle
GLYCINE
LYSINE
LEUCINE
ISOLEUCINE
VALINE
MAGNESIUM

Bone
HISTIDINE
LYDINE

Amino Acid needs by body location.

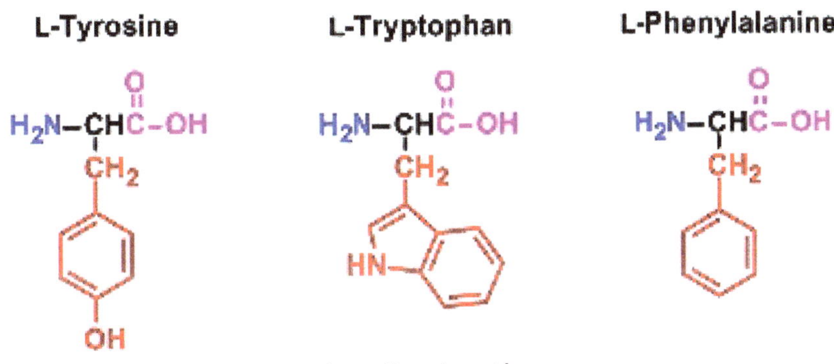

Aromatic amino acids.

The aromatic amino acids are precursors for important neurotransmitters. The same enzyme, L-aromatic amino acid decarboxylase is required for the synthesis of the monoamines serotonin and dopamine. If the amino acid precursors of one system dominate the enzyme in monoamine synthesis it could lead to an unbalance and depletion of the other monoamine.

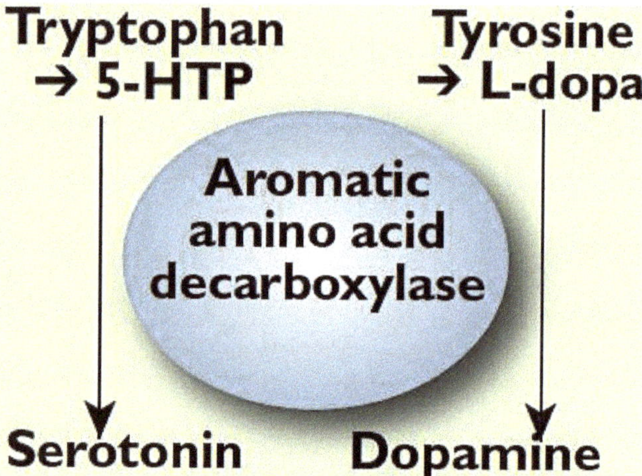

The same enzyme, L-aromatic amino acid decarboxylase (AAAD), is responsible for synthesis of the monoamines serotonin and dopamine.

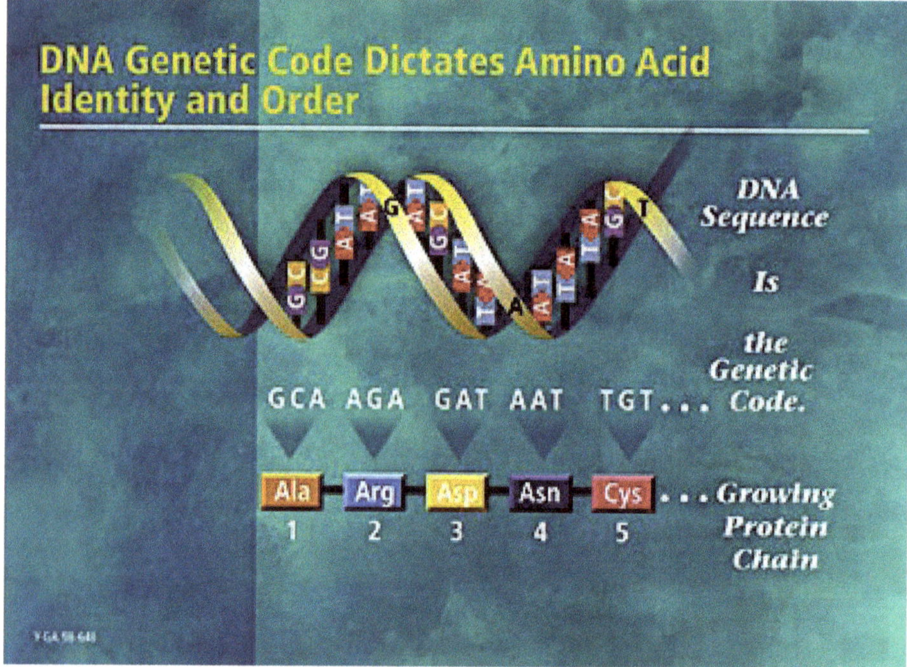

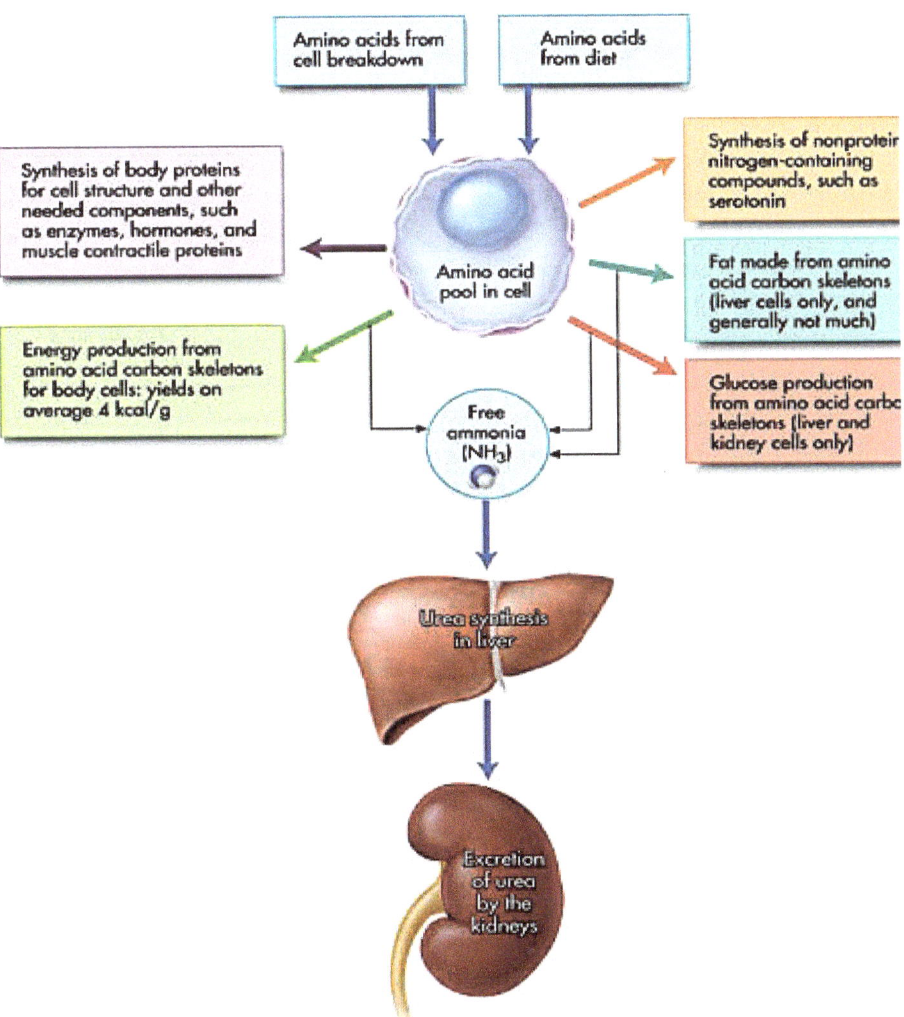

Amylase

Amylase is an enzyme that catalyzes the degradation of starches into sugars. Erhard Friedrich Leuchs (1800–1837) documented that starch was hydrolyzed and the active enzyme identified in the saliva was named amylase. You can see the effect of amylase in saliva by chewing on starchy food like potatoes for a few minutes. The salivary amylase breaks the starches down to glucose and the chewed starch begins to taste sweeter as the glucose is produced.

In addition to the salivary glands, the pancreas also produces amylase. The amylase enters the duodenum from the pancreatic duct via the Ampulla of Vater. It hydrolyzes the dietary starch into disaccharides and trisaccharides. These are further digested by other enzymes in the small intestine converting them to monosaccharides such as glucose, which can be more readily absorbed.

Plants, yeast, and some bacteria also produce amylase. Amylase also plays an important role in converting starches to sugars in the processing of bread and beer. For wheat, alpha-gliadins are seed-storage proteins, but also act as inhibitors of alpha-amylase activity.

Anus

The anal canal is the distal and terminal portion of the large intestine of the gastrointestinal tract, with the anus being the outlet for digestive waste. In the long tube like structure of the gastrointestinal tract, the term proximal means closest to the mouth, and distal means closest to the anus. In the intestines the term terminal means the end of the tube like structure. It is not used as the term for the end of life like the phrase terminal illness, it is more like the use of the word as in train terminal, where the travel line ends.

The proximal portion of the anal canal begins at the superior aspect of the pelvic diaphragm, where the rectal ampulla narrows. This is at the level of the U-shaped sling formed by the puborectalis muscle. The canal is approximately one and one-half inches (three and one-half centimeters) long. The distal aspect of the anal canal ends at the anus itself, the terminal outlet of the alimentary canal.

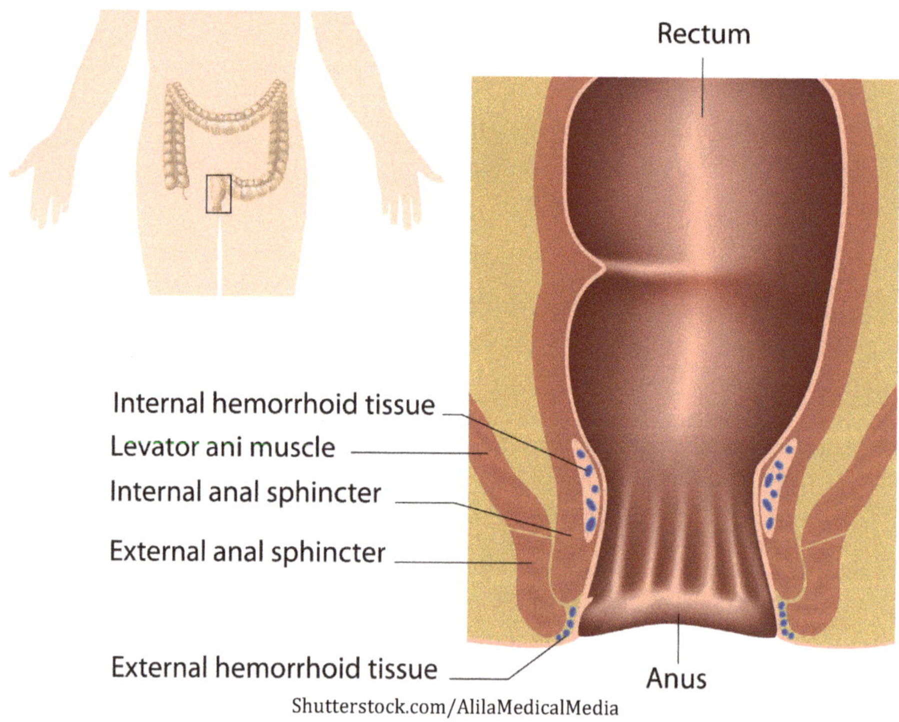

Shutterstock.com/AlilaMedicalMedia

Fecal continence is a function of the coordinated activity of the involuntary internal and voluntary external anal sphincters. The sympathetic nervous system maintains the tone of the involuntary internal sphincter. This tone allows it to remain closed, except during filling of the rectal ampulla. The rectoanal inhibitory reflex is the involuntary internal anal sphincter relaxation in response to rectal distention. This reflex is one reason why an enema can be promptly effective in stimulating a bowel movement. The loss of the tone of the internal anal sphincter leading to fecal incontinence with capital punishment is known to the executioner, but is rarely known to those who commit suicide by this means. Perhaps this knowledge would deter this form of suicide by those who believe they are selecting a very sanitary way of leaving the world behind. The greatest deterrent might be if they were aware of how much grief and pain they leave behind for their loved ones, and how a tragic suicide is all too often a permanent 'solution' for a temporary problem.

The anal sphincter tone may also be relaxed and inhibited during parasympathetic stimulation inducing contraction of the rectum. During these events, the closure must be maintained by voluntary contraction and heightened tone of the puborectalis and external anal sphincter, to prevent defecation before it is socially appropriate.

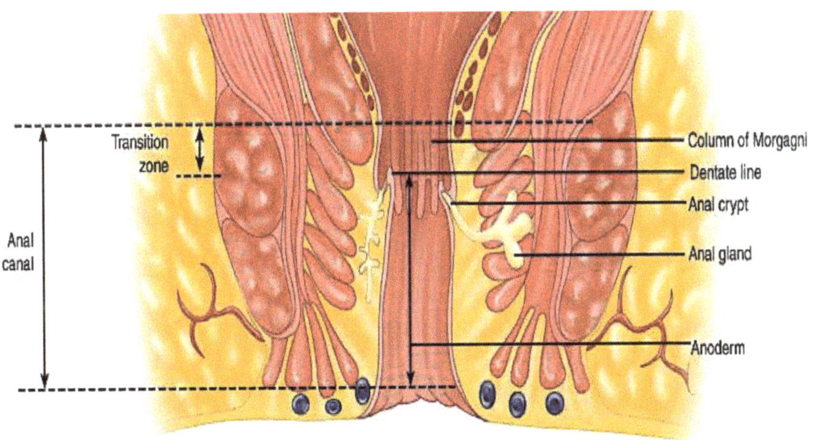

www.knowyourbody.net/wp- Creative Commons License

Internally the pectinate line is a visible landmark that demarcates the transition from visceral to somatic innervation and vascular supply. The canal is surrounded by superficial and deep venous plexuses, which normally have a varicose appearance. The hemorrhoidal vascular plexus contributes to the maintenance of fecal continence.

The external anal sphincter is usually under voluntary control. The sphincter is a large muscle forming a broad band across both sides of the lower two-thirds of the anal canal. The external anal sphincter is supplied through the inferior rectal nerve, which also serves the levator ani and puborectalis. They contract simultaneously to preserve continence when the internal sphincter is inhibited or relaxed, except during defecation. Internally the superior half of the anal canal has a series of longitudinal ridges called anal columns. Within these columns are the terminal vessels of the superior rectal artery and vein. The anorectal junction is demarcated by the proximal ends of the anal columns. It is at this point that the wide rectal ampulla narrows as it traverses the pelvic diaphragm.

The distal ends of the anal columns are bridged by anal valves. Proximal to the valves are small indentations called the anal sinuses. When compressed by feces the anal sinuses exude mucus, which aids in lubrication and the evacuation of feces from the anal canal. The distal limit of the anal valves forms an irregular line called the pectinate line. This line demarcates the junction of the superior and inferior portions of the anal canal.

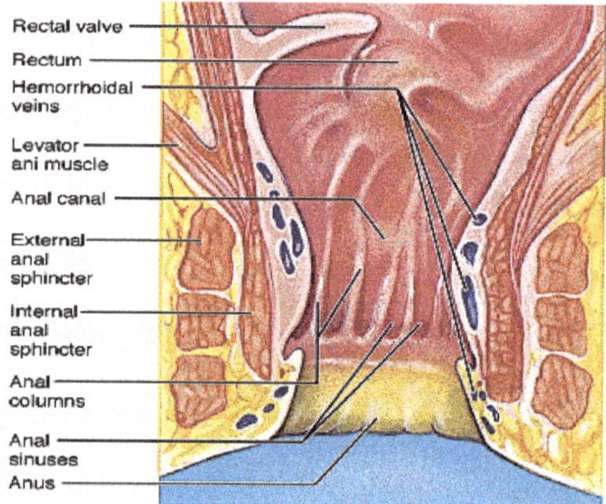

Anal canal anatomy http://www.webdicine.com Creative Commons License

The anal canal proximal to the pectinate line has significant differences from the part that is distal to this landmark. The pectinate line is the anatomical landmark that separates the arterial supply, innervation, venous circulation, and lymphatic drainage of the proximal and distal portions. These differences are the result of the separate embryological origins of the proximal and distal parts of the anal canal. The proximal portion is visceral and derived from the embryonic hindgut. The distal portion is somatic and is derived from the embryonic proctodeum.

Proximal to the pectinate line, the anal canal cannot sense pain, touch or temperature. The proximal anal canal is sensitive only to stretching, which evokes sensations at both the conscious and the unconscious reflex levels. For example, distension of the rectal ampulla inhibits and relaxes the tone of the internal anal sphincter. Distal to the pectinate line, the sensory nerves of the anal canal have somatic innervation. As somatic sensory nerves they are able to sense pain, touch, and temperature. This is why internal hemorrhoids that occur above the pectinate line are painless. External hemorrhoids that occur distal to the pectinate line can be excruciatingly painful. Efferent fibers of the somatic nerves cause contraction of the voluntary external anal sphincter when stimulated.

Based on the histology of cellular tissue the anal canal may be divided into three parts. The zona columnaris is the proximal portion of the anal canal and is lined by simple columnar epithelium. The distal half of the anal canal, below the pectinate line, is further divided into two zones separated by Hilton's white line. The two parts are the zona hemorrhagica lined by stratified squamous non-keratinized epithelium and the zona cutanea, lined by stratified squamous keratinized epithelium.

The anal glands or sacs are sebaceous glands located in the anal canal of many mammals including dogs and cats that secrete a liquid used in the marking of territory. The anal glands are emptied passively with the passage of solid feces. With soft or loose stools the glands may not be sufficiently emptied and impaction can develop. Humans have anal glands as well, and can identify the scent of their own feces and flatus.

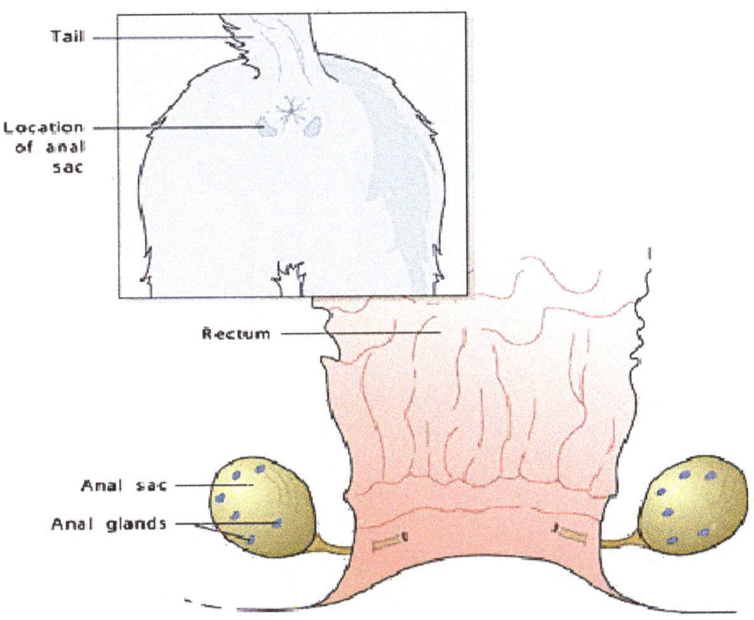

Anal glands. www.michigananimalhospital.com

Irritation or impaction of the glands can lead to pruritus ani (anal itching), perianal pain, and abscess formation. Perirectal abscess is a very painful and potentially dangerous condition that responds to antibiotics after surgical incision and drainage. Perirectal fistula may also develop and are often associated with an inflammatory bowel condition such as Crohn disease. Perianal disease such as abscess, fistula, and fissures are best treated early for pain relief and healing.

In dogs, these glands may be referred to as 'scent glands', and butt sniffing is a means of identification of territorial markers. If the anal glands are impacted it can lead to scooting its bottom on the ground or floor, tail chasing, or licking and biting the anus. Dog groomers often perform anal sac expression for the hygiene and comfort of the animal. In cats impacted glands can cause defecation outside of the litter box. Skunks anal glands generate the foul smelling spray they utilize as a defense mechanism.

Some humans find the scent of the anal glands attractive, and many people are surprised that they find the scent of their own farts particularly appealing. Perhaps even more unexpected is how many find the aroma of farts of others attractive. Musk (Sanskrit muskies - testicle) is a class of aromatic substances used in perfumery. It is also used in Ayurveda, the traditional medical healing system developed in ancient India, where it is considered a life-saving drug in cardiac, mental, and neurological disorders. Musk was obtained from a gland of the now endangered male musk deer. By weight it is has three times the value of gold. The organic compound responsible for the musk odor is mascon. Nearly all musk used in perfumes today is synthetic.

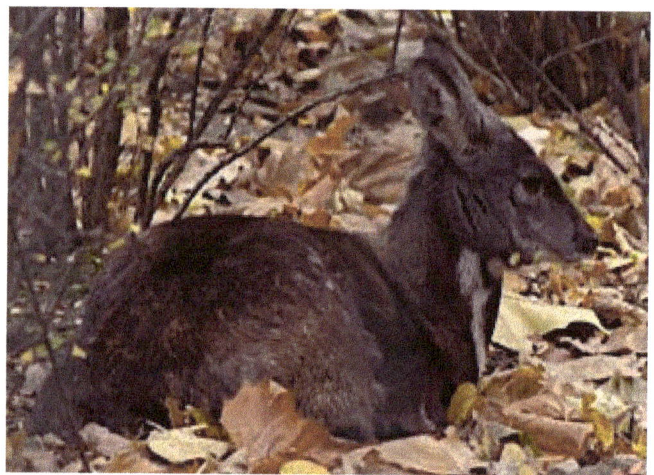

Deer Musk (Moschidae) Author: F. Spangenberg Creative Commons License

Throughout history high quality musk was stored in special containers and vessels made of gold, silver or brass. These were often placed in the royal palace for its intoxicating fragrance. Musk is produced in a special gland found in a hairy sac midway between the stomach and the genitals of the musk deer *Moschus moschiferus*. The name musk is derived from the Sanskrit term muska, which means testicle. This is actually a misnomer as the musk gland is not the testicle and the hairy sac in which it is anatomically located is not the scrotum.

The musk deer is a shy and nocturnal animal that is about three feet in length and one and a half feet tall. Hunters have historically resorted to entrapment to capture the musk deer. Its natural habitat is in the Himalaya Mountains, highlands, and forests of Tibet, as well as Siberia, and northwest China. Somewhat ironically for a product named after the testicle, the female of the musk deer species is the primary producer of black musk. This premier product is a high quality perfume additive.

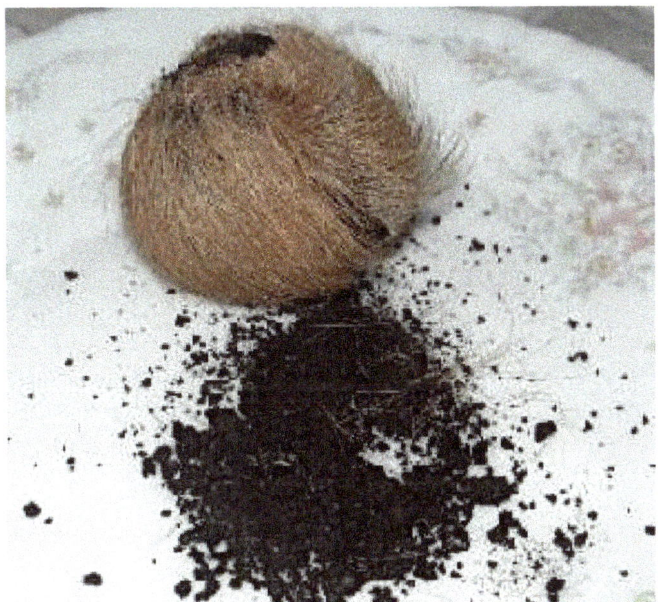

Musk sniffffffff.blogspot.com Creative Commons License

Historically, hunters would unnecessarily kill the deer for the musk sac, which is then dried under direct sunlight, or dipped in very hot oil. Musk can actually be harvested in the proper season without killing the animal. The musk deer whose life has been spared may be available for future musk harvesting. Musk comes from several countries including China, Tibet, Nepal, and Siberia in Russia.

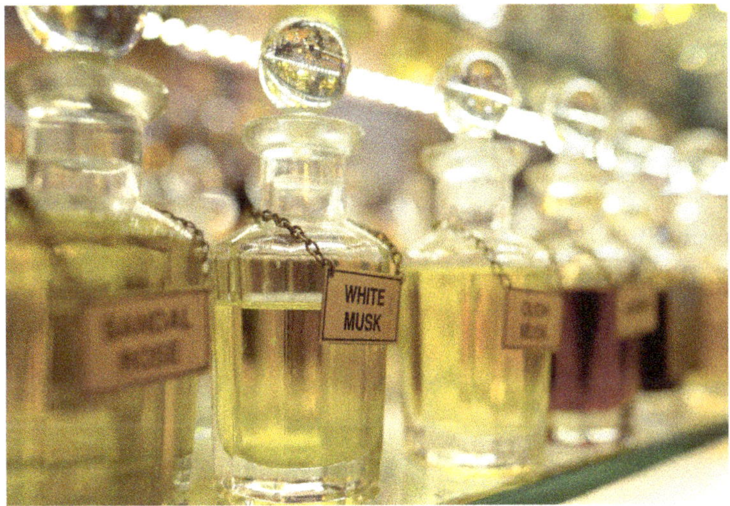

Shutterstock/jcfmorata

Skunks (also called polecats) are mammals related to the ferret, which spray a liquid with a strong offensive odor from their anal glands as a defense mechanism. The skunk can aim the spray, which contains sulfur containing thiols and mercaptans, accurately over a distance of over ten feet (three meters). They are generally reluctant to release their spray, as it takes them up to two weeks to replenish the supply once dispensed.

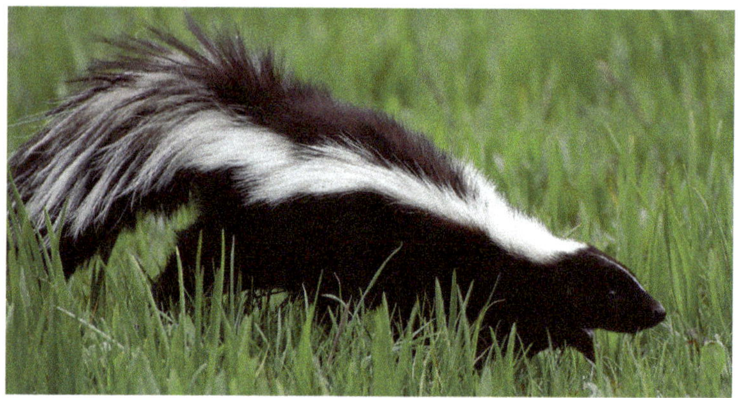

Shutterstock/JamesColeman

Anal cleansing after defecation was historically accomplished with sticks, leaves, stones, clay, corncobs, water, or literally whatever was available at hand. The ancient Greeks used clay and stone. Romans used a water soaked sponge on a stick. Toilet paper has been used for the cleaning of the anus and urethra after elimination for well over one thousand years. The first recorded use of toilet paper was in China in the sixth century.

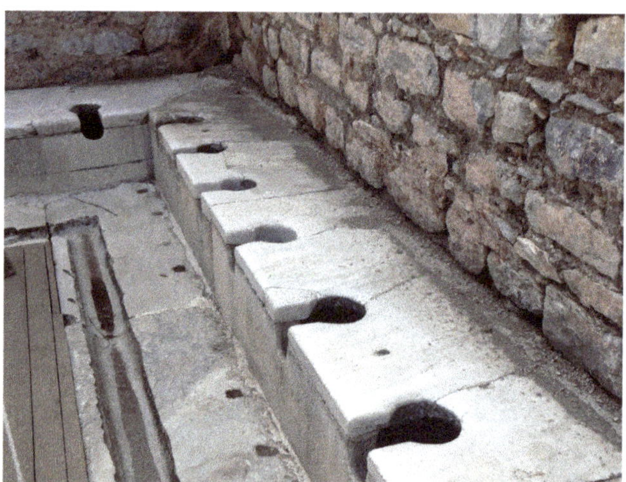

Toilets in ancient Rome had sophisticated sewer lines with running water to remove waste. Remarkably many countries around the world have more primitive systems in place today than the Romans had over two thousand years ago. shutterstock/AbelFeyman

Toilet is derived from the French word toilette meaning the act of washing, dressing, and preparing oneself. In Western society human feces waste management is usually a matter of a toilet with indoor plumbing, and a sewer or septic system. Anal cleansing after defecation was historically accomplished with sticks, leaves, stones, clay, corncobs, water, or literally whatever was available at hand. In many parts of the world only the left hand was used for wiping and cleansing after defecation. That may have contributed to the use of the right hand for social greetings and shaking hands. The Hongwu Emperor was the first ruler of the Ming dynasty (1368-1644). Chinese imperial court documents show that fifteen thousand sheets of 'thick but soft' perfumed toilet paper were ordered in 1393. The royal family was recorded as using 720,000 sheets of toilet paper a year. The large sheets of two feet by three feet were for general use at the court, but smaller and even better quality sheets that were three inches square were designed for the exclusive use of the imperial family.

In the United States toilet paper was often simply pages torn out of the Farmer's Almanac, or the catalog of merchants such as Sears, Roebuck. & Company. They often came with a pre-punched hole in the catalog for ease of hanging by wire in the bathroom or outhouse. A humorous spinoff on the Sears Roebuck catalog was the 'Rears and Sorebutt' catalog. New York entrepreneur Joseph Gayetty invented aloe-infused sheets of Manila hemp in 1857 that he claimed prevented hemorrhoids. The product was sold in 500 sheet packages and marketed as Gayetty's Medicated Paper. The name Gayetty was imprinted on each sheet of the patented paper, and he was happy to see his name so besmirched as his fortune increased every time his customers wiped. In 1872 John Kimberly, Charles Clark , and other investors started a paper manufacturing company in Wisconsin. In 1874 the brothers Thomas, Clarence, and E. Irvin Scott created a competing paper company and in 1890 popularized toilet paper on a roll. Scott advertised that "over 65% of middle-aged men and women suffered from some sort of rectal disease". The Scott brothers claimed that inferior toilet paper was responsible and that "harsh toilet tissue may cause serious injury". The advertisement went on to say "ScotTissue, Sani-tissue and Waldorf are famous bathroom tissues specifically processed to satisfy the three requirements doctors say toilet tissue must have to be safe: absorbency-softness-chemical purity".

In 1901 the Northern Paper Mills in Green Bay Wisconsin developed a toilet paper that was not made from hardwood pulp, but from softer pulp. They advertised it as the first toilet tissue that guaranteed you would not get wood splinters on wiping. The appeal of not getting wood splinters on wiping with toilet paper not surprisingly led to immediate market success. Competitors soon joined in the rush to market splinter free toilet paper. By 1925 the Scott brothers were the largest toilet paper manufacturers in the world. Acquired by Kimberly-Clark in 1995 for just under ten billion US dollars, the Scott brand name of toilet paper remains very popular. Twenty-six billion rolls of toilet paper are sold annually in the United States. Americans use an average of twenty-three and a half rolls per capita a year.

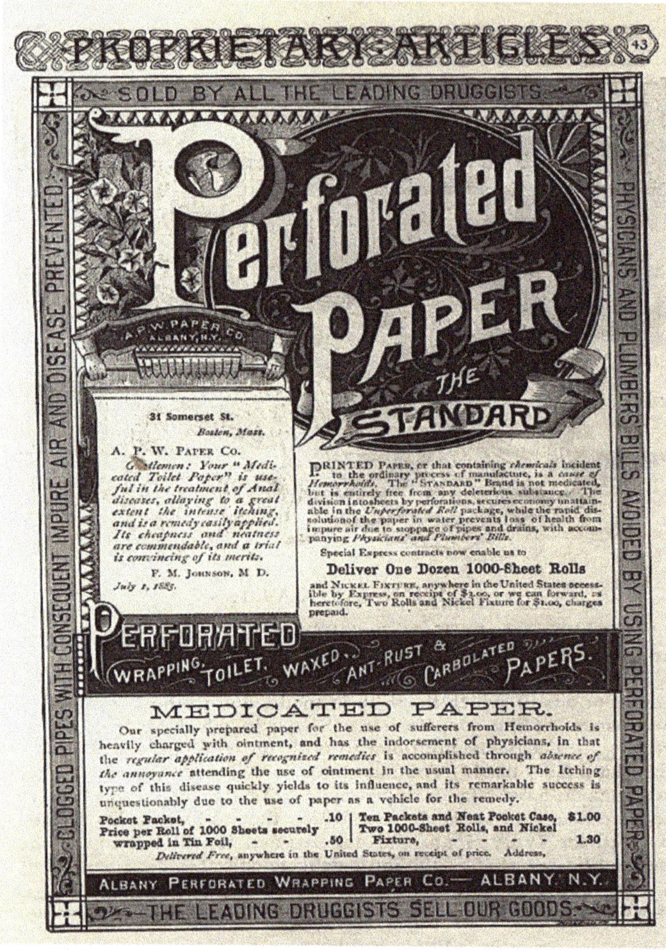

Toilet Paper was medicated, perforated, perfumed, and considered the state the art of anal hygiene in the mid-nineteenth century. Creative Commons License

One tree produces about one hundred pounds (forty-five kilograms) of toilet paper, and global production consumes twenty-seven thousand trees daily. Perforated toilet paper for ease of tearing off sheets was patented in 1871 by New York businessman Seth Wheeler. He established the Albany Perforated Wrapping Paper Company, and toilet paper in those days was more politely referred to as wrapping paper. The patent application specified that the end of the roll of toilet paper was to be on the outside or in the 'over' position. Although the subject of ongoing debate, controversy, and arguments within a household, the official patented invention specifies 'over', and seventy percent of the public dutifully complies. The toilet paper business in the United States is an enormous enterprise. The industry is innovative in finding ways to increase profit margins. According to the financial newspaper The Wall Street Journal in 2013 the Kimberley-Clark Corporation announced that it improved its toilet paper product by making it fifteen percent bulkier, but at the same time reduced the number of sheets by thirteen percent, a process the industry terms desheeting. Desheeting while making bulkier tissue is a money saver as Kimberly-Clark says it doesn't need additional material to make its sheets fluffier. Kimberly Clark is the largest manufacturer of toilet paper in the world with products sold in over 150 countries.

According to Kimberly-Clark's research, Americans use on average forty-six sheets of toilet paper a day over five bathroom trips. Over eighty-three million rolls of toilet paper are manufactured in the United States each day. In 2012 companies sold over ten billion dollars of tissue and toilet paper, a two percent increase over the previous year. Seven billion rolls of toilet paper are sold each year in the United States. In the U.S. more than fifty miles of toilet paper are produced every second. A roll of toilet paper will last five days in the average U.S. household. The average American uses one hundred rolls of toilet paper (twenty thousand sheets) per year, and will require the processing of 384 trees during their lifetime to create the toilet paper they will use. Most of the world has embraced the use of water cleansing for hygienic purposes wherever available. Approximately four billion people around the world do not use toilet paper. The use of only paper products for anal hygiene is counterintuitive, and is surprisingly still the procedure of choice in the United States and many Western countries. The last figures for toilet paper consumption by country were published over twenty years ago. The US led the world with 730 pounds of toilet paper consumption per resident each year. Other countries on the list with pounds of consumption per year for each resident included Finland 669, Belgium 565, Japan 526, Canada 505, Singapore 502, Taiwan 492, Switzerland 476, Denmark 471, New Zealand 468, Brazil 77, China 48, Indonesia 31, and Russia 28. Since the list was published Japan has moved into second place and China a rapidly rising third place.

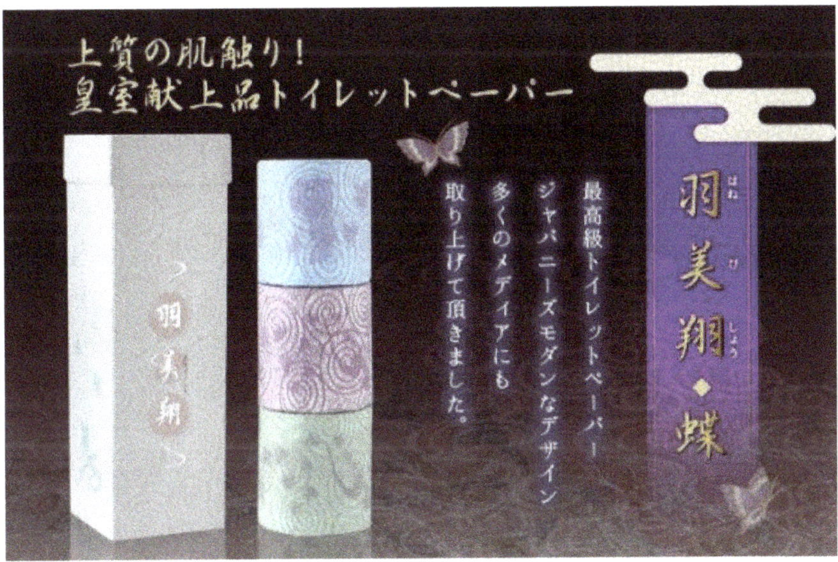

Designer toiler papers are very popular. They come in various colors, but white remain the most popular followed by beige, and peach. Some come with embossed patterns, and others with writings, poetry, and images. The most exclusive designer toilet paper comes from Japan, where the Hanebisho Company creates handcrafted toilet paper that sells for nearly $20 per roll. It is created from the highest quality wood fiber pulp from Canada, and treated with the purest water fin Japan from the Nyodo River. The special drying process is constantly adjusted for humidity and temperature. The paper is then decorated by highly trained artisans and carefully wrapped and packaged in special decorative boxes. The product has been delivered to the residence of the Emperor of Japan for years. If you were to take toilet paper in your bare hands to wipe your pet or child's behind after a bowel movement, you would probably instantly recognize the unhygienic nature of the activity and wash your hands thoroughly. If you did not know it before now you do, toilet paper has to be at least ten sheets thick to prevent bacteria from easily transiting through the porous paper. Even double and triple folding of toilet paper allows fecal bacteria to be in direct contact with the hands. After wiping the person touches the handle to flush. It should not come as any surprise that the toilet faucet or handle has four hundred times the number of bacteria per square inch than the toilet seat.

In the United States and Western society many people wipe after a bowel movement with only porous toilet tissue paper between their fingers and fecal material. These same fingers are then often used to prepare food or pick up finger food that is often shared with others. In the United States health department codes require that restaurant and food preparation employees wash their hands after using the bathroom. The best approach is to practice regular hand washing with an anti-microbial soap and water. The lack of hand washing after using the bathroom is commonplace, as is the lack of basic hand washing skills. The use of an ultraviolet backlight below demonstrates how the hands harbor pockets of potential sources of infection. The touching of a toilet handle and door knob on leaving the bathroom can allow the further transmission of infectious microbes.

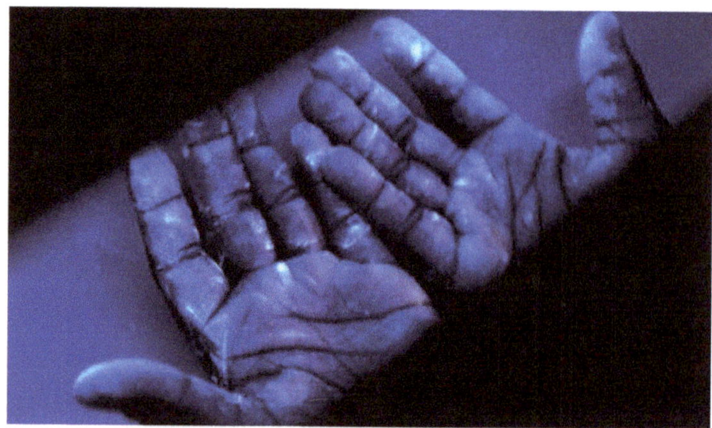

OUTFOXprevention.com. Used with Permission.

The United States Center for Disease Control publishes the following guidelines for proper hand washing. Wet the hands with clean, running water (warm or cold), turn off the tap, and apply soap. Lather the hands by rubbing them together with the soap. Lather the backs of hands, between fingers, and under the nails. Scrub the hands for at least twenty seconds. Rinse the hands well under clean, running water. Dry the hands using a clean towel or air-dry them. The U.S. CDC advocates washing hands before, during, and after preparing food, before eating food, before and after caring for someone who is sick, before and after treating a cut or wound, after using the toilet, and after changing diapers or cleaning up a child who has used the toilet. Hand washing is also recommended after nose blowing, coughing, or sneezing, after touching an animal, animal feed, or animal waste, after handling pet food or pet treats, and after touching garbage. Alcohol based hand sanitizers that contain at least sixty percent ethanol is also effective in reducing the transmission of contaminants and infective agents. Hopefully, the advent of high technology toilets incorporating automatic water washing features, as well as warm air blow-drying, obviating the need for toilet paper and touching the anogenital area will be more readily embraced by Western and other cultures.

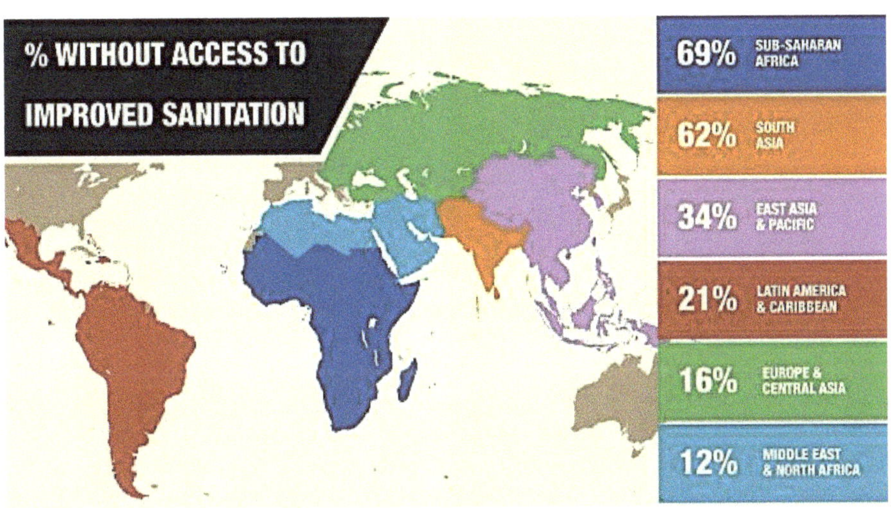

fastcompany.net Creative Commons License

Contrary to popular belief Thomas Crapper did not invent the indoor flush toilet. It had been developed hundreds of years before he established his manufacturing company in Victorian England. Credit for the flushing toilet is usually attributed to Sir John Harrington, a godson of Queen Elizabeth I. One rumor is that his first name is the source of the nickname 'john' for a toilet. Thomas Crapper had a successful plumbing business and the inventor Albert Giblin was an employee of his. Giblin patented a silent siphon valve and Crapper bought the patent and marketed the improved toilet from 1861-1904 at great profit and name recognition. The average person goes to the toilet 2,500 times per year, and spends a total of three years of their lifetime sitting on the toilet. For those musically inclined most toilets flush in the key of E flat. Other trivia of note, one third of Americans flush the toilet while still sitting on it, and there are 40,000 injuries a year while sitting on the toilet seat.

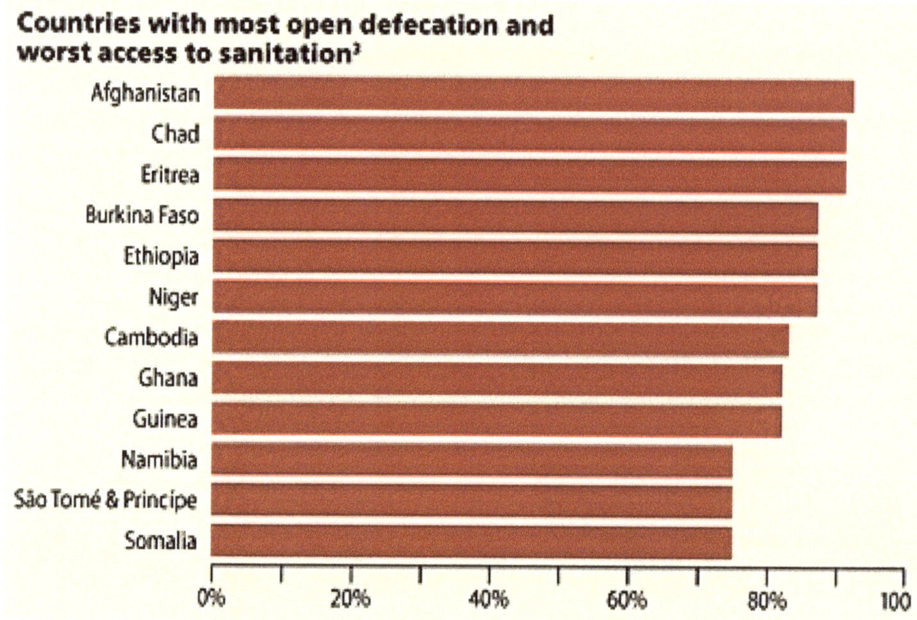

uwcm-geog.wikispaces.com/Food+Aid Creative Commons License

In France the invention of the bidet in the early eighteenth century made water cleansing popular. The word bidet means pony in French, and using the bidet required that one straddle the bowl of the bidet as if riding a pony. A bidet spray or health faucet is a hand held hose and nozzle that utilizes a water spray for perianal and genitourinary cleansing after defecation and urination. The bidet is commonplace in many countries including Spain (thirty percent), Portugal (seventy percent), Greece (eighty percent), Italy (ninety-five percent), and Japan (fifty percent). In Japan automated and high technology toilets incorporate water washing as well as air blow drying and other features. The water bidet is also very popular in the Middle East, and growing in popularity in the United States.

Although popular in Europe and elsewhere around the world, the United States has been very slow to adopt the preferable water based approach to anal hygiene. In addition to its increased efficacy it has environmental benefits in reducing forest product consumption and sewage disposal of paper waste products. The reluctance of Americans to adopt the use of the bidet may be related to a misconception on the part of American and British troops during World War I. When they were first exposed to the bidet in France they assumed its purpose was purely for the washing of the genitals after sexual intercourse. The bidet incorrectly became associated as a product developed to accommodate French sexual immorality.

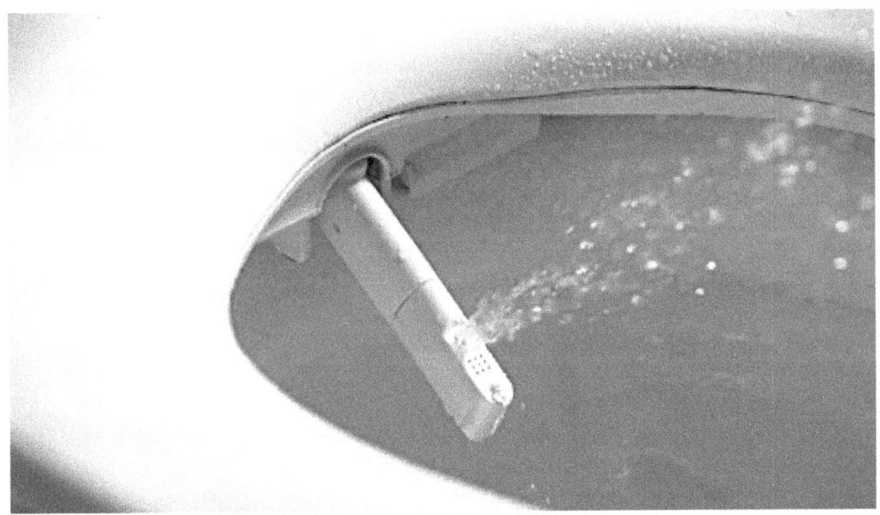

Although popular in Europe and elsewhere around the world, the United States has been very slow to adopt the preferable water based approach to anal hygiene. In addition to its increased efficacy it has environmental benefits in reducing forest product consumption and sewage disposal of paper waste products. Creative Commons License

Although there are some very expensive models of toilets combined with bidets, the cost of an aftermarket addition of a washlet feature to a toilet is very economical. Many bidet equivalent washlets cost less than one hundred dollars, and with the savings by reduced toilet paper usage the device rapidly pays for itself. On the Indian subcontinent, in spite of the lack of bidets, over ninety-five percent of the population use water for anal cleansing. Many also use soap with water for cleansing after defecating. Use of paper is rare in this region, and hand washing after cleansing is critically important to prevent illness. In Japan the technological innovation of combining the bidet and toilet into a single product was introduced and advanced. Rapid innovations included a heated seat, automatic deodorizing, automatic lid raising and closing, directed water jets for female and male anatomy, music playing during use, vacuum fan ventilation, and warm air blow drying to obviate the need for wiping or use of toilet paper.

Genital and anal infections do not come in contact with the toilet seat in normal use. The intact skin of your buttocks is an efficient barrier against most disease organisms. Most transmission of pathogens is via the fecal to oral route is usually accomplished by way of the hands. The flush handle, sink handles, and door knob are much more likely to be a source of contamination since they are much likely to have been touched by someone whose hands had just been used to wipe their bottoms with a thin piece of toilet paper. It would be a good precaution to use toilet paper or paper towels to prevent your hands from touching the flush, faucet, and doorknobs or handles.

Most transmission of pathogens is via the fecal to oral route is usually accomplished by way of the hands. The average human stool contains three trillion microorganisms. Wiping with toilet paper nearly guarantees that the hands will come into contact with fecal microorganisms. After wiping it is not uncommon to find brown streaks on underwear because of inadequate anal hygiene. The average man's underwear contains one-tenth of a gram of feces at laundering. Another infection risk from the toilet is the splashing and aerosol formation that can occur during flushing, particularly when someone with diarrhea has used that toilet. Surprisingly one-third of Americans remain seated on the toilet when they flush, and perhaps mistakenly find the misting of their anogenital region refreshing and hygienic. If they put paper toilet seat covers down before they sit on a public toilet seat for hygienic purposes, they should definitely get off the toilet seat before they flush.

The typical toilet flush creates a mist of contaminated water droplets that can travel up to twenty feet in all directions. It includes fecal matter and pathogens that settle on any exposed surface in the flush zone, including toothbrushes, drinking cups, bath toys, handles and doorknobs. The mist can stay airborne for up to two hours and be easily inhaled. The microbial pathogens can live on surfaces for up to a week. Before you flush, lower the lid to keep the aerosolization and spread to a minimum. Worldwide there are approximately two million fatalities every year due to diarrhea. The majority of these are in children under five years of age. Simple routine hand washing with soap and water could reduce the incidence of diarrhea by approximately fifty percent, and respiratory infections by about twenty-five percent. Hand washing also reduces the incidence of skin diseases, eye infections, and intestinal worms and parasites.

In most cultures and faiths food is not stored, prepared, or consumed in the vicinity of a toilet area. Both Islam and Judaism have a brief prayer of thanksgiving to be offered after the body functions of eliminating waste and the washing of hands. With the risk to health and wellness from exposure to human waste, religious customs and practices often offered practical guidance and hygiene to avoid disease. Istinja (Arabic: استنجاء), a component of Islamic hygiene practices, is the cleansing away of any residue and impurities (najasat) that remain after being passed from the urethra or anus. Istinja requires the use of water if available, and may be utilized with water alone or in combination with toilet paper. If water is not available stones, soil, or other natural material (other than bone or dung) may be utilized in the process known as 'istijmar'. The passage of intestinal gas alone does not require Istinja

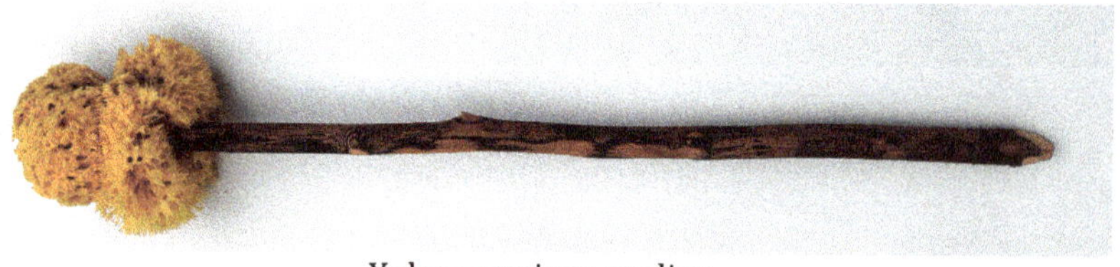

Xylospongium replica

Xylospongium, also known as *sponge on a stick*, is a device used to clean the perianal area after a bowel movement. It consists of a wooden stick (Greek: ξύλον, *Xylon*) with a sponge (Greek: Σπόγγος, *Spongos*) fixed at one end. In the *baths of the seven sages* in Ostia, a fresco from the 2nd century contains the Inscription *(u)taris xylosphongio* which is the first known mention of the term. Also in the early second century a papyrus letter of Claudius Terentianus to his father Claudius Tiberianus uses the term *xylospongium* in a phrase.

Shit stick is a thin stake or stick used for cleaning the perianal area after a bowel movement. It is used when water or toilet paper was not available for this purpose. The term has also been used in Chinese Buddhism and Japanese Buddhism. A well-known example is *gānshǐjué/kanshiketsu* (乾屎橛 "dry shit stick") from the Chan/Zen *gōng'àn/kōan* in which a monk asked "What is Buddha?" and Master Yunmen/Unmon answered "A dry shit stick". The presumed logic for such language was that most of the great masters of these schools did not directly state what they wished to convey. They often used a shout, or strike with a rod, or striking phrase as above to place their student in a state between comprehensibility and incomprehensibility. According to this logic it somehow promoted their development of enlightenment." Another explanation was that Zen Buddhist masters used the image of a dry shit stick to neutralize and balance of our image of a true person as sine thing other than pure or noble.
Ancient Roman latrines in Ostia Antica

Gaki zōshi 餓鬼草紙 "Scroll of Hungry Ghosts", a *gaki* condemned to shit-eating watches a child wearing *geta* and holding a *chūgi*, c. 12th century. People have used many different materials in the long history of anal cleansing, including leaves, rags, paper, water, sponges, corncobs, earthenware, pottery, and sticks. In ancient times, instruments made from bamboo, possibly in the form of spatulas ([*cèchóu*] 厠籌, [*cèbì*] 厠篦, or [*cèjiǎn*] 厠簡), may have been used with water for cleansing after a bowel movement. the assistance of water in cleaning the body after defecation. Japanese *chūgi* from the Nara period(710-784), shown with modern toilet paper for size comparison. When monks and missionaries introduced Buddhism into China and Japan, they also brought the Indian custom of using a *śalākā, a* small stake, stick, or rod for wiping away fecal residue after a bowel movement. Translators rendered this Sanskrit word into a number of different terms based on the words of *chóu* or *chū* 籌 "small stake or stick", or *jué* or *ketsu* 橛 "short stake or stick". Such terns included the Chinese *cèchóu* 厠籌 and Japanese *chūgi* 籌木. The custom of using shit sticks became popular and had the advantages of being inexpensive, washable, and reusable.

The Chinese invented paper around the 2nd century BCE, and toilet paper no later than the 6th century CE, when Yan Zhitui noted, "Paper on which there are quotations or commentaries from the Five Classics or the names of sages, I dare not use for toilet purposes". The earliest Japanese flush toilets date from the Nara period (710–784), when a drainage system was constructed in the capital at Nara. It was designed as squat toilets built over 4 - 6 inch (10–15 cm) wide wooden conduits that users would straddle. Archaeological excavations in Nara have also found numerous *chūgi* wooden sticks that were used for fecal cleansing. Ming Dynasty Xuande Emperorplaying *touhu*, 15th century. Chinese *Chóu* 籌 and chóumù or Japanese chū 籌 or *chūgi* 籌木 (with 木 "tree; wood") and *cèchóu* 厠籌 (with 厠 "toilet") "small stake; stick" are used as the equivalent terms meaning "shit stick". The Buddhist Sanskrit term *śalāka* or *śalākā* (Pali *salākā*) is its equivalent and may be a small stake, stick, rod, or twig. In Indian Buddhist contexts, *śalākā* can also represent a stick used for purposes other than anal hygiene. particularly meant "a piece of wood or bamboo used for counting or voting". *Salaka-Grahapaka* was the wood or bamboo sticks used in counting votes in general assembly. The Jain term *salakapurusa* "illustrious or worthy person" compounds *salaka* "stick used for voting" and *purusa* "person". *Chou* 籌 originally meant "arrow used in *tóuhú* (an ancient game wth competition on the number of arrows thrown into a pot)" or "tally stick (used in counting)". *Chóu* 籌 "shit stick" was first described in writing around the 3rd century CE. The Jin dynasty (265-420) *Yulin* 語林 by Pei Qi 裴啟 has stories about the ostentatious bathrooms of wealthy merchant Shi Chong 石崇 (249-300) who mocked the politician Liu Shi 劉寔 (220-310) for not being familiar with the perfumed shit sticks offered by two female bathroom attendants.

Chinese *jué* or Japanese *ketsu* 橛 "short wooden stake; stick; peg; post" is compounded with *shi* or *shǐ* 屎 (written with 尸 "body" and 米 "rice") "shit; excrement; dung" into Japanese *shiketsu* or Chinese *shǐjué* 屎橛 "shit stick". The famous term *gānshǐjué* or *kanshiketsu* 乾屎橛 "dry shit stick", modified with *gān* or *kan*乾 "dry, dried; hollow". Kan-shiketsu 乾屎橛 Excrement-wiping spatula. A Zen word of abuse for a person who clings to things. Kan-shiketsu Japanese, literally a "dry shit stick"; a Zen expression designating a person who is attached to the world of appearance. Chinese *bì* 篦 "fine-tooth comb; spatula" or Japanese *hera* 篦 "spatula; scoop" is compounded into Chinese *cèbì* 厠篦 "toilet spatula" and Japanese *kusobera* 糞篦 "shit spatula" or *kusokakibera* 糞掻く篦 "shit scratching spatula". While most Japanese "shit stick" words have Sino-Japanese roots such as *chūgi* from *chóumù* 籌木, both *kuso* 糞 "shit; crap" and *hera* 篦 "spatula; scoop" are native Japanese terms. Chinese *cèjiǎn* 厠簡 or 厕简 "toilet stick" is a synonym of *cèchóu* 厠籌 using the word *jiǎn* 簡 "bamboo and wooden slips". During the time of Queen Zhou the Elder (r. 961-964), a monk used a sharpened toilet stick to remove a tumor.

The English language has some *shit(e) stick* parallels in its lexicography parallel to these Asian language terms. The *Oxford English Dictionary* (shyte, shite, shit) quotes two early *shit-stick* examples: "a hard chuffe, a shite-sticks" (1598) and "a shite-sticks, a shite-rags, that is to say, a miserable pinch-pennie" (1659); and defines poop-stick as "a fool, ineffectual person", with the earliest usage in 1930.

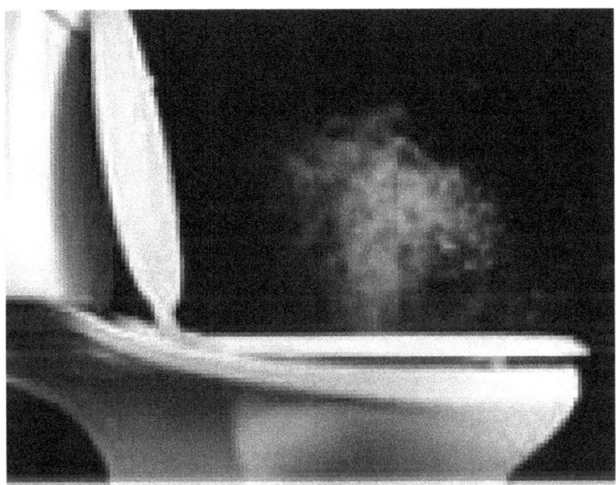

The microscopic mist that emanates with each flush of the toilet bowl distributes contaminated water droplets up to twenty feet in reach direction. Creative Commons License

Microbiological surveillance studies of *Escherichia coli* and other fecal bacteria have been performed in typical American household kitchens and bathrooms. The surprising finding was that toilet seats were one of the cleanest areas in the house with a very low microbe count. Faucets and refrigerator handles were more heavily contaminated. The highest concentration of microbes, more than two hundred times that of the toilet seat, were found on kitchen cutting boards. It was theorized this was from poultry, which often has fecal microbe contaminants in processing. Public toilet seats were also surveyed and less than two percent had any *Escherichia coli* or fecal contaminants. Even this small percentage was thought to represent contamination from the water mist that is generated by flushing. The best use of the toilet seat paper protector dispensed would be to use it instead of your bare hands to touch the faucets and door handles in the bathroom. In other public places some of the highest concentrations of fecal bacteria are found on sanitary napkin dispensers, hotel TV remote control units, vending machine buttons, and drinking water fountain controls.

The following twenty-five locations were surveyed in the United States for fecal contaminants with some surprising findings. Fast food restaurants in the US serve ice that had more bacteria than the toilet water in seventy percent of locations surveyed. Public restrooms have about two million bacteria per square inch, while the average toilet seat has only fifty per square inch. The average office desk has four hundred times more bacteria than a toilet. Keyboards can have up to two hundred times more bacteria than a toilet seat. Cell phones and mobile electronic devices can have ten times more bacteria than a toilet seat, and they are frequently in close contact with the fingers, face, and mouth. There are on average one hundred times more bacteria on restaurant menus than on restroom toilet seat. Raw meat carries a very high level of fecal bacteria, so food-chopping boards harbor more fecal contaminants than toilet seats. When the toilet is flushed the plume of toilet water with fecal contaminants often end up on toothbrushes left exposed. With two hundred thousand bacteria per square inch, carpets are four thousand times dirtier than a toilet seat. Humans shed one and one-half million skin cells every hour that helps feed the bacteria carpeting the carpets.

Most refrigerators test positive for the fecal contaminant *Escherichia coli* because thorough cleaning and disinfecting is an infrequent undertaking. Reusable shopping bags have more fecal matter than underwear and are rarely washed. In many households the television remote control is one of the most contaminated items handled. Hands are one of the dirtiest parts of the body, and they are frequently used to grasp and hold doorknobs, which are a reservoir of contaminants. Light switches can have up to two hundred and seventeen bacteria per square inch. The kitchen sink is usually dirtier than the bathroom and is often overlooked when cleaning. The bathtub, although thought of as a place to get clean, typically harbors nearly twenty thousand bacteria per square inch around the drain. Dead skins cells, dust mites, fungal spores, pollens, and other body secretions build up on the pillow, the place the head usually rests at night. After ten years a mattress will nearly double in weight thanks to the number of dust mites and dust mite feces that it has collected. The inside rim of a pet bowl alone contains over two thousand bacteria per square inch.

Currency bank notes can harbor up to two hundred thousand bacteria. It's a good idea to wash the hands after directly handling cash and currency. It brings new meaning to those having lots of money being known as 'filthy rich'. Draperies collect pet fur, mold, dander, debris, dust mites, and dust mite feces. The warm, dark, and moist insides of showerheads are popular breeding grounds for bacteria. Handbags contain cell phone, money, hairbrush, lipstick, cosmetics, and other items teeming with contaminants. Handbags are rarely cleaned and are a notorious source of potential contaminants. The kitchen sponge is nearly always the most heavily contaminated item in the house. With ten million bacteria per square inch the kitchen sponge is nearly a quarter of a million times dirtier than a toilet seat. The toilet seat is usually very clean, and the reason is really pretty simple, it gets cleaned often. A swimming pool visited by one hundred children can have over two pounds of feces floating around. Little kids can carry as much as ten grams of leftover feces around their anus after wiping their rear ends which just rinses off into the pool. Fecal contamination also occurs from adults with less than stellar anal hygiene. The U.S. Center for Disease Control (CDC) found that more than half of swimming pools in the U.S. test positive for the fecal bacteria *Escherichia coli*, which can cause gastroenteritis. Your best line of defense is to try not to swallow any water.

Restaurant menus have over one hundred times more bacteria than a toilet seat. They are held and fingered touched by dozens of people but only wiped down once a day, if that, and usually with a used rag. Instead of washing your hands before you sit down at the restaurant you may want to scrub up and use a hand sanitizer after you order. Be careful to never lay your silverware on top of the menu. Do you like a squeeze of lemon wedge with your water or beverage of choice? Researchers found that nearly seventy percent of the lemons had disease-causing microbes, including fecal contaminants such as *Escherichia coli*. Drinking fountains, especially public water fountains, have high bacteria counts, particularly on the faucet or push button. Ironically, the handles and push buttons on public restroom soap pumps are a breeding ground for bacteria, too. So scrub your hands for at least twenty seconds or better yet, carry your own personal hand sanitizer. And before you reach for that door handle leaving the restroom, think about how many people don't wash after going to the bathroom. The Center for Disease Control says only thirty-one percent of men and sixty-five percent of women do. Kitchen employees are supposed to always wash their hands after using the bathroom, and one can only hope that they do comply with this basic hygiene measure

Shopping cart handles can be swarming with millions of microorganisms, including ones from raw meat from a previous shopper, or fecal bacteria if a diapered child was sitting in the cart earlier in the day. A lot of grocery stores have antibacterial wipes handy, so use them, or put your items directly into paper or plastic bags or boxes. Many people are careful not to touch heavily contaminated door handles, including refrigerator and freezer handles, but are not as wary as they should be of push buttons on elevators, remote controls, computer or bank ATM keypads, etc. In hotel rooms the television remote control is the dirtiest object there and could use a disinfectant wipe before you channel surf. Other potential microbial hotspots include the bedside lamp switch, bedspread, hair dryer, telephone, and unwrapped drinking glasses.

If you take children to a playground, remember it is also a playground for microbes. Playgrounds are rarely cleaned and kids are continuously handling railings, handles, swings, slides. Your child would actually be in less contact with microbes if they were playing with public restroom toilet seats, which are at least cleaned frequently. The worse spot in the playground is the sandbox, with thirty-six times more germs than a restaurant tray. One organism found all too often in the sandbox is the parasitic protist *Toxoplasma gondii*. The U.S. Humane Society estimates that the wild feral cat population in the US exceeds fifty million, and the vast majority carry this dangerous and easily transmissible parasite. They look upon a playground sandbox as nothing more than a giant litter box and frequently defecate in them and mix their feces in with the sand.

Worldwide there are approximately two million fatalities every year due to diarrhea. The majority of these are in children under five years of age. Simple routine hand washing with soap and water could reduce the incidence of diarrhea by approximately fifty percent, and respiratory infections by about twenty-five percent. Hand washing also reduces the incidence of skin diseases, eye infections, and intestinal worms and parasites. In most cultures and faiths food is not stored, prepared, or consumed in the vicinity of a toilet area. Both Islam and Judaism have a brief prayer of thanksgiving to be offered after the body functions of eliminating waste and the washing of hands. With the risk to health and wellness from exposure to human waste, religious customs and practices often offered practical guidance and hygiene to avoid disease.

It is obvious that the transmission of contaminants from the feces of one person to the mouth of another is exceedingly common. Even taking great precautions and frequent hand washing the exposure possibilities are nearly limitless. Did your food preparer was their hands thoroughly after using the bathroom? How about after they touched the kitchen sink faucet or refrigerator door handle? Did you wash your hands after touching a drinking fountain knob, or after shaking someone's hands? Did you hold onto a stairway railing, open a door by turning a knob or touching a handle? Did you handle currency, share a pen, hold a child's hand, touch a computer keyboard, use a remote control, hold a restaurant menu?

Welcome to the world of overwhelming microbial presence. The number of bacteria and Archaea organisms on earth are estimated at five million trillion trillion (called a nonillion in short scale for English speaking countries and quintillion in long scale for non-English speaking countries). For those who prefer numbers in numerical form it is the number five followed by thirty zeroes written as 5,000,000,000,000,000,000,000,000,000,000. Over one half of the world's biomass are bacteria and Archaea, and they outnumber each human by many trillions of organisms. There are approximately ten trillion human cells in the body. The human gut microbiome alone, just the microbes living within the human intestinal tract is over one hundred trillion organisms, and outnumbers all human cells by more than ten to one. Adding in the quadrillions of viruses, prions, protist, fungi, parasites, and other life forms that have yet to be discovered humans are an extremely small minority.

The exposure to human and animal waste is nearly ubiquitous, in spite of our best efforts. Part of the challenge is the sheer quantity of waste generated by the human and animal. There are nearly one and a half billion cattle in the world today, each one producing an average of twenty-seven kilograms (sixty pounds) of feces a day. Fortunately, twenty-four kilograms is water, but that still leaves three kilograms (over six and one half pounds of feces by dry weight). Cows alone generate nearly one hundred billion pounds of feces per day. The world sheep population is one point two billion, each of which produces on average fifteen kilograms (thirty-three pounds) of feces, adding another forty billion pounds of feces a day to the waste challenge.

The world pig population is one billion, each producing seven kilograms (fifteen pounds) of manure a day. The world bird population is estimated at three hundred billion, horse population is sixty million, dog population is three hundred million, cat population is five hundred million. There are hundreds of billions of additional animals, ranging from the enormous blue whale and elephant to the diminutive mouse and termite adding trillions of pounds of feces into the environment every day. Of course, we should not forget our own contribution, with a world human population of over seven point three billion people ewe contribute over a billion pounds of feces per day. Fecal contaminants are commonly in the food and water supply around the world.

Atmospheric Pressure (Barometric Pressure)

Intestinal gas, like gasses everywhere, must comply with the laws of physics and the laws of nature. Boyle's law states that at a constant temperature, the product of the volume and pressure of a gas must remain constant. This requires that they maintain an inverse relationship, if one increases the other has to decrease. As such, an increase in pressure will result in the decrease of the volume of the gas, and vice versa.

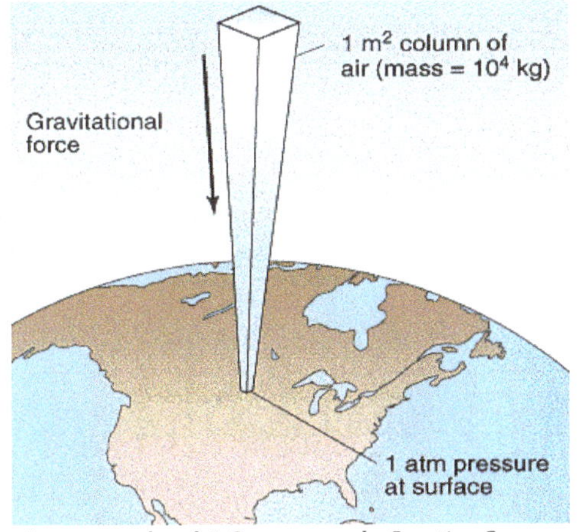

Atmospheric pressure hendrix2.uoregon.edu Creative Commons License

The atmospheric pressure on earth is defined as a standard of one atmosphere at sea level. As you go deeper down into the earth, such as happens in a mineshaft, or diving deeper into the oceans, the atmospheric pressure increases. As you go higher in elevation, whether climbing flights of stairs, ascending a mountain, or in a hot air balloon, the atmospheric pressure decreases. The atmospheric pressure is also not uniform, constantly changing along with the weather.

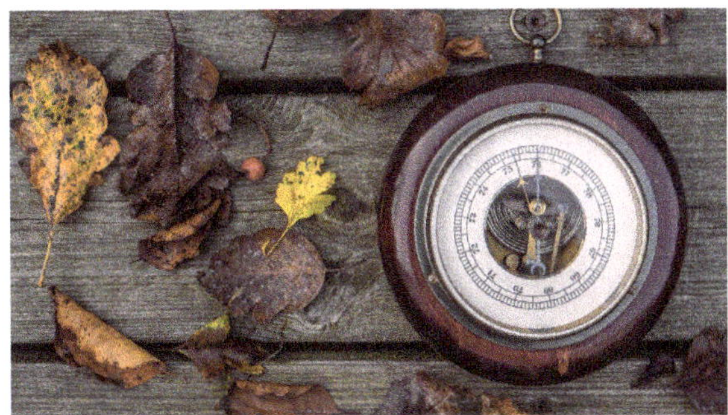

Atmospheric pressure and the weather are always changing. Shutterstock/polarpx

Using Boyle's law, you can calculate how much the volume will compress as you go deeper underground or underwater and atmospheric pressure increases. You can likewise calculate how much a gas will expand, as you go higher in altitude and the atmospheric pressure decreases. If you have ever gone diving into a swimming pool or scuba diving, you can feel the increasing atmospheric pressure on your eardrums.

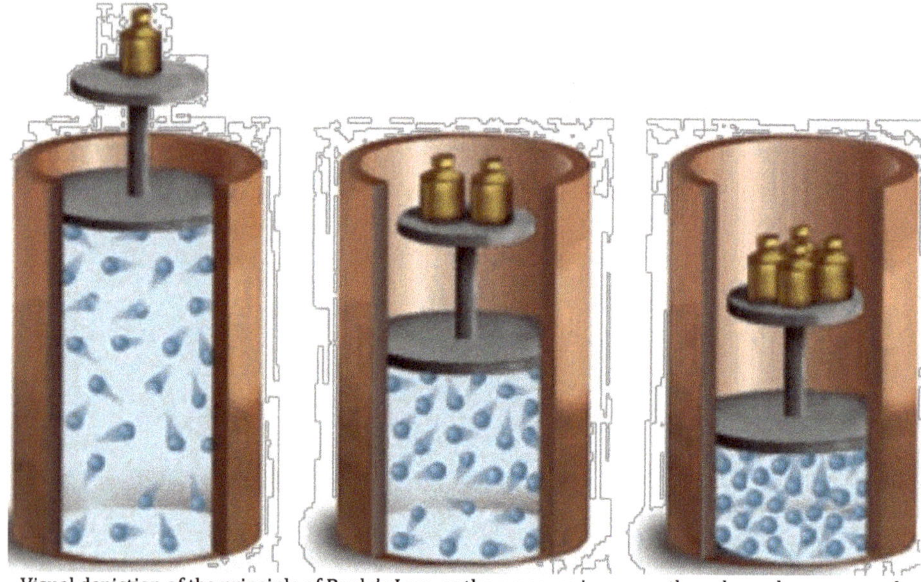

Visual depiction of the principle of Boyle's Law, as the pressure increases the volume decreases, and vice versa. Creative Commons License

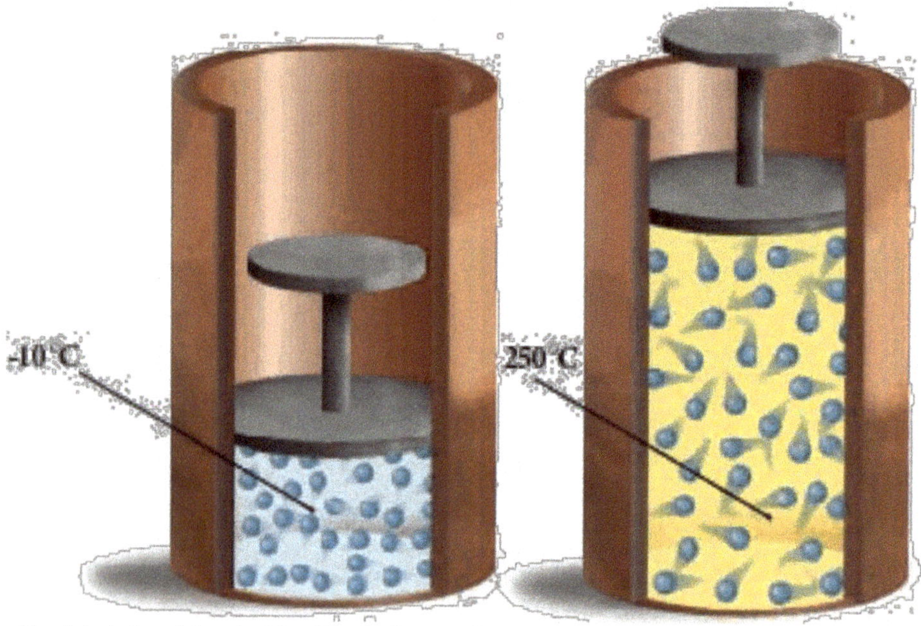

Visual depiction of the principle of Charles' Law, as the temperature increases the volume increases, and vice versa. Creative Commons License

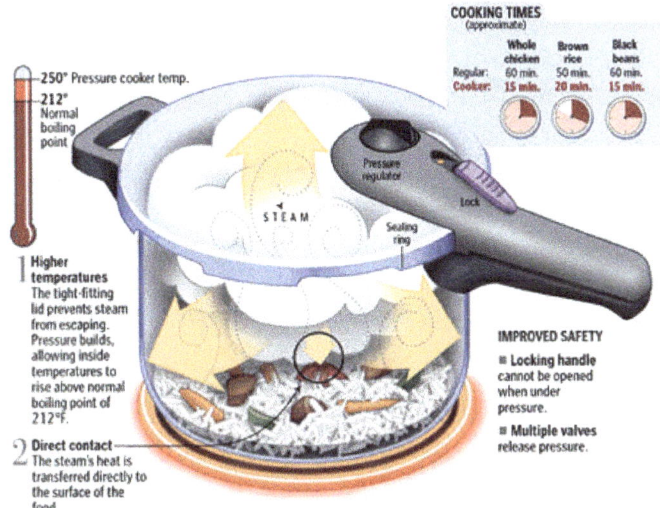

A pressure cooker is one example of the practical application of the laws of physics. As the pressure within the cooker increases the water can achieve a temperature higher than its boiling point. Creative Commons License

Aerospace

Intestinal gas, like gasses everywhere, must comply with the laws of physics and the laws of nature. Boyle's law states that at a constant temperature, the product of the volume and pressure of a gas must remain constant. This requires that they maintain an inverse relationship, if one increases the other has to decrease. As such, an increase in pressure will result in the decrease of the volume of the gas, and vice versa. See earlier entry on aerospace for more details.

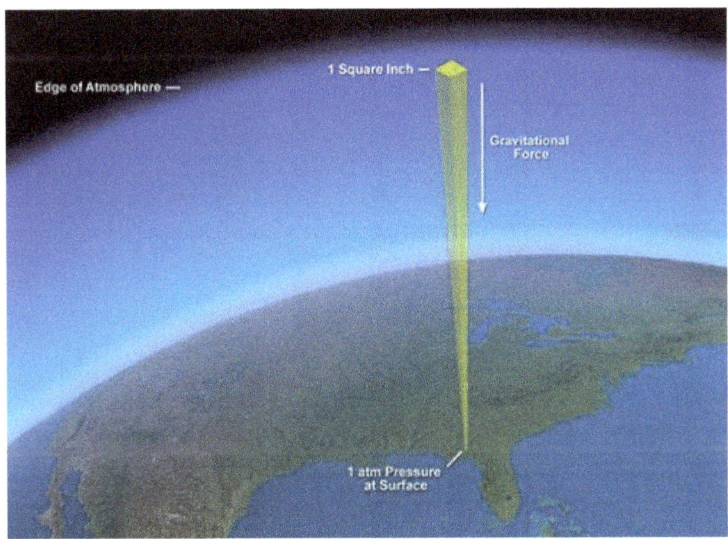

farm7.static.flickr.com Creative Commons License

Elevators

The sensation of the increasing volume of intestinal gas is most noticeable with the rapid decrease in atmospheric pressure experienced in airplane or space travel. A high-speed elevator comes close, and you may first sense the change in air pressure by the inequality of the pressure applied to the eardrums. You may have an ear 'popping' effect from a rapid ascent in the elevator. As you rapidly ascend by the elevator in a high-rise building, driving up a mountain road, or flying in an airplane, you may feel or hear your ears 'pop' as they adjust to the decreasing atmospheric pressure. If they do not 'pop' on their own, you may feel the discomfort of the unequal pressure as the eardrum begins to bulge. Since you are not underwater you can use the more comfortable maneuver of yawning, instead of the Valsalva maneuver (see page 432).

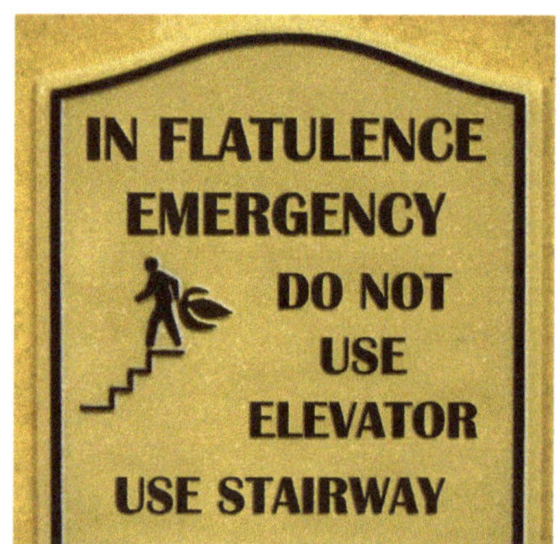
IN FLATULENCE
EMERGENCY
DO NOT
USE
ELEVATOR
USE STAIRWAY

www.flickr.com Kevin Trotman Creative Commons License

Unfortunately, with the elevator's rapid ascent comes the equally rapid expansion of intestinal gasses. This may lead to an increase in the passage of intestinal gasses in the confined space of the elevator. If the elevator is crowded there are lots of people to glare at to take the suspicion off of you. Fortunately, the same risk does not occur as the elevator descends. On the descent the increasing atmospheric pressure causes the volume of intestinal gas to decrease., and the risk of being subjected to your own or someone else's fart in the confined elevator decreases.

High Altitude Community

The majority of the world's population lives close to the seashore and have the standard atmospheric pressure of one atmosphere found at sea level. A significant percentage of the world's population lives at higher altitudes with atmospheric pressures less than one atmosphere. The higher above sea level you are, the lower is the atmospheric pressure you are subjected to. As a consequence, although the number of molecules of gas produced is identical, it will require a larger volume of space to contain it.

If you live in Denver Colorado, the mile-high city with an elevation of five-thousand one-hundred and eighty-three feet (one-thousand six-hundred and nine meters) feet above sea level, the volume will be larger than residing in Los Angeles or New York City. It is all relative as residing in Mexico City, which is at seven-thousand three-hundred and fifty feet (two-thousand two-hundred and forty meters), will produce a much larger volume than Denver.

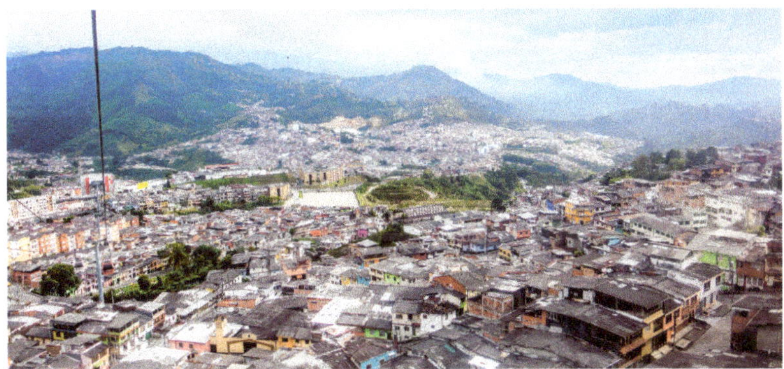

Manizales, Colombia is at an altitude of six thousand six hundred and ninety feet (2,021 meters) above sea level. Shutterstock/fotos593

For those flying at even higher altitudes the cabin pressure in commercial aircraft limits the reduction in atmospheric pressured to the equivalent of approximately eight-thousand feet above sea level high, much as if you were in Mexico City. With the atmospheric pressure at this altitude just over two-thirds of sea level, the gas volume expands by about forty percent. That is more than enough to cause a person to notice a significant increase in their flatulence and an increase in the flatulence of everyone else as well.

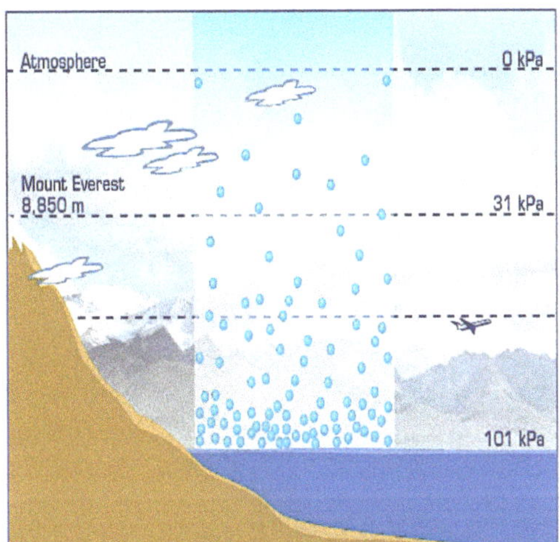

Atmospheric pressure arises from the weight of the air sitting above the observer. The mass of air in the column above the head of the observer is pulled down by the gravity of the Earth and exerts a pressure force on the observer. At the surface of the Earth at sea level the pressure is 14.7 pounds per square inch. This is also described in other measurement units as one atmosphere, 101,000 Pascals, 1kPa (kilopascal), or one bar. At higher altitudes, less air sits above an observer, so there is a lesser amount of atmospheric pressure. hendrix2.uoregon.edu Creative Commons License

High Rise Building

If you work or reside on the higher floors of an office building or residence tower, or if your place of work or residence is at a higher elevation in a mountain community the difference in atmospheric pressure may be significant. Whatever the reason for the change in altitude the resulting changes in atmospheric pressure affects intestinal gasses. They are subject to the same consequences of Boyle's Law as any other gas.

The heights of the tallest skyscrapers continue to reach new world records. Even coastal cities that are nearly at sea level will have buildings in which the changes in atmospheric pressure between those at the ground floor and those at the higher levels will be significant. This is most readily demonstrated by taking a high-speed elevator in a high-rise building. The rapid decrease in atmospheric pressure traveling from the lower to the higher floors often results in pressure changes on the eardrum (tympanic membrane). The equalization of pressure on both sides of the tympanic membrane may give rise to an ear popping sensation.

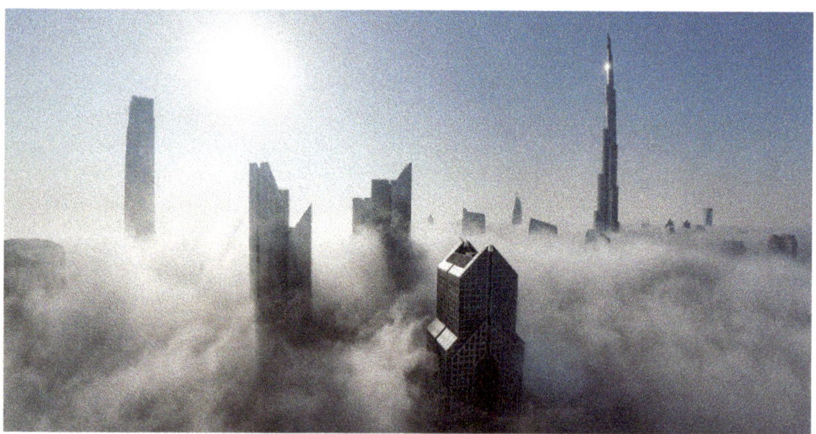

Burj Khalifa, Dubai, Tallest building in the world. Skyline is depicted above fog level.
Shuttertstock/NaufalMQ

Mountain Climbing

In rock or mountain climbing, the higher the altitude, the lower the atmospheric pressure. Although the number of molecules remain unchanged gastrointestinal gasses will expand by virtue of the laws of physics. The increasing volume of gas will lead to discomfort and ultimately will find a way to exit your digestive tract. Air in the stomach may be released, as a burp or belch, but the larger quantity of gasses in the colon will come out as flatus, commonly called a fart. The higher in altitude you go, the lower the atmospheric pressure, and the more flatus you will be passing.

As you go up the elevator in a high-rise building, or drive up a mountain road, or fly in an airplane you may feel or hear your ears 'pop' as they adjust to the decreasing atmospheric pressure. To relieve the discomfort you need to equalize pressure on both sides of the eardrum. As these pressure changes occur while not underwater, a simple yawn is easier and more comfortable the Valsalva maneuver to equalize the pressure difference.

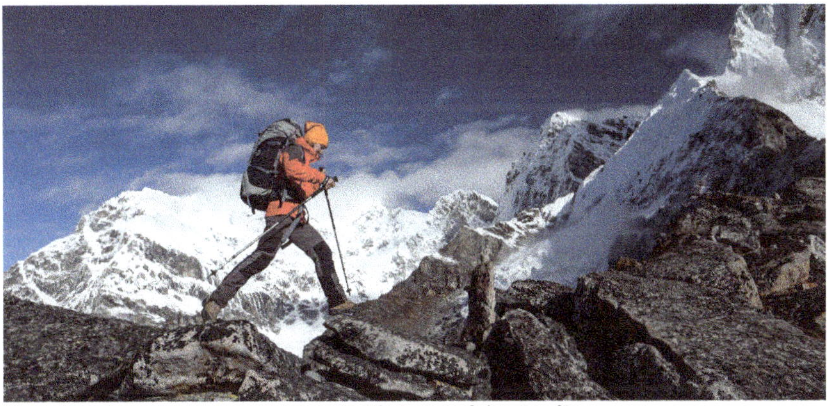

Mountain climber. Shutterstock/MyGoodImages

Scuba Diving

Using Boyle's law, you can calculate how much the gas volume will compress as you go deeper underground or underwater and atmospheric pressure increases. You can likewise calculate how much a gas will expand, as you go higher in altitude and the atmospheric pressure decreases. If you have ever gone diving into a swimming pool or scuba diving, you can feel the increasing atmospheric pressure on your eardrums., also known as the tympanic membrane. If you go deep enough, the atmospheric pressure increases to such a degree that it may become painful.

To relieve the discomfort, you have to equalize the pressure on both sides of your eardrums. This equalization of air pressure is usually accomplished by performing the Valsalva maneuver. This procedure can be initiated by attempting to exhale against a closed epiglottis, much like straining during a bowel movement. The open Eustachian tube from the pharynx allows equalization of the atmospheric pressure on both sides of the eardrum.

If unrelieved, or if pressure is increased further, it may exceed the ability of the tissue to withstand it resulting in rupture or perforation. A perforated eardrum is very painful and is more likely to occur if the Eustachian tubes that must be open to equalize the pressure on both sides of the eardrum are swollen shut by infection, inflammation, or other conditions. For this reason activities, which rapidly or excessively apply pressure on the eardrums, should be avoided if the individual has an upper respiratory or nasal congestion, such as sinusitis, head cold, ear infection, etcetera. The use of a nasal and sinus decongestant may be helpful but caution is still required. Scuba diving, flying, mountain climbing, and other activities require awareness of their potential effects on human health.

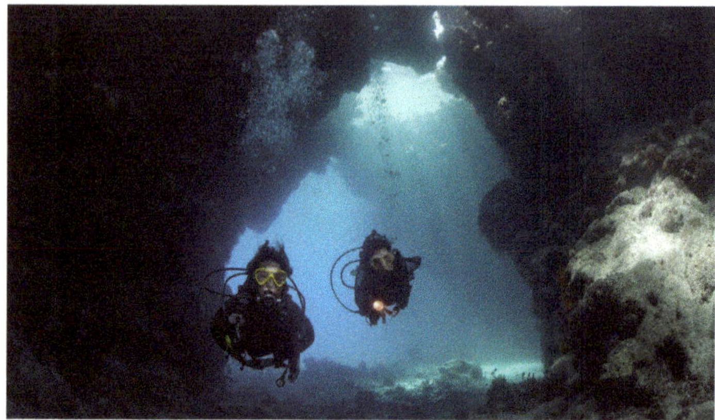

Shutterstock/timsimages

Other effects of pressure changes on the gasses within human tissue are less frequent but of even greater concern. Scuba divers know better than to eat a gas producing meal, such as chili with beans and carbonated beverages, before a dive. The gas bubbles generated within the gut while at a one hundred foot dive depth are compressed into a relatively small volume by the high atmospheric pressure. Upon returning to the surface at the conclusion of the dive that small gas bubble will rapidly expand to a much larger volume as the high atmospheric pressure is reduced back to normal at the surface. As the gas bubble expands the pressure on the intestinal tract wall dramatically increases and can lead to a rupture as the result of barotrauma. Unlike a perforated eardrum, a perforation and rupture of the gut is life threatening and may lead to peritonitis and death if the perforation is not sealed or corrected surgically.

Another gas pressure related condition has to do with nitrogen dissolved in the blood under high pressure, leaving solution and forming actual physical bubbles circulating in the bloodstream. The bubbles can lead to catastrophic effects if they prevent circulation of oxygen carrying blood to vital organs as an air or gas embolism. This condition was first recognized in deep sea divers and is known as caisson disease, decompression sickness, as well as 'the bends' because it often lead to a doubling over because of joint pain within hours of returning to the surface after prolonged dives. The limitation of dive length is calculated by dive tables or computers, and is typically based on the depth of the dive and the composition of the air or inhaled gasses in the dive tanks.

Nitrox was developed to reduce the incidence of nitrogen narcosis, which can lead to dangerous changes in mental awareness because of the buildup of dissolved nitrogen gas in the bloodstream. The term narcosis has the same Greek word root as the word for narcotic. The Greek word *αρκωσις* (narcosis) is derived from *narke*, which means a decline or loss of senses and movement.

Nitrogen narcosis has also been called 'raptures of the deep', inert gas narcosis, and the 'Martini effect'.

During ascent all gases increase in volume as the atmospheric pressure decreases. As the gases in the gastrointestinal tract increases in volume they may produce symptoms including cramping colicky abdominal pain, distension, belching, flatulence, and vomiting. Rare cases of rupture of the stomach and other portions of the gastrointestinal tract have occurred. Severe stomach pains have been reported during chamber dives after the divers drank carbonated beverages while under high atmospheric pressure.

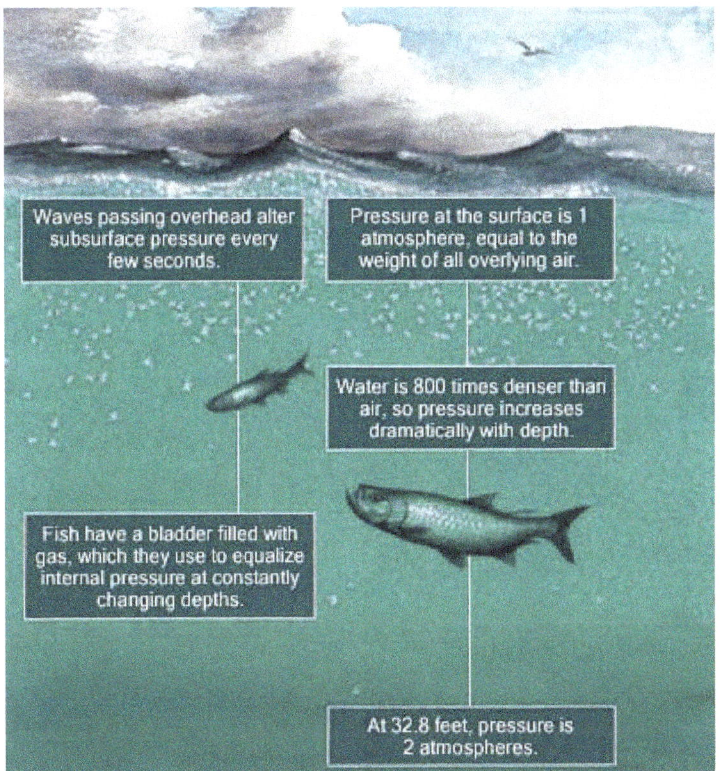

Waves passing overhead alter subsurface pressure every few seconds.
Pressure at the surface is 1 atmosphere, equal to the weight of all overlying air.
Water is 800 times denser than air, so pressure increases dramatically with depth.
Fish have a bladder filled with gas, which they use to equalize internal pressure at constantly changing depths.
At 32.8 feet, pressure is 2 atmospheres.

Atmospheric pressure rises quickly with greater underwater depths. Artist Jonathan Milo media.midcurrent.com.s3.amazonaws.com/wp Creative Commons License

One informative episode occurred with the grand opening of a brand new hyperbaric facility. The grand opening was toasted with champagne that was consumed while sixty feet (twenty meters) deep. The hosts and guests were disappointed that the champagne appeared to be flat without much carbonation. They decided to celebrate by drinking it even though it was flat because it tasted good. Their discomfort on ascent was exceeded only by their embarrassment. During ascent the gas in the 'flat' champagne (which was present in the normal amounts) came out of solution and expanded in their stomachs leading to uncontrolled belching.

Another unusual way to experience the effect of a prolonged dive was part of a research effort of the National Space and Aeronautic Administration (NASA) OCEAN project to assess the effects of long term space travel, comparing the similar exposures of space travel and underwater living. The research facilities have since remained open as a tourist hotel in Key Largo, Florida, where guests enter the hotel by scuba diving over twenty feet to the entrance. The hotel maintains and atmospheric pressure of approximately one and one half atmospheres.

For those who enjoy scuba diving, you are already familiar with the effects of increased atmospheric pressure. The pressure on the ears can become intense unless you are able to equalize the pressure regularly in descent and ascent. To be a certified scuba diver you must be knowledgeable about the risk of potentially life threatening illness and conditions that can be associated with these pressure changes. When inhaled at pressures higher than four atmospheres nitrogen can act as an anesthetic agent causing nitrogen narcosis. This is a temporary semi-anesthetized state of mental impairment similar to that caused by nitrous oxide, commonly known as laughing gas.

Nitrogen also dissolves in the bloodstream and body fats. Rapid decompression in the case of divers ascending too quickly, can lead to life threatening decompression sickness formerly known as caisson sickness or the bends, when nitrogen bubbles form in the bloodstream, nerves, joints. Most scuba divers also know not to ingest carbonated beverages or legumes and other gas producing foods during a dive. It is not the descent that is a problem. Remember from Boyles law that as you go deeper underwater the atmospheric pressure is increasing and the gas bubbles are getting smaller and smaller in volume. The problem is on the ascent where after a half hour of diving time at one hundred feet underwater, you begin your ascent. Your bowel has a modest size bubble of gas at that depth, but during the ascent this bubble expands and expands and can cause significant discomfort

Even though most experienced scuba divers know better than to fly shortly after a dive, even experienced scuba divers sometimes forget the same process can occur on land. Occasionally scuba divers will travel by land in an automobile from sea level after a dive, up a mountain road to a community or destination at a much higher elevation. Various gas mixtures have been developed for divers to reduce these risks. Trimix consists of oxygen, helium, and nitrogen, and Heliox is nitrogen free with just helium and oxygen. Hydrox is hydrogen and oxygen, an explosive combination if ignited. Nitrox is nitrogen and oxygen but is usually enriched for dives to increase the oxygen content and reduce the risk of decompression sickness.

Similar conditions can occur in miners when the mine shaft is pressurized to prevent ground water from entering, flying in unpressurized or depressurized aircraft at higher altitudes, and in space travel when the pressure in a spacesuit used for extravehicular activity is lower than the ambient pressure within the spaceship. An unusual but particularly dangerous combination is a novice scuba diver returning from a diving holiday unaware than a recent dive followed by even further reduction of atmospheric pressure by flying can lead to catastrophic consequences. Even though the dive table may suggest the risk period has ended, dive tables are calculated for a return to sea level, not the common commercial aircraft pressurization at an equivalent of an eight thousand foot elevation. See separate entry entitled Scuba Diving for more information.

Spelunking

Spelunking, the exploration of caves, has become an increasingly popular activity and can take place above or below sea level altitudes. Some of the deepest explored caves have vertical drops in excess of one thousand feet. Although changes in atmospheric pressure are noticeable, this effect is one of the least dangerous aspects of the sport activity. The exploration of underwater caves known as cave diving, combines spelunking with scuba diving, and is a particularly demanding and challenging activity. In this activity understanding the potential effects of atmospheric pressure changes becomes critically important.

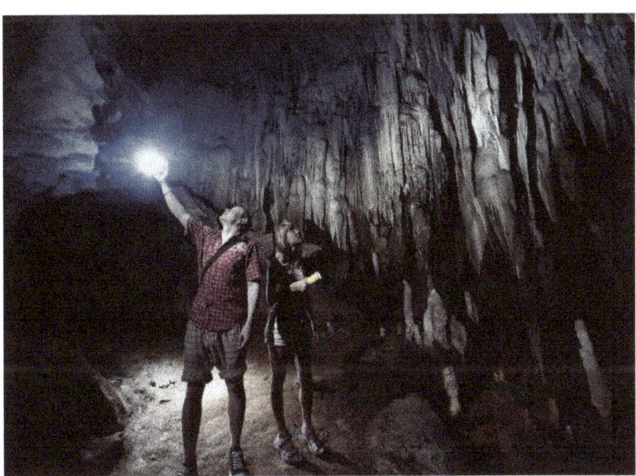

Shutterstock/DudarevMikhail

Underground Miner

Mines have been present from prehistoric times but the depth of mines continues to increase. The deepest mineshaft in commercial operation to date extends two and one-half miles below the surface. As one goes deeper into the interior of the planet the atmospheric pressure increases. Just like in the diving experience, the great depth of the mine can lead to significant reduction in the volume of gasses with the increasing atmospheric pressure. In addition some mines are pressurized to prevent ground water from entering the mineshaft. The danger is on the return to the surface as the higher atmospheric pressure is reduced back to normal. With the reduction in atmospheric pressure the volume of the gasses increases, and may leave solution causing bubble formation in the blood stream.

One of the additional occupational hazards of miners is the exposure to toxic gasses, including methane. The technology has now advanced to sophisticated monitoring for such gasses, but the miner's canary still carries an image into present day folklore and humor. Canaries and similar birds were taken into the mines as an early warning sign of methane toxicity. The birds are extremely sensitive to methane and die promptly on exposure to the toxic gas. If the miner's canary suddenly toppled off its perch in an episode of sudden death the miners knew that they had to quickly evacuate the mine. Bathroom humor would have the canary as a warning of toxic methane fumes emanating from flatus. If the canary died someone farted.

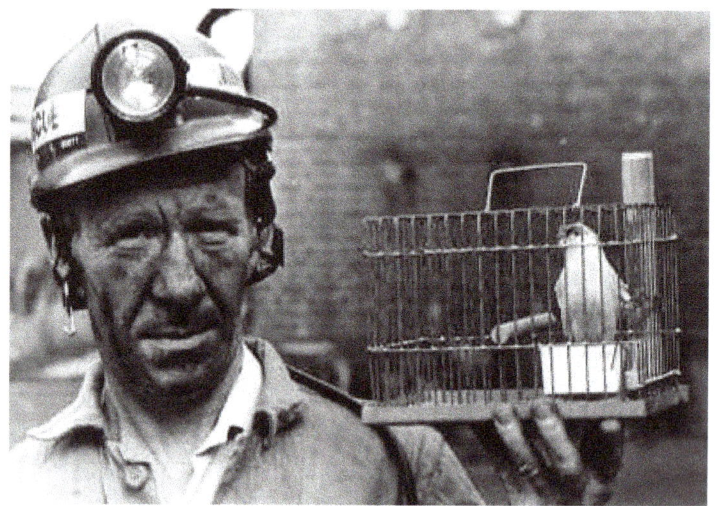

Public Domain Creative Commons License

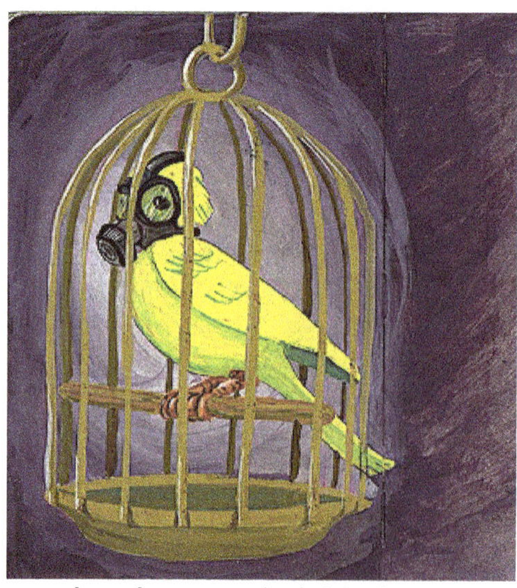

lunar.thegamez.net/coalmining/canary

Ayurveda Medicine

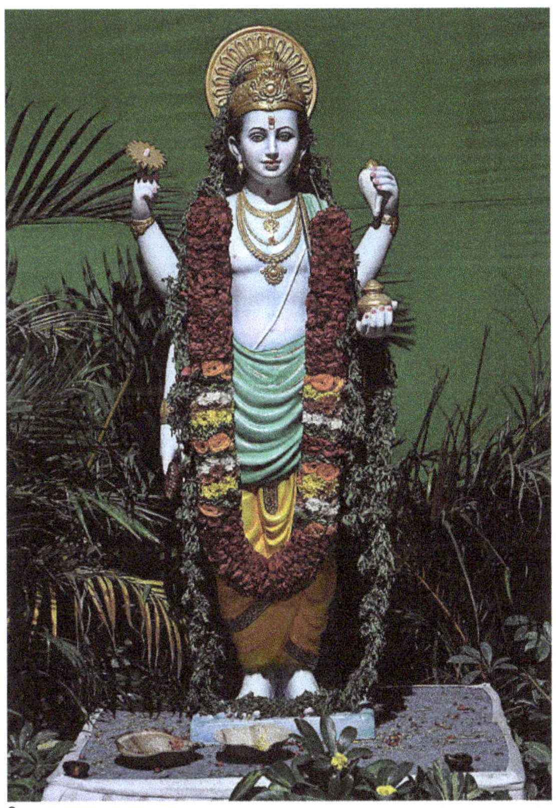

Dhanvantari (धन्वंतरी), known as an avatar of Vishnu is the Hindu god associated with Ayurveda. The above photo was taken at a recent Ayurveda expo in Bangalore titled 'Arogya'. Author HPNadig Creative Commons

Ayurveda (Sanskrit आयुर्वेद life-knowledge) also known as Ayurveda medicine is the oldest known system of traditional medicine, and is native to the Indian subcontinent. In Western cultures, Ayurveda medicine is considered a form of alternative or complementary medicine. The *Suśruta Saṃhitā* and the *Charaka Saṃhitā* are the oldest known Ayurveda texts. These classical Sanskrit encyclopedias of medicine are considered a formal compilation of the historical works of Ayurveda. A general overview of Ayurveda is offered in the introduction to this volume, on pages nine through sixteen.

Ayurveda medicine approaches health and wellness in a holistic approach, and has enjoyed renewed popularity in Western culture. It has a keen focus on digestive health. Ayurveda teaches that the human body digests not just physical nutrients, but the totality of all experiences, emotions, and sensory input. The sense of smell, touch, taste, sight, and hearing have a significant influence on digestion and health.

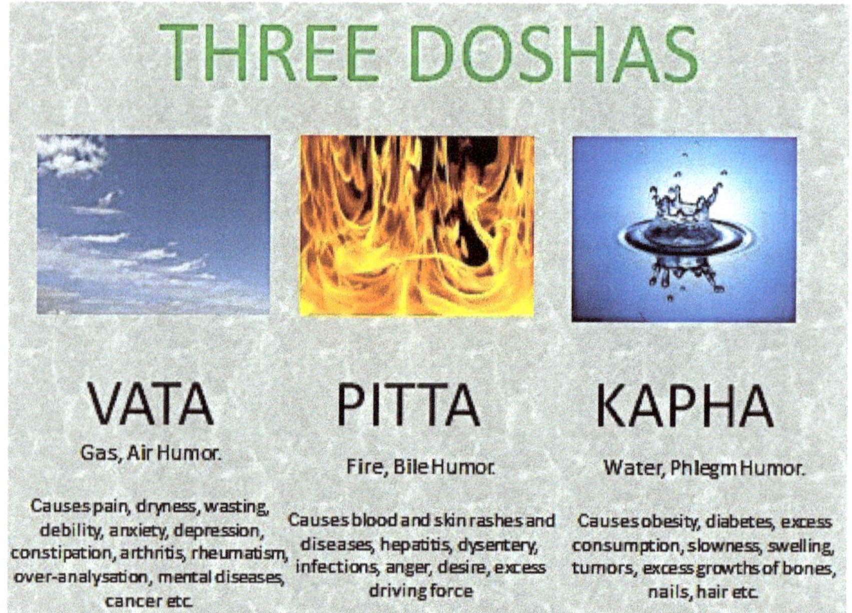
THREE DOSHAS
VATA
Gas, Air Humor.
Causes pain, dryness, wasting, debility, anxiety, depression, constipation, arthritis, rheumatism, over-analysation, mental diseases, cancer etc.
PITTA
Fire, Bile Humor.
Causes blood and skin rashes and diseases, hepatitis, dysentery, infections, anger, desire, excess driving force
KAPHA
Water, Phlegm Humor.
Causes obesity, diabetes, excess consumption, slowness, swelling, tumors, excess growths of bones, nails, hair etc.

In Ayurveda, a dosha is one of three bodily humors that in combination create an individual's constitution. Ayurveda medicine advocates that to be in good health one must achieve a balance between three doshas, known as Vata, Pitta and Kapha. Vata is required to activate and sustain the function of the nervous system. It affects rheumatism, gout, the windy humor, flatulence, etc. Pitta is the transforming bilious humor that is secreted through the digestive tract. It flows through the liver and in Ayurveda medicine it is believed to permeate the spleen, heart, eyes, and skin. Its primary quality is the heat and energy of bile to direct digestion and metabolism. Kapha is the body fluid associated with mucus, lubrication, nourishment and is the carrier of nutrients.

The strength and health of digestion in Ayurveda is ascribed to the Agni, a Sanskrit term for the "digestive fire". The digestive process metabolizes the food as well as environmental senses that are internalized. The body assimilates that which is useful, and produces a vital essence called Ojas, a Sanskrit word meaning strength. Ojas is the basis of physical well-being, strength, mental clarity, and immunity to illness. The digestive process also produces waste, which must be eliminated for health and wellness. When the digestive energy of Agni is weakened through physical inactivity, poor health, excess stress, or negative emotions the digestive process is impaired. The digestive process produces waste and toxins known as Ama that causes poor health and disease.

In the Ayurveda approach to digestive health the root cause of poor Agni is addressed, not just the symptoms that result. Ayurveda incorporates health practices designed to strengthen the digestive fire of Agni to improve the metabolism of food and minimize uncomfortable digestive symptoms such as gas, indigestion, bloating, and constipation. These holistic approaches include portion control to avoid overeating. The stomach should not be filled more than three quarters full as it needs internal space to allow room for the digestive process of acid, enzymes, the churning process and the gases produced. Overfilling the stomach can lead to reflux, indigestion, heartburn, and nausea.

Daily movement such as short walks, yoga, swimming, or exercise stimulate the digestive processes and enhance the peristalsis moving digestive material through the gastrointestinal tract. It also helps to maintain blood glucose levels without after meal spikes that nay cause difficulties especially for diabetics. Meditation on a regular basis for thirty minutes twice each day can be very beneficial in reducing stress and improving the Agni. Clearing away negative emotions and the deep relaxation of meditation is a practice that may provide many health benefits.

Ginger is a helpful carminative and is known in Ayurveda as the "universal remedy" due to its many benefits including relaxing the smooth muscle of the intestines. It also stimulates saliva, bile, and digestive enzyme production aiding in the digestive process. Ginger contains phenolic compounds such as gingerol, shogaol, and other volatile oils that are responsible for its potent properties. It may be taken during the day in the form of a refreshing and easy to prepare ginger tea.

The timing of meals is also important with the major meal of the day best consumed at midday. Having lunch as the major meal instead of dinner is a healthful approach allowing activity through the rest of the day to assist in the digestive process. The typical approach in the US of a large evening meal followed by inactivity and the recumbent position for sleeping leads to a propensity to reflux and a sluggish digestive process.

The Ayurveda focus on proper digestion and its central role in physical and emotional health is summarized in its philosophy. According to Ayurveda we are not what we eat, but we are what we digest. The wisdom of Ayurveda has withstood the test of many thousands years of experience well. Each individual can best judge what approaches provide benefit and chose selectively from a variety of health care disciplines.

In Sanskrit literature, Ayurveda is called "the science of eight components" (Sanskrit *aṣṭāṅga* अष्टांग). This system of classification became the basic canons of Ayurveda medicine.

Kāya-chikitsā - cure of diseases affecting the body (general medicine)
Kaumāra-bhṛtya - treatment of children (pediatrics)
Śhalya-chikitsā - removal of any substance, which has entered the body such as the extraction of darts, of splinters, etc. (surgery)
Śālākya-tantra - cure of diseases of the eye or ear etc. by sharp

instruments (ophthalmology/ENT)
Bhūta (past)-vidyā - treatment of mental diseases supposed to be produced by past experiences (psychiatry)
Agada-tantra - doctrine of antidotes (toxicology)
Rasayana-tantra doctrine of Rasayana (elixirs)
Vājīkaraṇa tantra (aphrodisiacs)

Ayurveda medicine advocates that these ancient concepts based on the knowledge discovered by the Rishis and Munis long ago remain timeless. Ayurveda examines the homeostasis of the whole body system, and approaches good health as the ability to exist in harmony with physical reality. While people may be of a predominant dosha, it is common to have variable displays of all of their elements. The dominance of the doshas within an individual are likewise variable, and Ayurveda medicine attempts to modify the doshas to achieve the correct balance needed to achieve and maintain health.

Bacteria (see Microbiome, Pathogen)

Bacterial Overgrowth, Small Intestine

Small intestinal bacterial overgrowth (SIBO) is a condition characterized by excessive bacterial growth in the small bowel. This results in alteration of the gut flora and microbiome. Risk factors include motility or anatomical changes that lead to stasis, immune deficiencies, and the reflux of colonic bacteria into the small bowel.

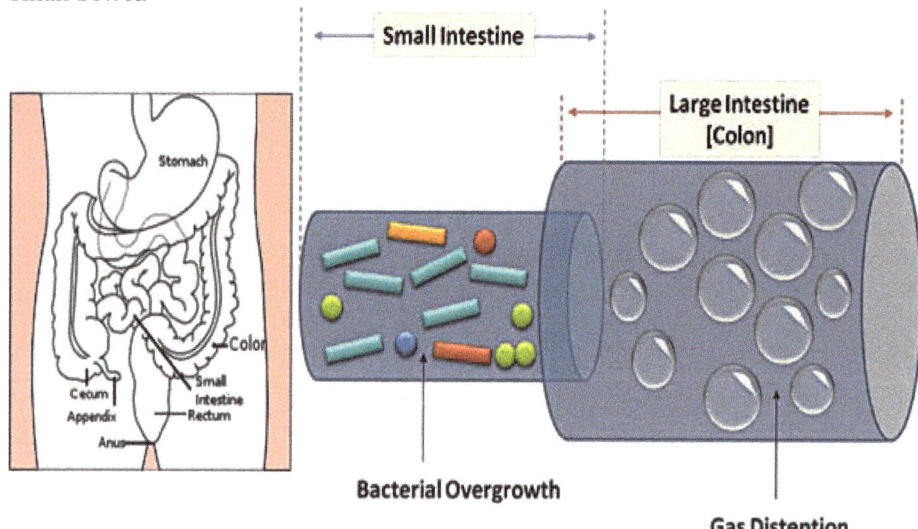

Anatomical changes, such as the surgical removal of the ileocecal valve, may predispose to small bowel bacterial overgrowth. The symptoms of bacterial overgrowth may include nausea, vomiting, bloating, flatus, chronic diarrhea, constipation, abdominal discomfort, weight loss, malnutrition, and anemia from vitamin B_{12} deficiency.

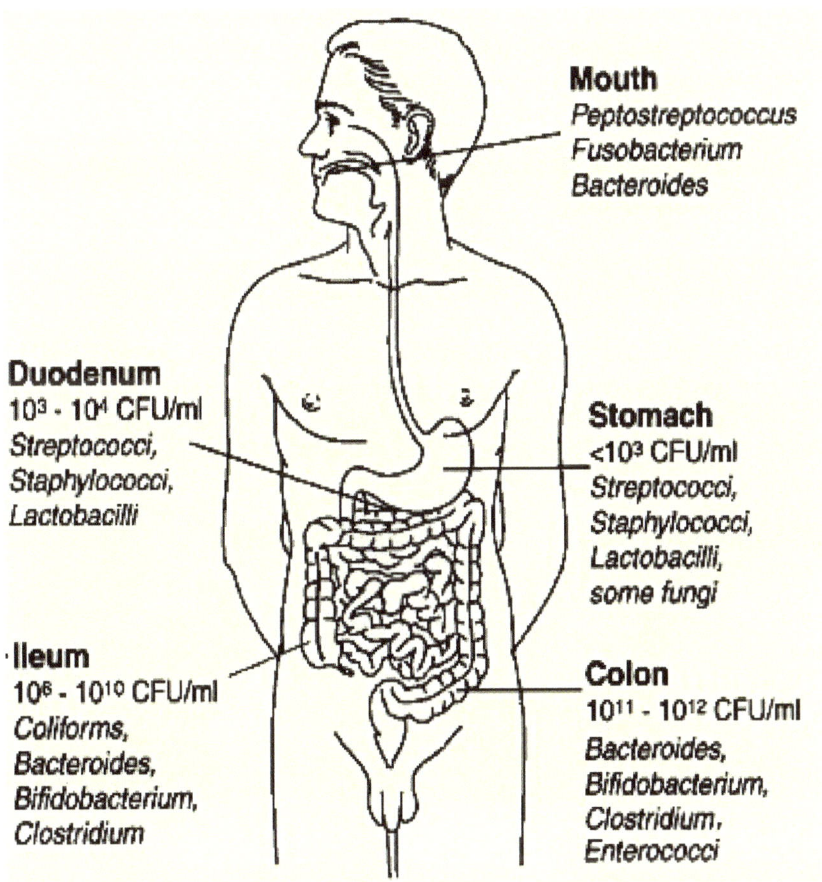

Irritable bowel syndrome (IBS) may have an association with SIBO with some studies showing improvement after treatment. Rosacea, a dermatological condition, also appears to have an association with improvement after treatment. Small bowel bacterial overgrowth syndrome is often treated with antibiotics. If retreatment is required, various antibiotics may be given in a cyclic fashion. Probiotics may also be of benefit in an attempt to return the microbiome to normal flora and balance.

Bariatric (Weight Loss) Surgery

Bariatric (Greek bar- weight, iatr - treatment) is the field of knowledge that deals with obesity including diet, exercise, behavioral therapy, pharmaceuticals, hormones, and surgery. Overweight and obesity are defined in relationship to the Body Mass Index, commonly referred to by its initials BMI. They are commonly associated with complicating co-morbid conditions including heart disease, diabetes, cancer, asthma, sleep apnea, and chronic musculoskeletal problems that lead to higher mortality rates.

Diet, exercise, behavior therapy, and anti-obesity drugs are first-line treatment. Bariatric surgery is the term for the surgical treatment of morbid obesity and gastric bypasses are one class of such operations. Gastric bypass surgery divides the stomach into a small upper pouch and a larger lower "remnant" pouch and then reconnects the small intestine to both. There are a variety of anatomical variations that have been developed, but all result in a marked reduction of the volume of food the stomach can receive during a meal.

Bariatric weight loss surgery is usually reserved for those who have failed more conservative approaches. It generally results in greater weight loss than conventional treatment and may lead to improvement in quality of life and obesity related disorders such as hypertension and diabetes. Unfortunately, surgical complications may occur and a poorly motivated patient may defeat the limitation of the size of their meals by continuing to ingest excess calories by increasing their daily meal frequency. The combination of approaches is best tailored to each individual patient.

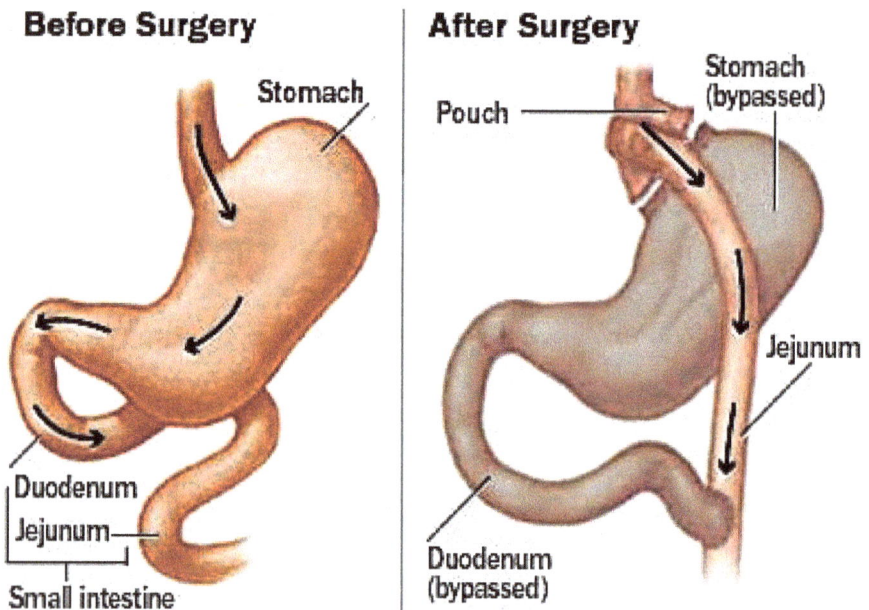

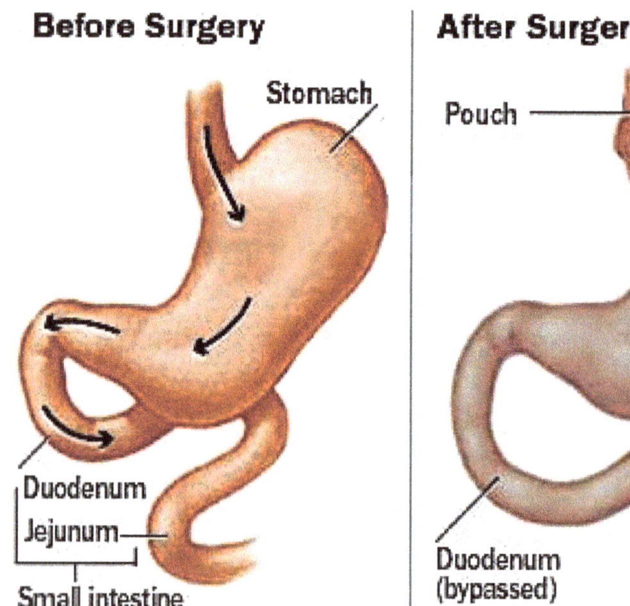

The surgery is usually undertaken to treat morbid obesity, defined as a body mass index greater than forty, when traditional dietary therapy has failed. Morbid obesity complications include type 2 diabetes, hypertension, and sleep apnea, and the rapid weight loss following surgery often results in improvement of these conditions a well. Although there are risks and complications with any surgery the benefits of weight loss can be very significant and each case must be individualized to every persons unique situation.

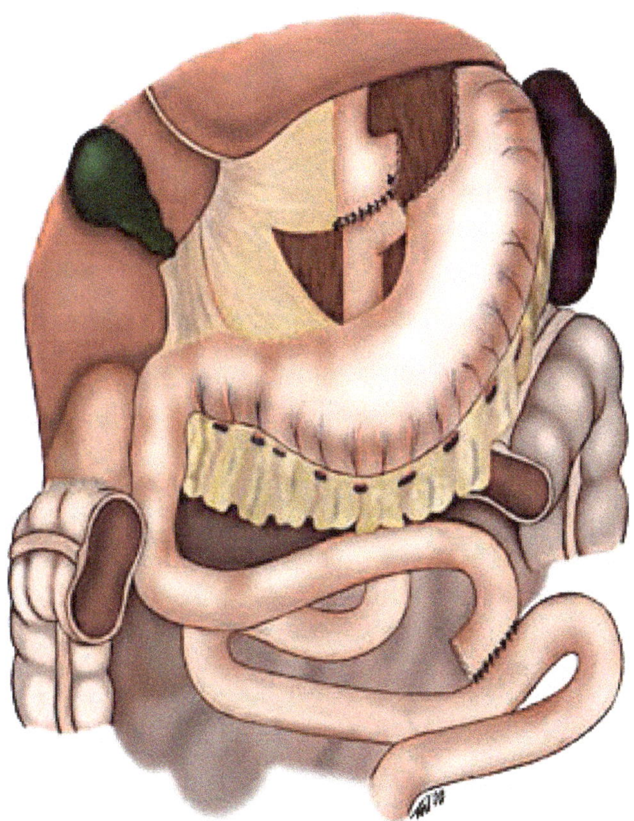

Graphic of a gastric bypass using a Roux-en-Y anastomosis. The transverse colon is not shown so that the Roux-en-Y can be clearly seen. The variant seen in this image is *retrocolic, retrogastric*, because the distal small bowel that joins the proximal segment of stomach is behind the transverse colon and stomach. Author: Courtesy of Ethicon Endosurgery, Inc.

Weight loss of sixty-five to eighty percent of excess body weight is common after surgery in the large series of gastric bypass operations reported. Hyperlipidemia and hypertension is corrected in over seventy percent of patients. Obstructive sleep apnea is markedly improved. Type 2 diabetes is reversed in up to ninety percent of patients. Gastroesophageal reflux disease is relieved in nearly all patients. Research publications show that overall there was an eighty-nine percent reduction in mortality over the five years following surgery in comparison to a matched group of patients treated without surgery. Surgical complications rate is approximately fifteen percent with a mortality rate of approximately zero point five percent.

With the volume the stomach can stretch reduced by approximately ninety percent when even a small amount of food is eaten it creates a feeling of fullness and satiety. For many people with morbid obesity the normal sensation of fullness and satiety does not stop compulsive overeating. After the gastric bypass surgery, they quickly learn that overeating results in nausea, vomiting and increasing discomfort. Post-operative gastric bypass patients also develop a lowered tolerance for alcoholic beverages, which are absorbed at a faster rate after surgery.

The reasons gastric bypass surgery works is multifactorial. It appears to be a combination of reduced caloric intake, behavioral changes to eating patterns and diet, and physiological changes related to the digestive process and the hormones that control appetite and satiety. More recent research suggests it leads to important changes in the gut microbiome. Human beings are creative and complex individuals and a number have managed to regain the weight loss accomplished after expensive and not without risk surgery. This often requires an excessive number of frequent small meals throughout the day. Research to elucidate the causes and approaches to obesity and eating disorders is an ongoing process.

Bean (Legume)

Beans are a legume native to the Americas that have a well-deserved reputation for contributing to intestinal gas production. The bean is rich in the sugars raffinose, verbascose, and stachyose. As humans do not produce the enzyme required for its degradation, alpha galactosidase, these sugars undergo fermentation by the gut flora.

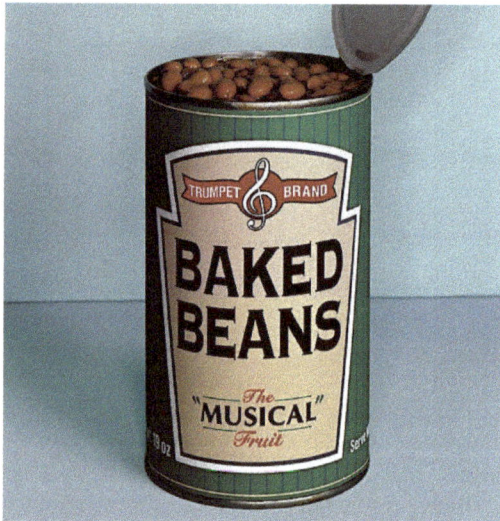

"Beans, Beans, The Musical Fruit" is a schoolyard saying and children's song about the capacity for beans to contribute to flatulence.

Beans, beans, the musical fruit
The more you eat, the more you toot
The more you toot, the better you feel
So we have beans at every meal!

There are also several alternative versions, such as the one below:

Beans, beans, they're good for your heart
The more you eat, the more you fart
The more you fart, the happier/better you feel
So let's eat beans with every meal

The US Department of Agriculture is working on the development of a bean with lower levels of these sugars and so far the Anasazi bean has been the leading candidate, but no breakthrough yet. Thankfully there are alpha-galactosidase enzyme supplements that can provide relief. The enzyme is not heat stabile, so it will be inactivated with the heat of cooking. The enzyme should be added to the first bite of the beans consumed and if a large portion is ingested additional enzyme intake during the course of the bean meal is recommended.

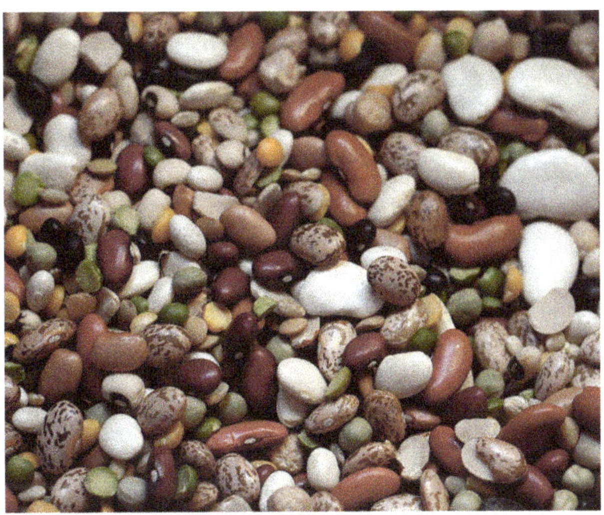

An alternative approach is to soak the beans for several hours, leeching out some of the sugars into the water, which is discarded. The best approach is to soak the beans until they begin to germinate. With germination the bean itself begins to release alpha-galactosidase to break down its complex sugar content for the nutritional use of the newly germinated bean plant. With germination approximately eighty percent of the complex sugars are digested.

A legume is a plant in the family Fabaceae (or Leguminosae), grown agriculturally for their food grain seed, livestock forage and silage, and soil-enhancement. Most legumes harbor the symbiotic bacteria Rhizobia in their root nodules, which convert nitrogen in the atmosphere into ammonia and ammonium. This source of nitrogen contributes to the legumes production of amino acids and high protein content. Legumes include alfalfa, clover, peas, beans, lentils, lupins, soybeans, and peanuts and a number of trees and shrubs.

In farming crop rotation or growing legumes near non-legumes is common. Legumes are sometimes referred to as "green manure" because their symbiotic bacteria enrich the soil with nitrogenous products. A legume fruit is typically a pod that opens along a seam. They are an excellent source of protein but contain lower quantities of the essential amino acid methionine.

Beer (see Carbonation, Nitrogenation)

Belch (see Burp, Eructation)

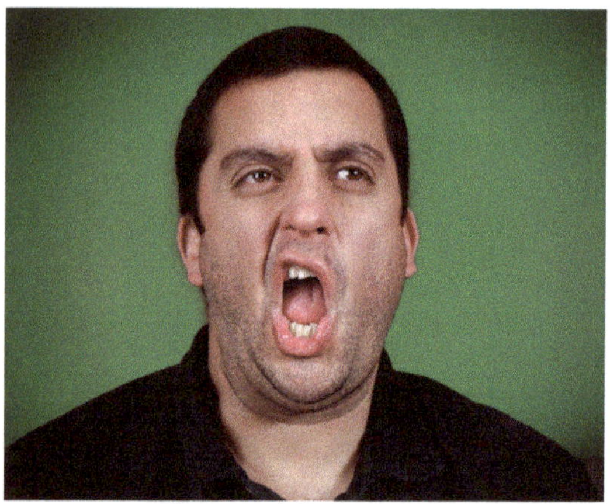

Shutterstock/Catherine Lall

Bicarbonate Secretion

Sodium bicarbonate secretion is stimulated by the hormone secretin. Sodium bicarbonate is produced and released from the Brunner glands of the proximal duodenum as well as secreted by the pancreas. The pancreatic juices flow through the pancreatic duct, sphincter of Oddi, and ampulla of Vater into the second portion of the duodenum. The sodium bicarbonate neutralizes the acidic chyme, which has entered the duodenum from the stomach. When sodium bicarbonate interacts with and neutralizes acid, water results and carbon dioxide is released as a gas. The large quantity of carbon dioxide released when the gastric acid is neutralized in the duodenum by the addition of sodium bicarbonate may lead to temporary bloating and distension. As carbon dioxide easily diffuses across the cell lining of the small intestine, it is rapidly absorbed into the bloodstream and carried to the lungs where it is released from the bloodstream at the alveolus, and eliminated from the body by exhaling the carbon dioxide in the breath.

Baking soda and baking powder are both used to make dough rise with bubbles of carbon dioxide. Baking soda is pure alkaline sodium bicarbonate that when mixed with an acid releases CO_2 gas. That's why sodium bicarbonate is a long-standing treatment for 'acid or sour stomach' and indigestion as its alkaline nature neutralizes the stomach acid and generates carbon dioxide gas in the process.

Baking powder contains sodium bicarbonate and the acid cream of tartar, which will react when dissolved in water. A drying agent, normally a starch, is also in the mix to prevent moisture from starting the reaction prematurely. Baking powder is fine for baking but it would not be an effective antacid as it also contains acid that would consume all of the sodium bicarbonate's neutralizing capacity.

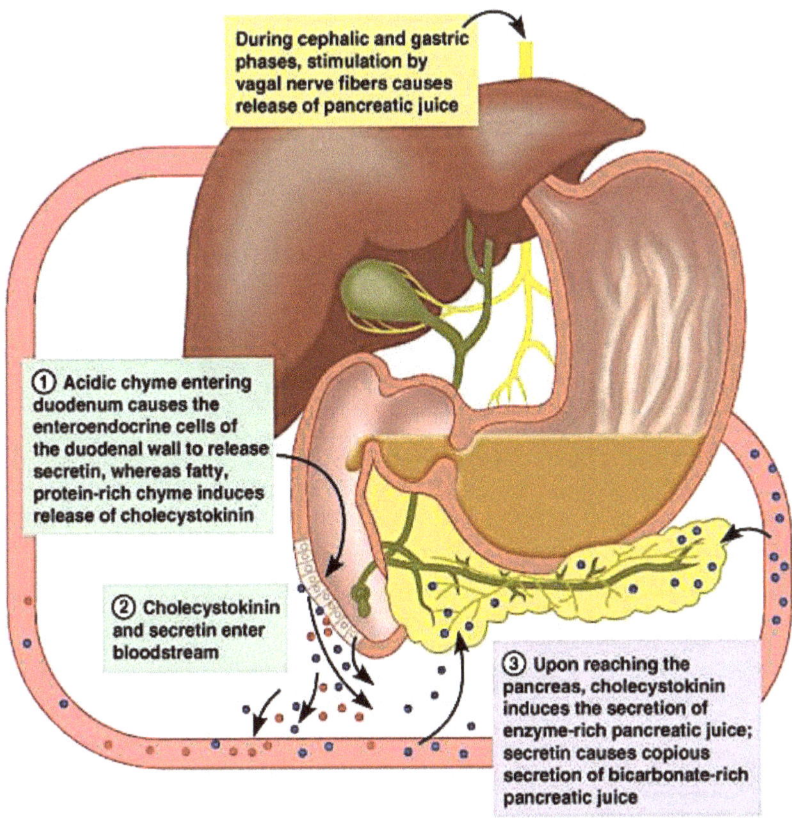

Bifidobacteria (see Probiotic)

Bifidobacteria (previously called *Lactobacillus bifidus*) is a Gram-positive anaerobic symbiotic bacterium, which is commonly found in the gastrointestinal tract, vagina, and mouth. Some bifidobacteria have a long history of being used as probiotics. In 1899 Henry Tissier, a French pediatrician at the Pasteur Institute in Paris, identified dominant bacteria shaped like the letter Y in the bowels of healthy infants that he named Bifidobacterium. He recommended treating infants suffering from diarrhea with the bacteria. In 1907 Elie Metchnikoff at the Pasteur Institute proposed that lactic acid bacteria are beneficial to human health. He observed that the longevity of Bulgarian peasants was the result of their consumption of fermented milk products such as yogurt. He suggested that oral administration of healthful organisms would improve the intestinal microflora.

A number of Bifidobacterium strains are important probiotics and are used in the food industry. Beneficial effects may include regulation of intestinal microbiome, inhibition of pathogens, modulation of immune responses, repression of pro-carcinogenic activity, production of vitamins, and the bioconversion of dietary compounds into bioactive molecules.

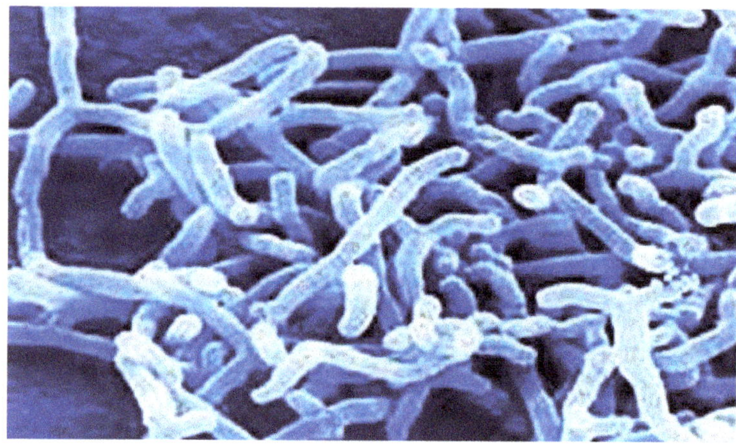

Mother's milk contains high concentrations of lactose and lower quantities of phosphate a pH buffer. When bifidobacteria and other lactic acid bacteria in the infant's GI tract ferment the mother's breast milk, the pH is reduced making it more difficult for Gram-negative bacteria to grow. The genus Bifidobacterium possesses a unique fructose based pathway to ferment carbohydrates. The sensitivity of members of the genus Bifidobacterium to oxygen generally limits probiotic activity to anaerobic habitats.

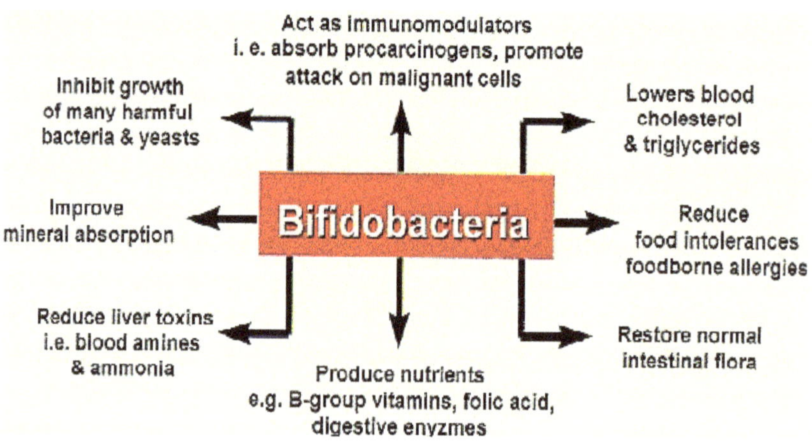

Bismuth

Bismuth is a chemical element, number eighty-three on the periodic table, which has long history of being used in preparations designed to treat gastrointestinal complaints. It is a heavy metal with a low level of toxicity. Its various compound have also been used historically to treat syphilis and the severe diarrhea from cholera. Bismuthinite is a mineral consisting of bismuth sulfide (Bi_2S_3) and is an important ore of bismuth.

Bismuth subgallate, with a chemical formula $C_7H_5BiO_6$, is the active ingredient in Devrom, an over the counter product described as an internal deodorizer. The term 'sub' refers to the high oxygen content in the molecule and the presence of bismuth oxygen compounds. It is used to reduce the fecal odor arising from flatulence and fecal incontinence. Those with gastric bypass bariatric surgery, inflammatory bowel disease, irritable bowel syndrome, and ostomy appliances commonly use it. It has also been used to treat *Helicobacter pylori* infection and is also used in wound therapy.

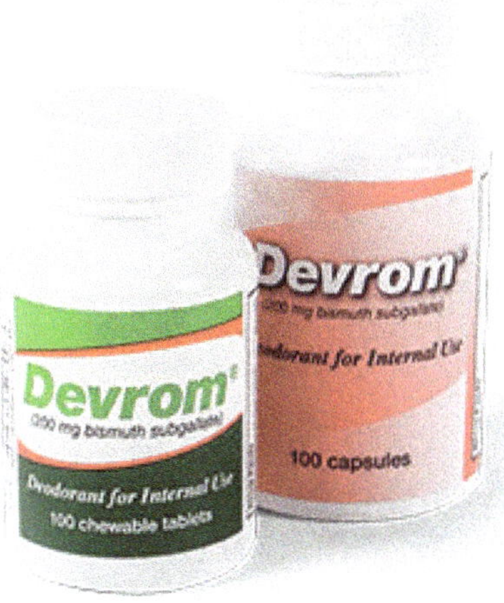

The mechanism by which bismuth works is uncertain. It may be related to its known antimicrobial activity, perhaps inhibiting the microbes that generate some of the more offensive gasses that contain sulfur as well as aromatic and volatile organic compounds. Bismuth also reacts directly with sulfur producing bismuth sulfide, a dark black insoluble compound. Bismuth sulfide may cause darkening or blackening of the tongue if sulfur is found in high concentrations in the saliva. It will also cause blackening of the stool as it binds with the sulfur that would otherwise give rise to hydrogen sulfide and other offensive sulfur gasses. The dark black color of the stool may be mistaken for melena, a sign of internal bleeding that results from the digestive process on blood cells and hemoglobin. The black coloration is not a health concern and is temporary, clearing with cessation of bismuth intake.

Bismuth subsalicylate has a bismuth oxide core structure with salicylate ions attached to its surface. It is used as an antidiarrheal and is the active ingredient in Pepto-Bismol, as well as the U.S. version of Kaopectate since it was reformulated in 2004. It is a popular remedy for indigestion, nausea, heartburn, and as a preventative for traveler's diarrhea. It is also used to treat some other gastrointestinal diseases and infections including the microorganism *Helicobacter pylori*, which is associated with peptic ulcer disease and stomach cancer.

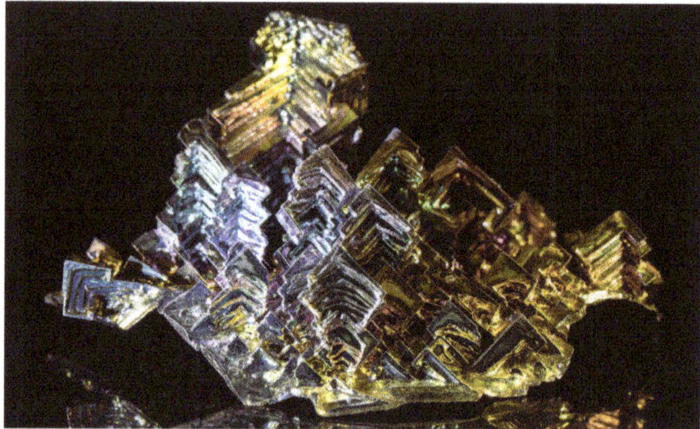
Bismuth in crystalline form. Shutterstock/MiriamDoerr

The antimicrobial property may be as a result of an oligodynamic effect, where toxic small doses of heavy metal ions are toxic to microbes. Another antimicrobial effect may arise from the release of salicylic acid as the compound is hydrolyzed. It is believed that the salicylic acid acts as an antimicrobial for toxigenic *Escherichia coli*, a principal cause of traveler's diarrhea.

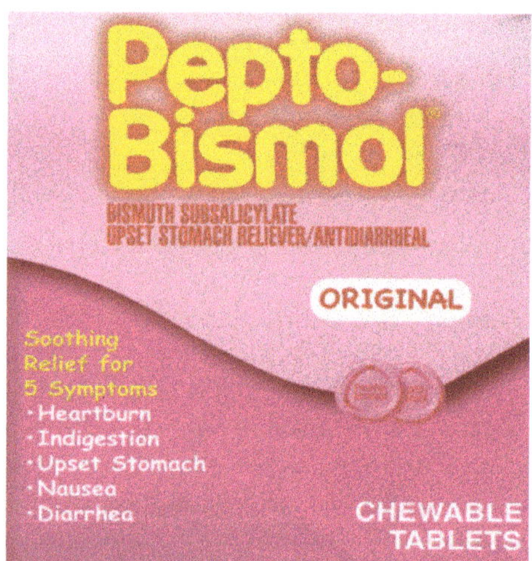

As a derivative of salicylic acid, bismuth subsalicylate also displays anti-inflammatory properties as well as some of the adverse effects of salicylates. Because salicylate levels can accumulate and lead to toxicity any use beyond a few weeks length is discouraged. Children should not take bismuth subsalicylate while suffering from a viral infection between of the associated risk of acquiring Reye's syndrome and liver failure. Nursing mothers should not use bismuth subsalicylate as it is excreted in breast milk and may pose a risk of Reye's syndrome in nursing children.

Bloat

Bloat is the common sensation that the abdomen is distended or overly full. There are many causes of bloating ranging from simple overeating and the normal production of intestinal gasses to abdominal ascites fluid buildup from an underlying tumor. Common causes of abdominal bloating include overeating, gastric distension, lactose intolerance, fructose intolerance and other food intolerances, food allergy, aerophagia (air swallowing), irritable bowel syndrome, partial or complete bowel obstruction, gastric dumping syndrome or rapid gastric emptying, gas producing foods, constipation, visceral fat and obesity.

Less common causes include splenic flexure syndrome, menstruation, dysmenorrhea, premenstrual syndrome, polycystic ovary syndrome and ovarian cysts, Alvarez' syndrome, intestinal parasites (e.g., *Ascaris lumbricoides*), diverticulosis, celiac disease, prescription medications such as phentermine, intra-abdominal tumors such as cancer of the ovary, liver, uterus, stomach, and colon.

Temporary bloating is common after gastrointestinal endoscopic procedures. Rarely a megacolon, which is an abnormal dilation of the colon, can be caused by ulcerative colitis or Chagas disease caused by the parasite *Trypanosoma cruzi*. After surgical repair of a hiatal hernia or treatment for gastro esophageal reflux with a procedure known as a Nissen fundoplication, the ability to burp and belch is restricted resulting in uncomfortable bloating and distension.

Common Foods that Cause Bloating/Gas:

- Cabbage
- Cauliflower
- Beans
- Oats
- Apples
- Milk
- Fluffy Wheat
- Broccoli
- Onions
- Corn
- Potatoes
- Pears
- Soft Cheese
- Peaches

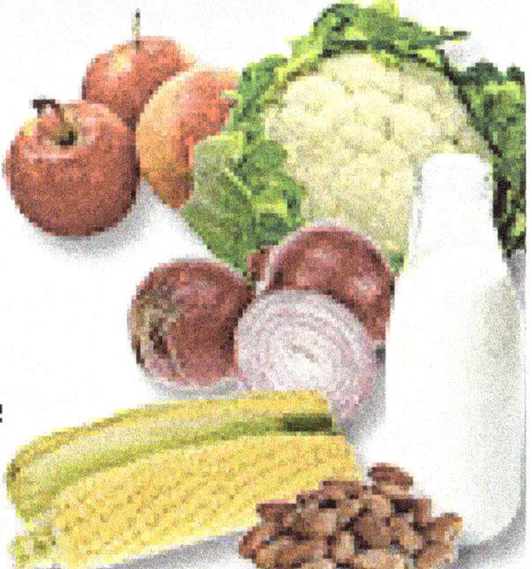

A number of lifestyle and dietary factors can also affect the frequency and intensity of the sensation of bloating. Exercise stimulates the releases of hormones that encourage peristaltic activity in the bowels. In a similar fashion, caffeine containing beverages and food such as coffee, tea, cola, and chocolate also stimulate peristalsis and improve the transit time of food through the digestive tract. This gives the gut flora less time to ferment the material in the lumen of the bowel, with a resultant decrease in the total volume of gas produced by bacterial fermentation. Even a walk after a meal may help to move the contents along helping to ease the volume of gas produced. If nothing else, it at least allows you to release it outdoors!

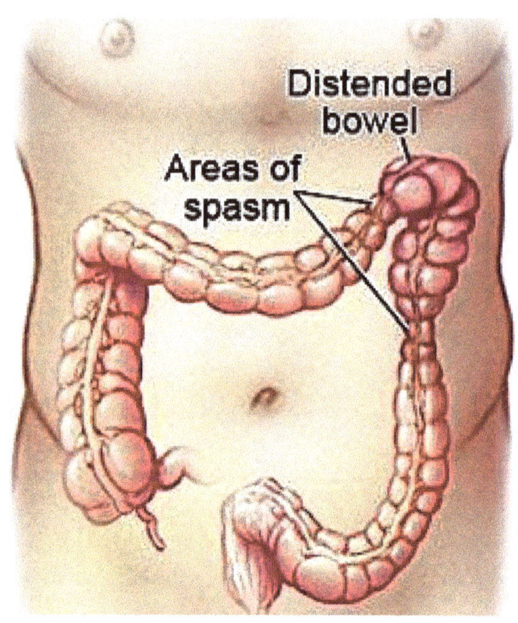

Meals that are high in fat create the exact opposite effect, as fat causes the release of hormones and slows down gut motility. As the food spends more time in the digestive tract continued bacterial fermentation produces increasing quantities of gas. In addition, foods that are extremely hot or cold tend to be swallowed in smaller quantities resulting in more swallows being necessary to eat or drink the same volume at a moderate temperature. As each swallow contributes an additional quantity of air entering the esophagus and digestive tract, more swallows results in more air ingestion. Foods or snacks that require excess chewing with resultant excess swallowing of saliva, such as chewing or bubble gum, also contribute to excess air ingestion.

Certain types of vegetables and fruits contain sugars and starches, which may be poorly digested by people but happily fermented by bacteria comprising the gut flora. The most common food intolerance is lactose intolerance. The treatment is always directed at the underlying cause. Empiric trials of carminatives, probiotics, dietary restrictions, enzyme replacement therapy, simethicone etc. can be attempted. Alternative health approaches to treat bloating include acupuncture, homoeopathy and hypnosis. Sometimes the underlying bloat is not bloating from air but from the increased body fat of obesity. Now that is a real challenge, but the benefits of eliminating that bloat can be profoundly beneficial to health and longevity.

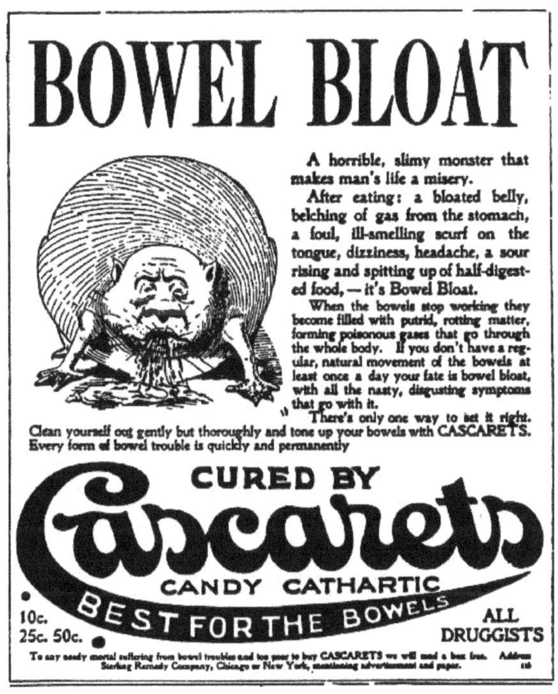

With the increasing popularity of surgery to correct hiatal hernia and reflux the gas bloat syndrome is occurring more frequently. This is a postoperative consequence of hiatal hernia repair, typically called a Nissen fundoplication. With the correction of the hiatal hernia and increasing tightness around the lower esophageal sphincter the ability to burp and belch is impaired. The inability to release swallowed air or gasses forming in the upper digestive tract can lead to bloating, distention, and discomfort. At times dilation of the lower esophageal sphincter can be performed as an outpatient to provide relief, or reoperation may be necessary if the gas bloat is intolerable.

Bariatric surgery is the term for the surgical treatment of morbid obesity, and gastric bypasses are one class of such operations. Gastric bypass surgery divides the stomach into a small upper pouch and a larger lower "remnant" pouch and then reconnects the small intestine to both. There are a variety of anatomical variations that have been developed, but all result in a marked reduction of the volume of food the stomach can receive during a meal. The surgery is usually undertaken to treat morbid obesity, defined as a body mass index greater than forty, when traditional dietary therapy has failed. Complications of morbid obesity include type 2 diabetes, hypertension, and sleep apnea, and the rapid weight loss following surgery often results in improvement of these conditions a well. Although there are risks and complications with any surgery the benefits of weight loss can be very significant and each case must be individualized to every persons unique situation.

Weight loss of sixty-five to eighty percent of excess body weight is common after bariatric surgery of the gastric bypass type operation. Hyperlipidemia and hypertension is corrected in over seventy percent of patients. Obstructive sleep apnea is markedly improved and Type 2 diabetes is reversed in up to ninety percent of patients. Gastroesophageal reflux disease is relieved in nearly all patients. Research publications show that overall there was an eighty-nine percent reduction in mortality over the five years following surgery in comparison to a matched group of patients treated without surgery. The surgical complications rate is approximately fifteen percent, with a mortality rate of approximately one-half of one percent.

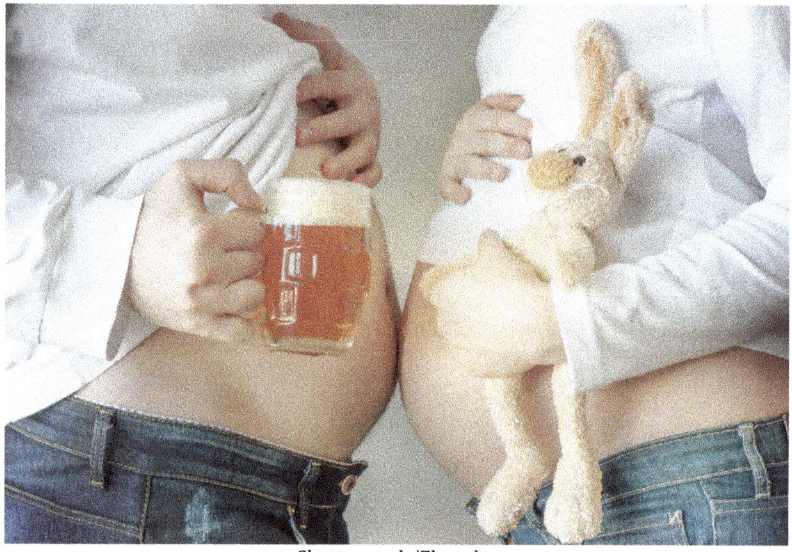

Shutterstock/Zhoozha

With the volume the stomach can stretch reduced by approximately ninety percent when even a small amount of food is eaten it creates a feeling of fullness and satiety. For many people with morbid obesity the normal sensation of fullness and satiety does not stop compulsive overeating. After the gastric bypass surgery, they quickly learn that overeating results in nausea, vomiting, and increasing discomfort. Post-operative gastric bypass patients also develop a lowered tolerance for alcoholic beverages, which are absorbed at a faster rate after surgery.

The reasons gastric bypass surgery works is multifactorial. It appears to be a combination of reduced caloric intake, behavioral changes to eating patterns and diet, and physiological changes related to the digestive process and the hormones that control appetite and satiety. More recent research suggests it leads to important changes in the gut microbiome. Human beings are creative and complex individuals and a number have managed to regain the weight loss accomplished after expensive and not without risk surgery. This often requires an excessive number of frequent small meals throughout the day. Research to elucidate the causes and approaches to obesity and eating disorders is an ongoing process.

Bloat, Veterinary

Bloat, a critical veterinary medical condition also known as gastric dilatation volvulus occurs when the stomach becomes over distended by gas and cannot release it by eructation. It can also be a gastric torsion if the stomach is also twisted on its mesentery. The condition occurs in domesticated animals, especially ruminants and certain dog breeds. In dogs, gas accumulation in the stomach is usually associated with volvulus of the stomach, which prevents gas from escaping. In cattle eating in a young pasture of legumes such as alfalfa with the air bubbles becoming trapped in the rumen often causes bloating. Signs of bloat in cattle are abdominal distention, cessation of grazing, lethargy, and difficulty in urinating or defecating, and rapid breathing.

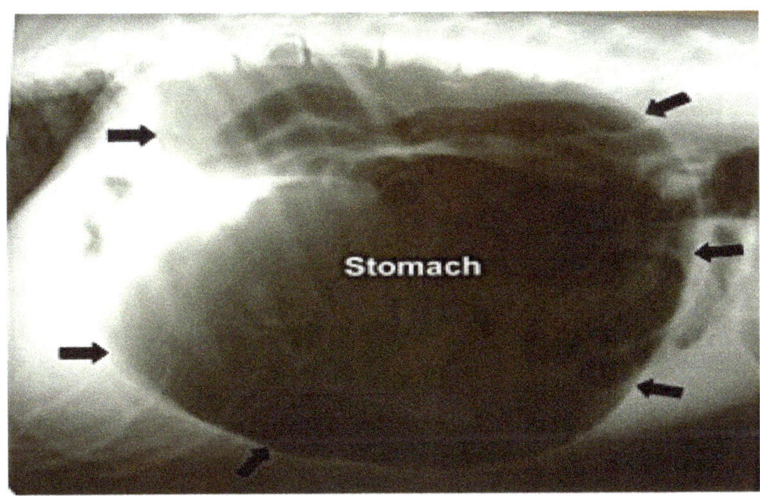

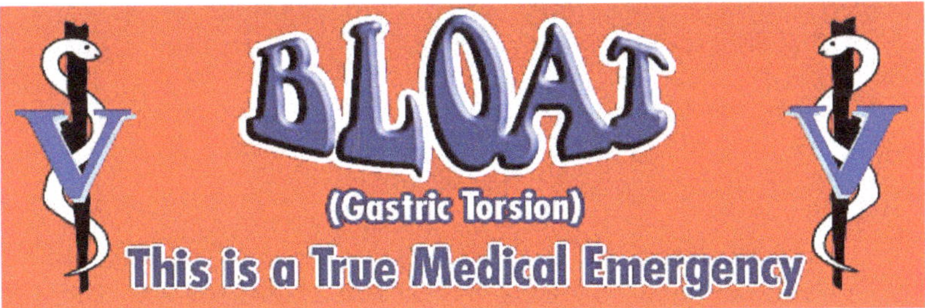

A stomach tube may be inserted to release the trapped air or a surgical incision into the flank to open the rumen and manually remove the froth and air may be required. Bloat is an emergency veterinary medical condition and has a high mortality even under professional care.

Borborygmus

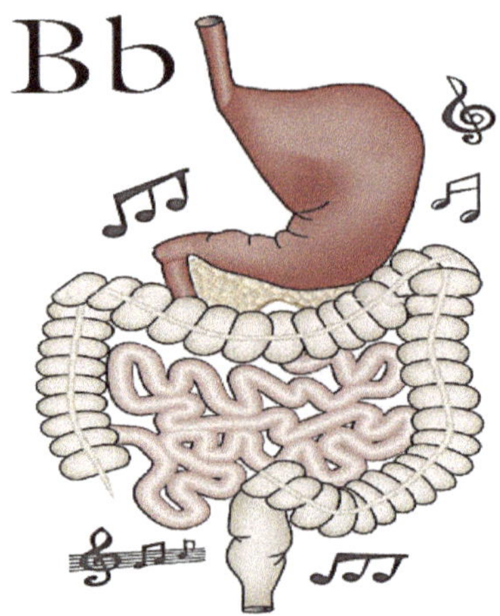

borborygmus

Borborygmus (Greek βορβορυγμός borborygmós). The Greeks created this onomatopoetic word to imitate its sounds. In humans and animals peristaltic activity with the mixing, churning, and propulsion of chime, liquids, solids, and gasses can create intestinal noises audible to oneself and others nearby. The noises are described as rumbling, growling or gurgling and louder sounds may also occur with hunger. The actor Humphrey Bogart gives an Academy Award worthy demonstration of borborygmi in the 1951 movie *The African Queen*.

Bowel sounds are normally always audible with a stethoscope over a brief period of time. Partial obstruction of the intestines may also contribute to more borborygmi; the audible bowel sounds that can be heard by the unaided ear. When listening with a stethoscope the bowel sounds in early obstruction are often hyperactive, and become quiescent and diminished with longer standing obstruction. The absence of bowel sounds is frequently noted for a few hours after anesthesia, but can also be a sign of serious bowel injury or obstruction. It is common after anesthesia that eating or drinking is not allowed until the bowel sounds have returned, and the individual begins to pass gas proving that the bowels have resumed their normal motility and movement.

The word borborygmus is a type of word called an onomatopoeia. Onomatopoeia. Comes from the Greek word ὀνοματοποιία ὄνομα for "name" and ποιέω for "I make". Although its origin describes a word that literally means making up a name, in the English language it is defined as a word that imitates or phonetically reproduces the sound that it is defining. A more accurate word would be echo mimetic, from the Greek words from Ηχώ meaning "echo or sound" and μιμητικό meaning "mimetic or imitation". Common onomatopoeias are echomimetic words that reproduce animal sounds such as "oink", "meow", "roar" or "chirp". Onomatopoeias vary with languages, for example the sound of a clock may be described as tick tock in English, dī dā in Mandarin Chinese or katchin katchin in Japanese.

In the case of a frog, the variation of echo mimetic onomatopoeia are not due to the frogs speaking foreign languages but because different species of frogs make different sounds. Ancient Greece marsh frogs went brekekekex koax koax (as in Aristophanes' comic play The Frogs), English ribbit for species of the American pond frog said ribbit, ribbit, and the common English frog went "croak".

Bowel Movement (Defecation, BM)

Defecation, a bowel movement or often named for its abbreviated initials BM, is the elimination of fecal waste material from the digestive tract via the anus. The stimulus to defecate is the distention of the rectum or sigmoid colon with feces. This reflex can be triggered by manual stimulation of the rectal wall stretch receptors. Voluntary control of defecation is part of the toilet training process and is typically mastered during childhood. This control can be lost again with neurological, psychological or senescent changes. The involuntary release of feces is known as fecal incontinence, often called encopresis in children.

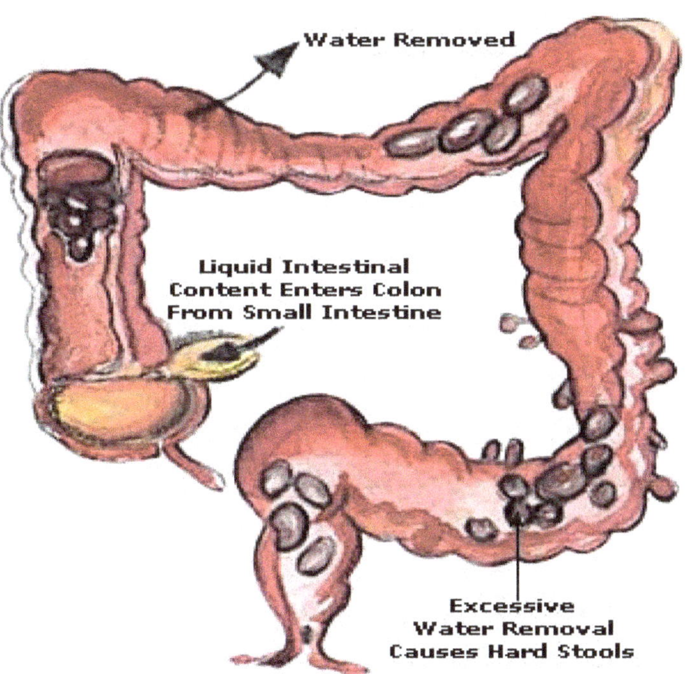

Creative Commons License

Defecation is a complex reflex coordination of neuromuscular activity that relaxes the puborectalis muscle straightening the normally ninety-degree anorectal angle and initiates the relaxation of the internal anal sphincters. There is a strong urge to defecate but the external anal sphincter contracts to prevent defecation until voluntarily released to initiate the process. Colonic contractions, along with increased intra-abdominal pressure by performance of the Valsalva maneuver (attempting to exhale against a closed epiglottis), then push the fecal material out of the rectum via the anus.

The frequency range of normal bowel movements is variable and can range from two bowel movements per day to once per week, often dependent on diet. The squatting position is most conducive to defecation. Using Western style sitting toilets, as opposed to squat toilets found in non-Western locales, can be problematic especially if the feet cannot reach the ground, as in young children. An elevated footrest to allow the thighs and legs to be flexed can greatly assist in the ease of elimination for both children and adults.

The puborectalis sling forming the anorectal angle is responsible for gross continence of solid stool. The internal anal sphincter is an involuntary muscle that contributes about fifty-five percent of the resting anal pressure. Together with the hemorrhoid vascular cushions, the internal anal sphincter maintains continence of flatus and liquid during rest.

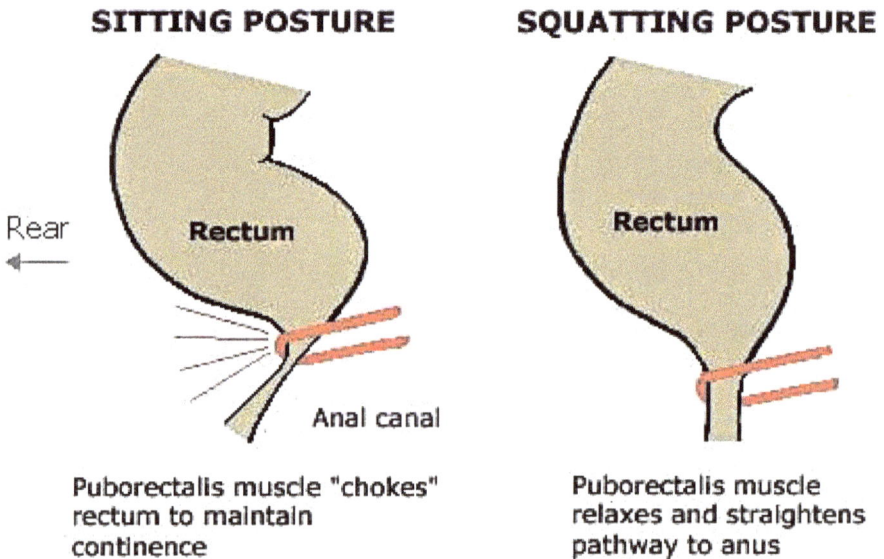

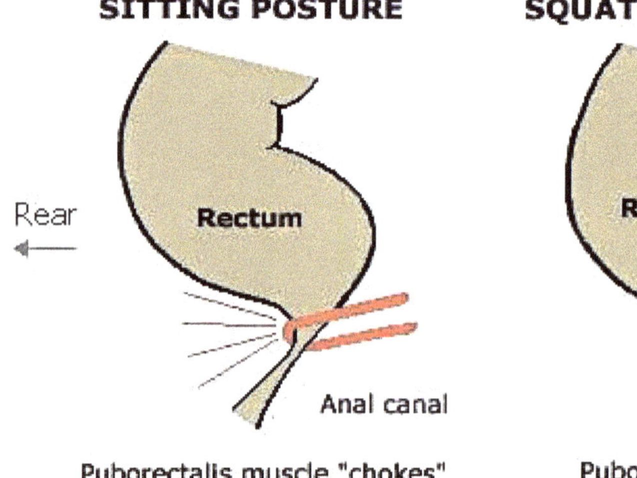

The external anal sphincter is a voluntary muscle, doubling the pressure in the anal canal during contraction. The rectoanal inhibitory reflex is an involuntary internal anal sphincter relaxation in response to rectal distention. This allows a sampling of some of the rectal contents to descend into the anal canal. Here it is brought into contact with specialized sensory mucosa to detect consistency. The rectoanal excitatory reflex is an initial semi-voluntary contraction of the external anal sphincter and puborectalis, which returns tone following the rectoanal inhibitory reflex.

Other factors include the specialized anti-peristaltic function of the last part of the sigmoid colon, the sensory ability of the lining of the rectum and the anal canal to detect the consistency and quantity of stool when present, and the normal rectoanal reflexes and defecation cycle that completes evacuation. Humans can defecate in a number of different postures. The two most common are the squatting posture and the sitting posture. The squatting posture is used for squat toilets and is also commonly used for defecation in the absence of toilets or other devices. It is commonly used in non-Western cultures. The sitting defecation posture is used in Western toilets with either a leaning forward posture or a ninety-degree sitting upright posture. The posture chosen appears to be largely a cultural decision although there is evidence that the squatting posture is more efficacious and induces the least bodily strain.

The sitting position can cause the defecating human being to repeat the Valsalva maneuver (see page 432) many times and with great force. This can lead to diverticulosis, hemorrhoids, hernias, and cardiovascular stress with defecation syncope. For those with underlying cardiac disease the additional stress induced by defecating in the sitting position as opposed to the more natural squatting position may be surprisingly life threatening. The magnitude of straining during sitting defecation is at least three times greater than with the squatting posture. Difficulty with the seated position is particularly true if the feet cannot reach the floor, as is commonly seen when small children are placed on adult height toilets. The adults may become frustrated that it is taking the child so long to defecate, not realizing that without being able to brace their feet and apply resistance that an individual is unable to generate the intra-abdominal pressure needed to promote defecation.

The affectionate term 'potty' is often used with children especially during toilet training. The term potty is also used to describe the child-size chamber pot type toilets that are at the appropriate height with a child-size seat. When a child sits on an adult-size toilet seat they may have a genuine fear of falling in, which can inhibit having a bowel movement. Regular adult toilets, which have an opening that is normally too large and frightening for a child, may be used if a child seat adapter is provided. To put in perspective that their fear is not unjustified American adults suffer forty thousand toilet related injuries per year. Falling off a toilet directly contributed to the death of King George II of Great Britain. Because the height of the adult toilet does not allow their feet to touch the ground, a foot stool can be a great help. This gives their feet a place to rest and to assume the squatting posture. This eases the initiation of a bowel movement and can accelerate toilet training.

Bowel Sound

Bowel sounds, also known as abdominal sounds, if audible at a distance by the unaided ear are known by the onomatopoeia borborygmi. Onomatopoeia is a word created to imitate the sound it is meant to describe. Bowel sounds may also have a bubbling, gurgling, rushing fluid sound and are generated by the peristaltic movement of the contents along the gastrointestinal tract.

Most bowel sounds are usually audible only by placing the listening ear on the abdominal wall or with the aid of a stethoscope. The presence of bowel sounds indicates that peristaltic activity is occurring. Changes in the bowel sounds, such as hyperactivity or absence may be indicative of a gastrointestinal disorder such as bowel obstruction or ileus. The return of bowel sounds after anesthesia are commonly required before food or drink is reintroduced.

Brain Fart

Brain fart is the popular phrase for a mental lapse, which usually results in an error while doing a repetitive activity. The actual physiological event that triggers the error has been recorded on brain scans by scientists approximately thirty seconds before the event was observed by the patient. The scientists suspect that the brain is trying to enter a more restful state to conserve energy, and have given the brain fart the more scientific name of 'maladaptive brain activity change'. The findings were published in the *Proceedings of the National Academy of Sciences* in April 2008. Brain fart may also be used to describe a brief episode of absent-mindedness, impulsivity, or temporary inability to recall a name, word, or memory. Interestingly enough, the exact opposite of a brain fart is best described by an unusual word in the English Language, afflatus.

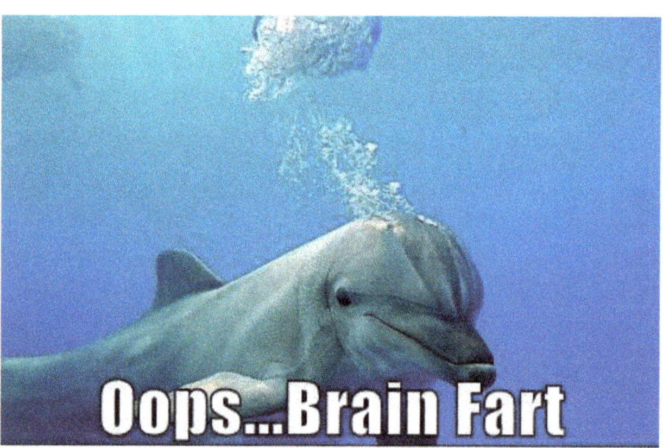

www.flickr.com/photos/ Creative Commons License

Afflatus incorporates the root word flatus, which is a commonly used as a synonym for fart. Perhaps surprisingly the definition of the word afflatus has nothing to do with a fart. Flatus is Latin for a blowing, breathing, or a wind. Afflatus is first used by Cicero in his volume *De Natura Deorum (The Nature of the Gods)*. In his book, it is used as a phrase for a sudden rush of unexpected breath or fresh inspiration. The word inspiration is derived from the term inspire, to breath as well as to have a creative thought or new idea. Afflatus thus can mean a divine inspiration. The only way to properly associate the word afflatus with a fart is to consider it to be the exact opposite of a brain fart.

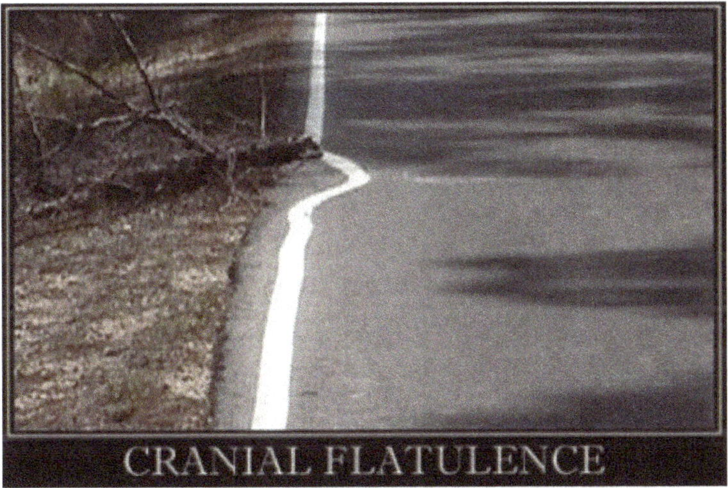

Bubble (see Nitrogenation, Surface Tension, Simethicone)

A bubble is a collection of gas, usually surrounded by a thin layer of fluid. The term gastric bubble is also used to describe the normal collection of gas within the stomach, and can be visualized on an abdominal radiograph (x-ray). Bubbles of gas within the digestive tract are called a burp or belch on eructation via the esophagus, or a fart or flatus on being passed out of the lower intestinal. The actual physical properties of a bubble are due to a physical property known as surface tension. This is also visually demonstrated in watching a water glider walk across water, in water forming droplets, the tears of wine in a wineglass, the water bulging without spilling above the brim of a glass, and other physical phenomena. Please see the entry on surface tension for more details.

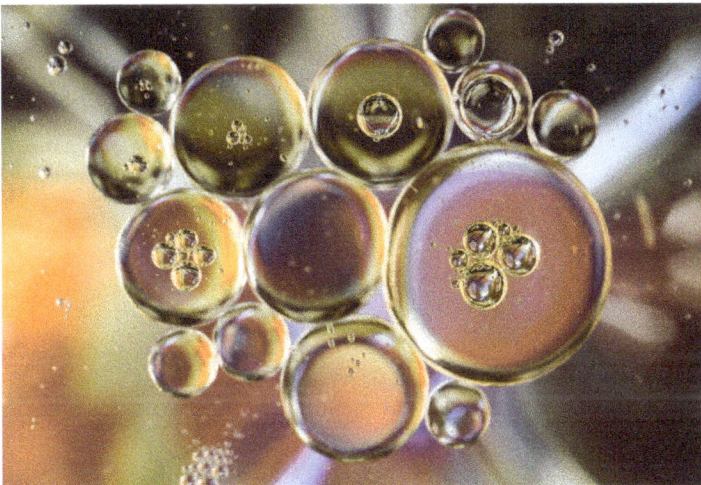

Bubbles created by surface tension. Shutterstock/GiulianoDelMoretto

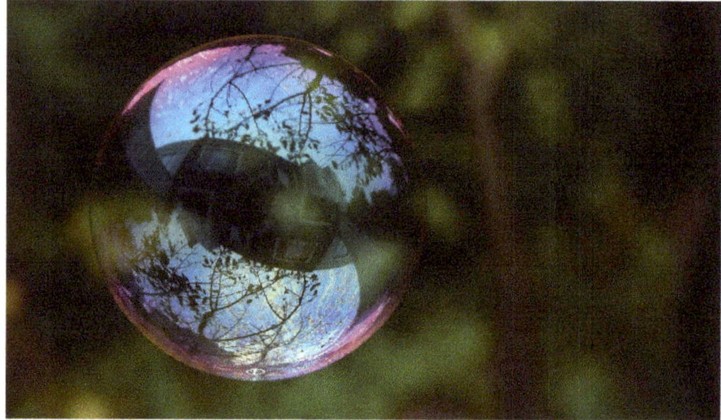
Bubble. Brocken Inaglory editing user:Alvesgaspar Creative Commons License

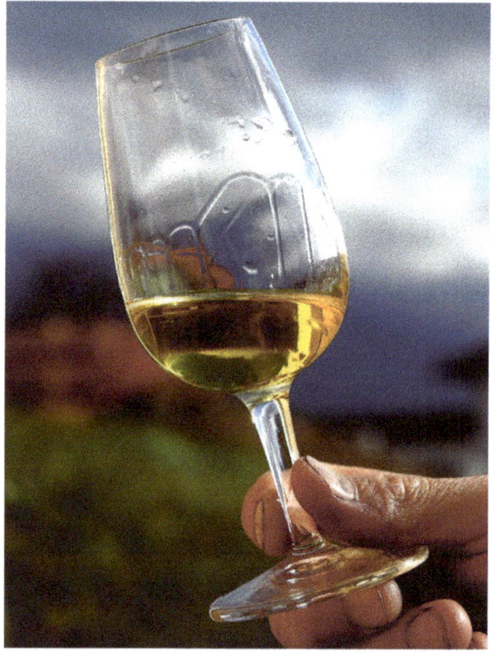
Tears of wine, also known as Marangoni effect. Shutterstock/mountainpix

Burp / Belch (see Eructation, Gastroesophageal Reflux Disease)

The words burp and belch are the common terms used to describe the more scientific term eructation. Please see the entry on eructation as well as Gastroesophageal Reflux Disease (GERD) for more details about this common physiological event that. Other interesting word pairs of the common words with the less commonly known scientific terminology include chew for mastication, sneeze for sternutation, cough for tusis, pee for micturition, itch for pruritis, skin for integument, smell for olfaction, taste for gustation, and many others that fill a medical dictionary. When the medical rather than the common terms are used by the health care provider, proper communication may require a dictionary to translate the foreign language of medicine.

If a doctor wanted to know if you chewed your food well he might ask if you masticated a lot with every meal. Most people would respond incredulously "Masticate a lot with every meal? Are you crazy, do you think I want to go blind. I never masticate!". Medicine and English are virtually two separate and foreign languages. You need to insist that your doctor speak to you in a language you can understand. There is a famous quotation attributed to Sir Winston Churchill, a British statesmen, former Prime Minister, and Nobel Laureate for Literature. He said affectionately that the American and British people are divided only by a common language.

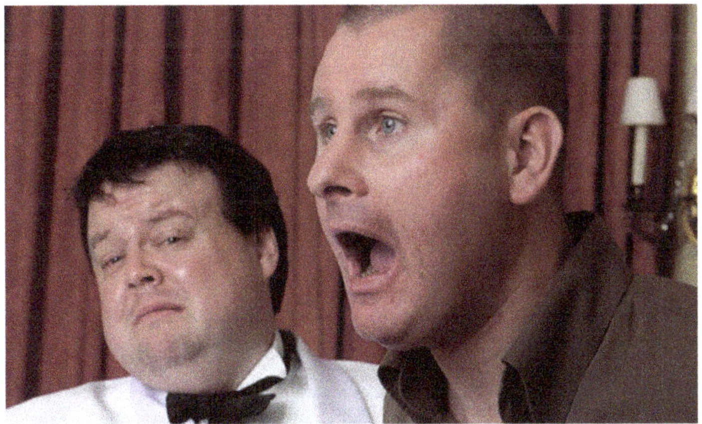

Loudest burp at 109.9 decibels youtu.be/Zt9rvaijpPY

The World Burping Federation located in Geneva Switzerland holds the annual World Burping Championship. The *Guinness Book of World Records* has a listing for the loudest burp on record. The record holder is Paul Hunn of the United Kingdom. His burp achieved a measurement of just under one-hundred and ten decibels, equivalent to a car horn. The world record for the longest burp is over eighteen seconds, held by Tim Janus. To achieve this record, he consumed approximately two gallons of Diet Coke and Mountain Dew. Imagine what would have happened if he swallowed a few Mentos tablets at the time of the competition (see photograph on page 33).

Butt Breathe

To butt breathe is a common term used to describe the ability to air fart. An air fart is the ability to control the anus and muscles of abdomen and respiration, to cause air to be aspirated into the colon and then released voluntarily as a fart. It is also known in more enlightened society as an air enema. The air enema has been practiced for hundreds of generations as an advanced yoga practice and as a means of achieving colonic hygiene.

Although usually considered under involuntary control, these muscles can be trained. Yogis have attained remarkable proficiency at controlling what has previously been considered involuntary muscles. At the turn of the twentieth century, the performer Joseph Pujol, under the stage name Le Pétomane, became an international sensation by demonstrating his prowess at butt breathing. This ability is not limited to trained yogi and stage performers. An internet-based survey on farting performed in 2001, had over one thousand three hundred participants. Although not a scientifically validated survey, over fifteen percent of respondents reported that they were able to fart on command.

Fart survey question for men: Can you fart on command also called "Butt Breathe"?

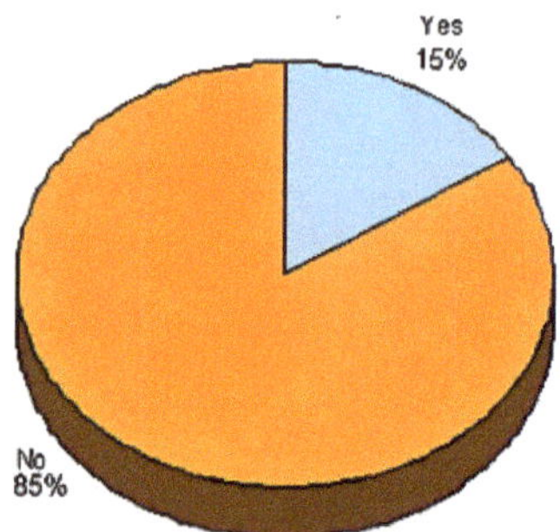

Only fifteen percent of the men surveyed can fart voluntarily by suctioning air into the colon. One-third of all men did not even know that this is possible!

Fart survey question for women: Can you fart on command also called "Butt Breathe"?

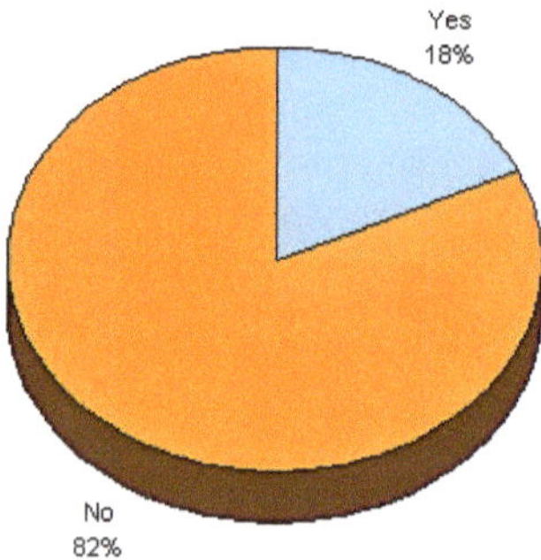

Only eighteen percent of the women surveyed can fart voluntarily by suctioning air into the colon.

Although rarely thought of as a form of butt breathe, the rare freshwater Fitzroy river turtle, *Rheodytes leukops*, found in Queensland, Australia has a unique ability. This species of turtle can breathe through its anus equivalent, the cloaca. It inspires air or, if submerged, oxygenated water into its cloaca. Through specialized highly vascular bursae it can absorb oxygen into its bloodstream. The Fitzroy turtle can obtain over two-thirds of its oxygen supply through the cloacal bursae. It pumps water in and out of the cloaca up to sixty times per minute.

Some turtles have a remarkable anaerobic capacity and can be without oxygen for up to thirty-three hours and survive. Although they are usually air breathing, they can also breathe underwater with the cloacal bursae acting like the equivalent of gills in removing oxygen from the water. This rare ability is shared with only a few other organisms, including the dragonfly nymph and the sea cucumber.

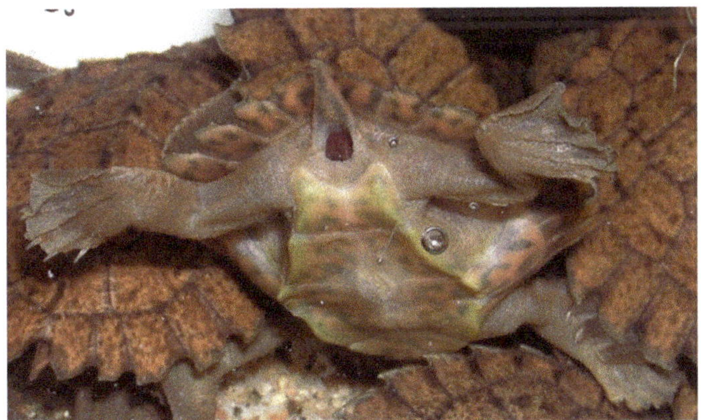

Photo by Craig Latta, freshwater turtle expert. www.tutles.net.au Used with permission.

The sea cucumber has a few other unique digestive tract features. Its anus serves as a defense mechanism and can eject sticky threads that entangle an enemy. If in danger it will expel its entire digestive and respiratory tracks that are also sticky and can ensnarl the enemy. These disgorged internal organs continue to move about independently, distracting the predator while the sea cucumber makes its escape. It then regenerates brand new respiratory and digestive tracks.

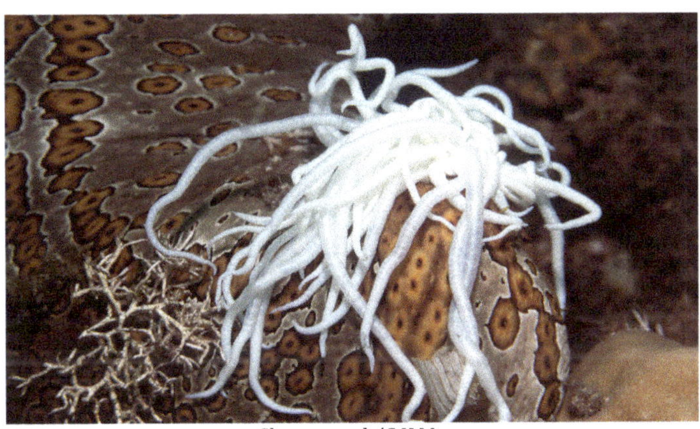

Shutterstock/C.K.Ma

Carbohydrate

A carbohydrate is an organic compound of carbon, hydrogen, and oxygen. The term is synonymous with saccharide (Greek σάκχαρον (sákkharon) "sugar". The carbohydrates are divided into monosaccharides, disaccharides, oligosaccharides, and polysaccharides. The smaller monosaccharides and disaccharides are commonly referred to as sugars ending with the suffix -ose, such as the monosaccharide glucose, the disaccharides sucrose and lactose.

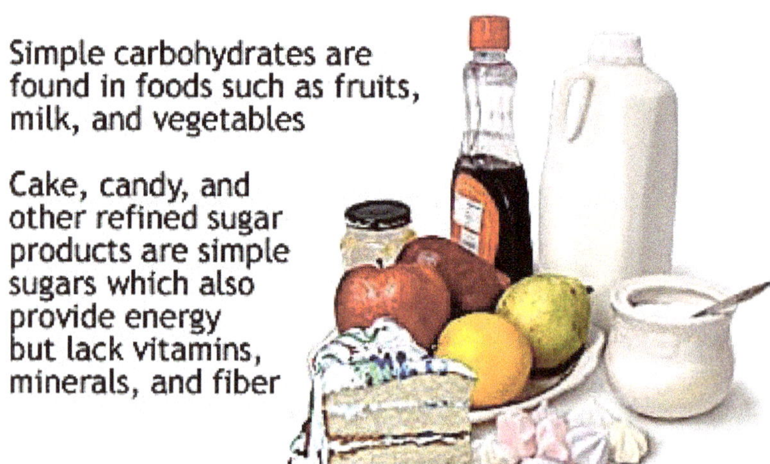

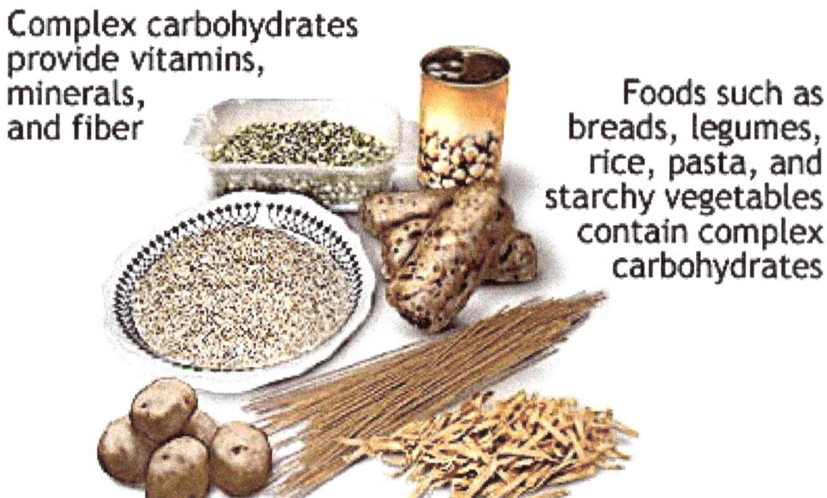
Complex carbohydrates provide vitamins, minerals, and fiber
Foods such as breads, legumes, rice, pasta, and starchy vegetables contain complex carbohydrates

Polysaccharides store linked chains of the simple sugars in the form of glycogen or starch, or as structural components such as cellulose in plants and chitin in arthropods. The monosaccharide ribose is important in coenzymes, and in the molecules of RNA and DNA dealing with protein synthesis and genetics.

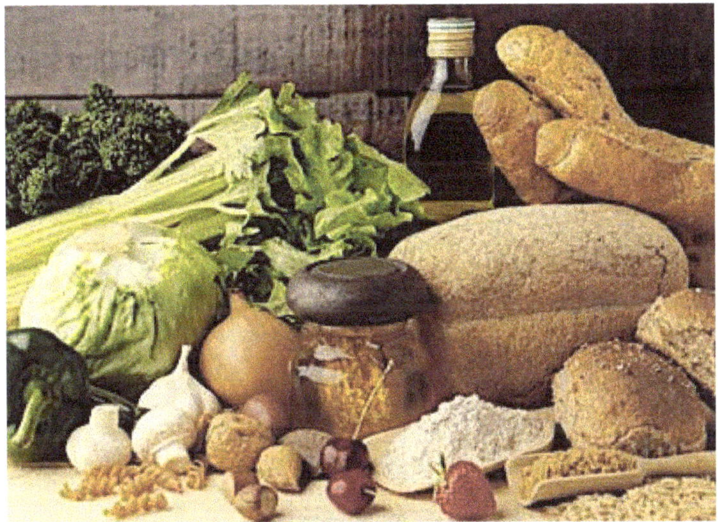

Carbohydrates. www.articlesweb.org Used with permission

Monosaccharides such as glucose are the major source of fuel for metabolism. The two joined monosaccharides of a disaccharide can be released by specific enzymes such as sucrase for sucrose and lactase for lactose. Foods high in carbohydrates include fruits, breads, pastas, beans, potatoes, bran, rice, and cereals. Carbohydrates are not essential for humans as the body can obtain all its energy from protein and fats. The brain and neurons generally use glucose or ketones as an energy source.

<u>Monosaccharides</u>

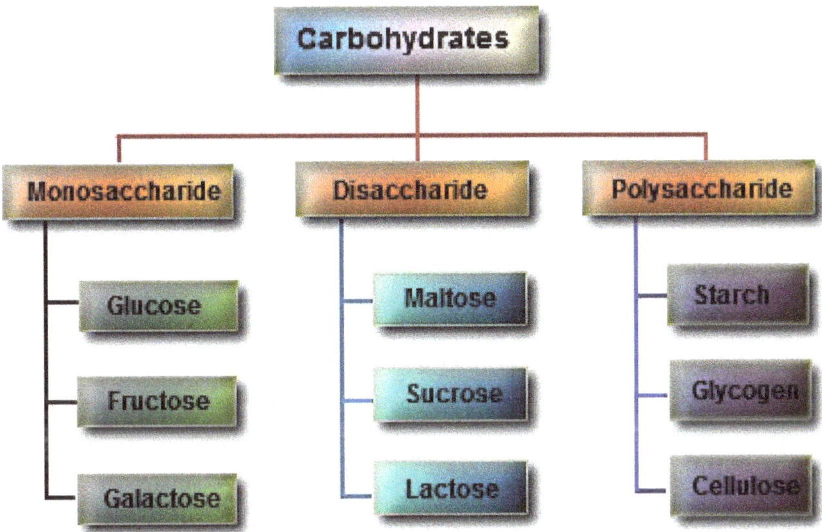

Monosaccharides (Greek monos-single, sacchar-sugar) are simple sugar carbohydrates that are water-soluble crystalline solids, a number of which have a sweet taste. Examples include glucose (dextrose), fructose (levulose), galactose, xylose, and ribose. Monosaccharides are the building blocks of disaccharides (such as sucrose) and polysaccharides (such as cellulose and starch). Monosaccharides can be classified by the number x of carbon atoms they contain: diose (2) triose (3) tetrose (4), pentose (5), hexose (6), heptose (7), and so on. The most important monosaccharide, glucose, is a hexose.

There are a number of isomeric forms all with the same chemical formula. Most stereoisomers are chiral and therefore distinct from their mirror images. Those that rotate the direction of linearly polarized light to the right are called D dextrorotatory (rotates the polarization axis clockwise) and to the left called L is levorotatory (rotates it counterclockwise) or sys for sinister.

The Latin words dexter means right sided and laevus means on the left. Another Latin word sinister, also means on the left-hand side and in ancient times left handedness was considered a sinister (negative) characteristic. Mirror-image isomers usually have very different biochemical properties and occurrences in nature.

<u>Disaccharides</u>

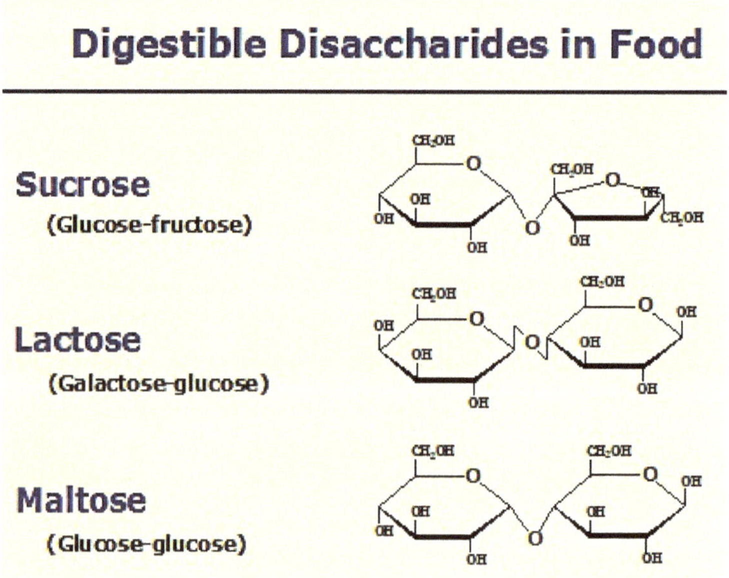

A disaccharide is the carbohydrate formed when two monosaccharides undergo a dehydration reaction and a molecule of water is removed and a glycosidic bond is formed. Like monosaccharides, disaccharides form an aqueous solution when dissolved in water. Three common examples are sucrose, lactose, and maltose. 'Disaccharide' is one of the four chemical groupings of carbohydrates (monosaccharide, disaccharide, oligosaccharide, and polysaccharide). Depending on the monosaccharide components a disaccharide may be crystalline, water-soluble, sweet and/or sticky.

Disaccharide
Sucrose: Glucose & Fructose
Lactulose: Galactose & Fructose
Lactose: Galactose & Glucose
Maltose: Glucose & Glucose, maltose is a hydrolysis product from starch
Trehalose: Glucose & Glucose
Cellobiose: Glucose & Glucose, cellobiose is a hydrolysis product of cellulose

<u>Oligosaccharide</u>

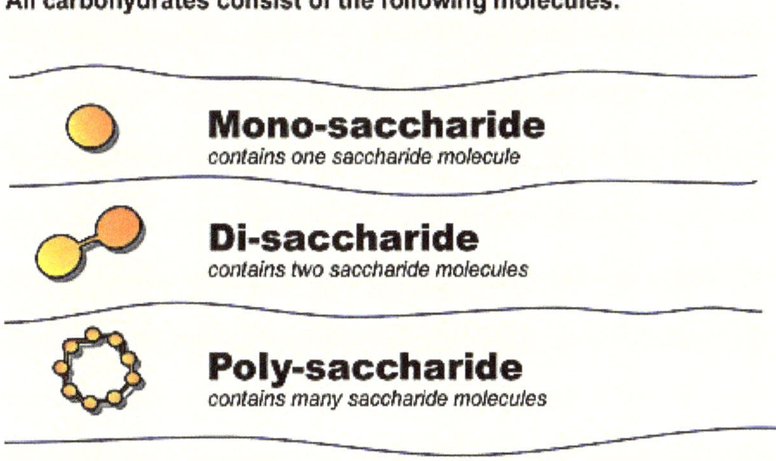

Oligosaccharides are carbohydrates composed of between two and ten monosaccharides joined by glycosidic linkage which can be hydrolyzed by acid to release the monosaccharide units. Some examples include maltose, sucrose, and lactose. An oligosaccharide (Greek oligos -few, and sacchar -sugar) is a saccharide containing two to ten monosaccharides. Oligosaccharides are a frequent component of glycoproteins and glycolipids and are often used as chemical markers for cell recognition. An example is ABO blood type markers where the A and B blood types have two different oligosaccharide glycolipids in the cell membranes of the red blood cells, the AB-type blood has both, while the O blood type has neither.

Fructo-oligosaccharides are also found in many vegetables and consist of short chains of fructose molecules. Naturally occurring galacto-oligosaccharides consist of short chains of galactose molecules. These compounds can only be partially digested by humans with microbial fermentation processing the residue. Mannan oligosaccharides are used in animal feed to improve digestive health, energy levels and performance. They differ from other oligosaccharides in that they are not fermentable. Other undigested oligosaccharides are fermented by the intestinal microflora and depending on the type of oligosaccharide, different microbial groups may be stimulated or suppressed. Clinical studies have shown that administering fructo-oligosaccharides, galacto-oligosaccharides, or inulin enhances the populations of symbiotic microorganisms and suppresses the populations of pathogens.

Fructo-oligosaccharides and inulin are found naturally in Jerusalem artichoke, burdock, chicory, leeks, onions, and asparagus. Fructo-oligosaccharides products derived from chicory root contain significant amounts of the polysaccharide inulin, a fiber frequently found in fruits, vegetables and other plants. Fructo-oligosaccharides can also be commercially synthesized by enzymes of the fungus *Aspergillus niger* acting on sucrose. Galacto-oligosaccharides is naturally found in soybeans and can also be synthesized from lactose. Fructo-oligosaccharides, galacto-oligosaccharides, and the polysaccharide inulin are commercially available as nutritional supplements in capsules, tablets, and as a powder.

Besides being components of glycoproteins or glycolipids some oligosaccharides, such as the raffinose family, act as storage or transport carbohydrates. Other oligosaccharides such as maltodextrins or cellodextrins, are the result of the microbial breakdown of larger polysaccharides such as starch or cellulose. Carrots can be an excellent source of oligosaccharides but this occurs only after they have been cooked for an hour as the starches need to be broken down into the shorter chains needed for bioavailability.

<u>Polysaccharides</u>

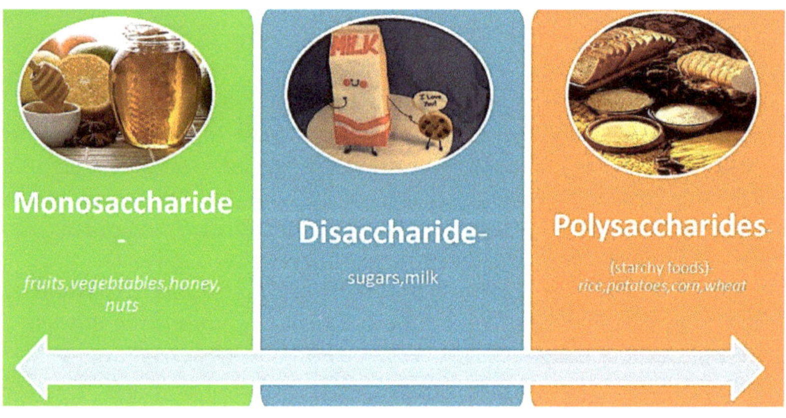

Polysaccharides are polymers containing ten or more monosaccharide residues. Two common examples are cellulose the main component of the cell wall in plants, and starch, a word derived from the Anglo-Saxon stercan, meaning to stiffen. For a polysaccharide composed of a single type of monosaccharide the ending "-ose" of the monosaccharide is replaced with "-an". For example, a polymer of glucose is named glucan, a polymer of mannose is named mannan, and a polymer of galactose is named galactan. Inulin has the capacity for a much higher degree of polymerization than fructo-oligosaccharides and is categorized as a polysaccharide. It is frequently found in fruits and vegetables and is a significant source of nutrition worldwide.

Polysaccharides are sources of energy for organisms that can convert starches into glucose, however most cannot metabolize cellulose. Ruminants and termites use bacteria and protist to process cellulose. Although not digestible, dietary fiber plays a major role in digestive health by acting as a prebiotic for the gut microbiome.

Carbohydrate Digestion

The digestion of carbohydrates, which are broken down into monosaccharides like glucose, begins in the mouth with the enzyme amylase found in saliva. The pancreatic enzymes and brush border enzymes of the small intestine continue the breakdown of the various carbohydrates into monosaccharides in the lumen of the bowel. These enzymes include lactase, maltase, sucrase, dextrinase and glucoamylase. The monosaccharides are then absorbed across the mucosal surface by intestinal epithelial cell facilitated cotransport with sodium ions and facilitated diffusion. They enter the capillary bed of the villi and are then transported to the liver via the hepatic portal vein.

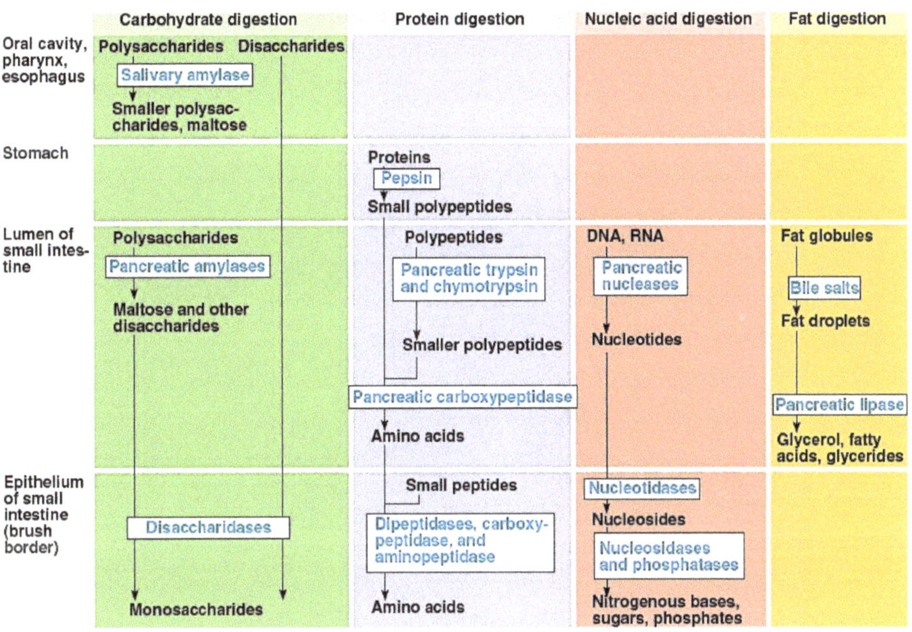

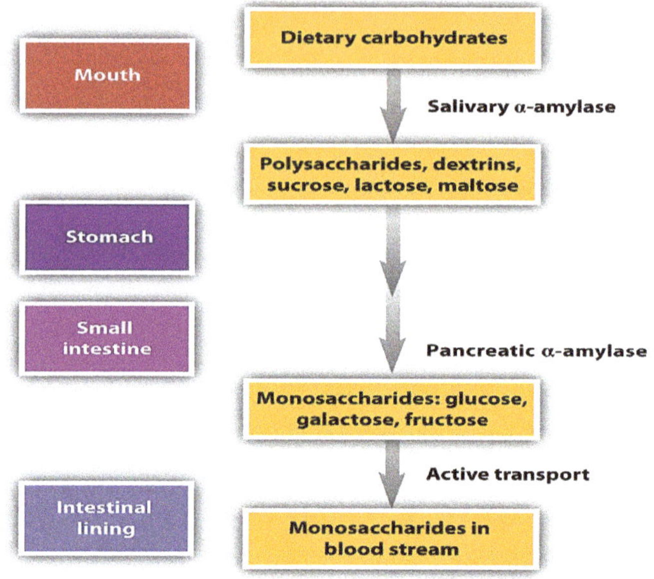

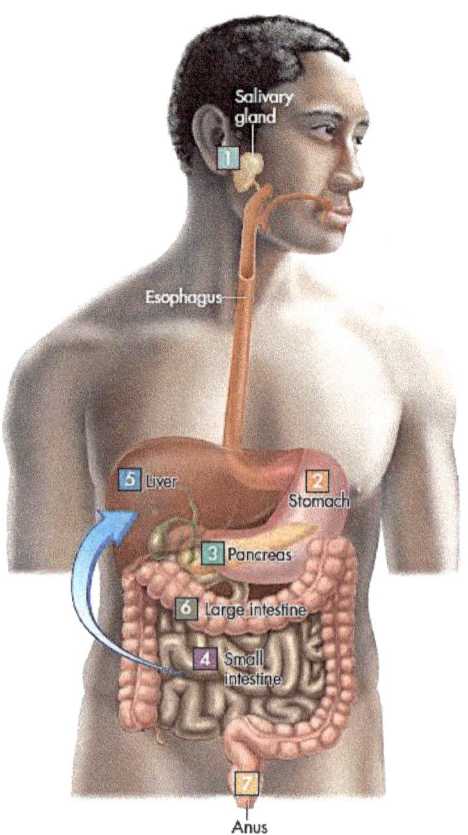

Carbohydrates

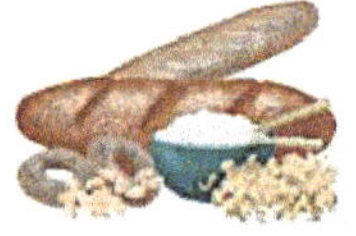

1. Some starch is broken down to maltose in the mouth by salivary amylase.
2. Salivary amylase is inactivated by strong acid in the stomach.
3. Pancreatic amylase breaks down starch into maltose in the small intestine.
4. Enzymes in the wall of the small intestine break down the disaccharides sucrose, lactose, and maltose into monosaccharides glucose, fructose, and galactose.
5. Glucose, fructose, and galactose are absorbed into blood to be taken to the liver by a portal vein.
6. Some soluble fiber is fermented into various acids and gases by bacteria in the large intestine.
7. Insoluble fiber escapes digestion and is excreted in feces, but little other dietary carbohydrate is present.

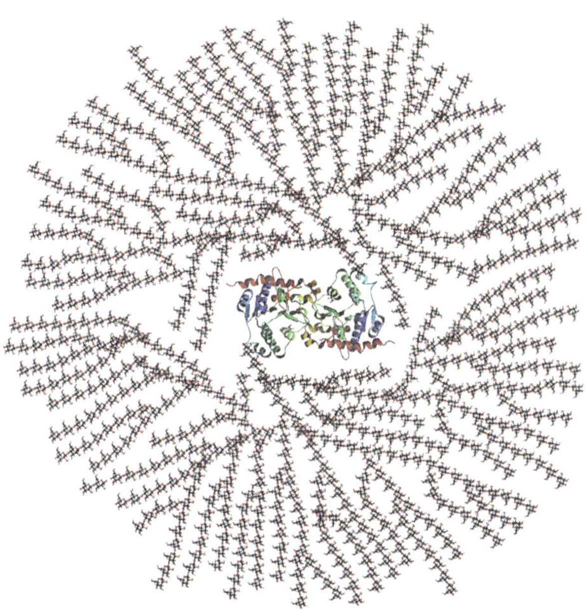

2-D cross-sectional view of glycogen: A core protein of glycogenin is surrounded by branches of glucose units. The entire globular complex may contain approximately thirty thousand glucose units. 2009 Author: Mikael Häggström Public Domain

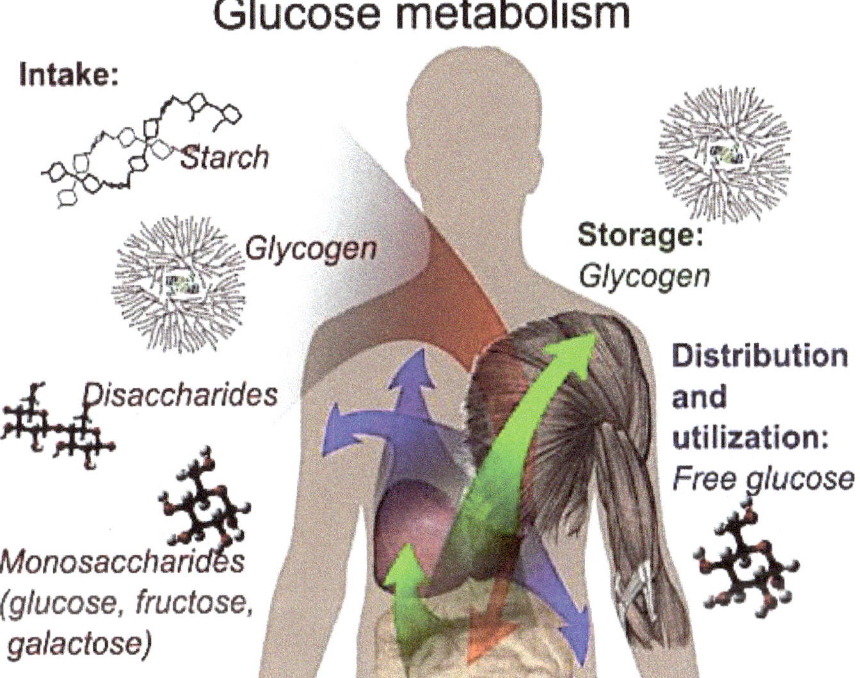

Glycogen is a polysaccharide of glucose that serves as a major form of energy storage in humans, animals, and fungi. This polysaccharide structure is the most important storage form of glucose in the body. In humans the liver and muscle are the main locations in which glycogen is made and stored. It functions as the secondary form of long-term energy storage. The primary form of energy stores are the fats held in adipose tissue. Muscle glycogen can be converted into glucose for use by the muscle cells. Liver glycogen can be converted to glucose for use throughout the body including the central nervous system.

Glycogen serves a function similar to the starch of plants. The glycogen polymer is much more extensively branched than starch allowing it to store energy in a more compact form. Glycogen is found in the form of granules in the cytoplasm of many cell types and forms an energy reserve that can be quickly mobilized to meet a sudden need for glucose. After a meal up to eight percent of the total weight of the liver cells may be composed of glycogen stores. The glycogen stored in the liver is accessible as an energy source to other organs, and for most organs is its only source of energy. An exception is muscle, which has its own limited stores of glycogen found in a lower concentration of one to two percent of the muscle mass. The muscle tissue of the uterus also stores glycogen during pregnancy to nourish the embryo.

During a meal containing carbohydrates, as the food is eaten and digested, the blood glucose levels rise. In response to the rising blood glucose levels the pancreas secretes insulin. Blood glucose from the portal vein enters the liver cells called hepatocytes. Insulin acts on the liver cells to stimulate the action of several enzymes including the key enzyme in glycogen production, glycogen synthetase. Under the influence of glycogen synthetase glucose molecules are continuously added to the chains of glycogen for storage as long as both insulin and glucose remain plentiful. In the postprandial (after meal) or fed state the liver takes in more glucose from the blood than it releases and stores the excess as glycogen.

Once a meal has been fully digested and absorbed the glucose levels begin to fall back to normal. With blood glucose returning to normal the insulin secretion is reduced and glycogen synthesis stops. When energy is required the stored glycogen is broken down and converted back to glucose. The glucose is released into the blood stream for the energy needs of other organs and cells. Glycogen phosphorylase is the primary enzyme of glycogen breakdown. For the next eight to twelve hours, glucose derived from liver glycogen is the primary source of blood glucose used by the rest of the body for fuel.

Glucagon is another hormone involved in glucose metabolism and is also produced by the pancreas. It serves as an opposite and balancing hormone to insulin. When blood levels of glucose begin to fall below the normal range the pancreas secretes glucagon in increasing amounts. Glucagon stimulates both glycogenolysis (the breakdown of glycogen), as well as gluconeogenesis (the generation of glucose from non-carbohydrates such as fatty acids). The glycogen stored in muscle cells functions as an immediate reserve source of available glucose. Muscle cells lack the enzyme glucose-6-phosphatase which is required to release glucose into the blood. As such the glycogen they store is only available for internal use by the muscle cells themselves, and cannot be shared with other cells.

Carbonation (see Nitrogenation)

Carbonated beverages are very popular worldwide. In the United States sales of carbonated beverages exceed twenty billion dollars per year, four times the sales volume of dairy products. The majority consumed today already comes carbonated with large amounts of carbon dioxide forced into solution under high pressure. As the pressure seal of the can or bottle is released the carbon dioxide forms bubbles and comes out of the solution, giving a pleasant tickling sensation on the palate, and a full at times bloated feeling in the stomach and gut.

Many soft drinks have high concentrations of simple carbohydrates such as glucose, fructose, and sucrose. Oral bacteria ferment these carbohydrates and produce acidic products, which can erode the tooth enamel beginning the dental decay process. A large number of soft drinks are already acidic and have phosphoric acid added in the manufacturing process bringing their pH level to three or lower. To put this value in perspective, neutral water has a pH of seven and gastric hydrochloric acid has a pH of two. Many dentists advocate that one should avoid the brushing of teeth shortly after an acidic beverage because the tooth enamel is more vulnerable to abrasions after being softened by acid.

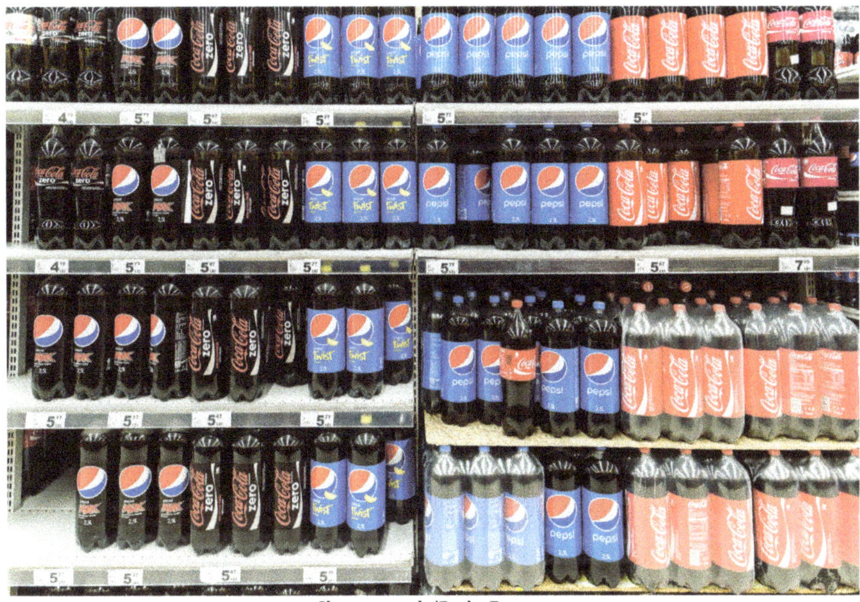

Shutterstock/Radu Bercan

Mineral water cures were very popular in the middle ages and beyond. Going to the source of mineral springs and the drinking of its contents was referred to as 'taking the waters'. The waters had a variety of mineral content depending on source locale and included various salts and sulfur contents. The sites of such resources became well known as spas, baths, and wells and developed into destinations for the ill and infirm, as well as those who wished to preserve their good health. The term Seltzer water was originally a trademarked name for the German town of Selter that had a famous mineral spring.

The bottling of mineral waters became a profitable enterprise by offering people the opportunity to partake of the presumed beneficial waters in their own locales. An attempt to imitate the effervescent effect of the mineral waters was made by Joseph Priestley in 1767. Some fans of carbonated beverages believe this should be his claim to fame rather than his discovery of oxygen. J. J. Schweppes of Switzerland commercialized the process in 1783, moving his factory and enterprise to England in 1783.

Before the commercial availability of already carbonated beverages, a device for home use was popular and remains commercially available. It uses canisters of carbon dioxide under pressure that are then added to and dissolved in the beverages to create the carbonation effect. The soda siphon bottles with the carbon dioxide cartridges are making a retro look comeback in today's higher technology environment. Carbon dioxide can diffuse through the plastic container over time, which is why carbonated beverages in plastic bottles go flat and lose their carbonation over a few month's time. Glass and aluminum containers hold the carbonation for longer time periods.

Have you ever wondered how much carbon dioxide gas is released from a soft drink or carbonated beverage. You have already gotten a visual demonstration if the bottle or can was dropped or shaken before being opened. This agitation accelerates the release of the carbon dioxide, and it can form a jet stream of gassy bubbles to be sprayed on everyone within a dozen feet of the demonstration. This social activity is very popular amongst preadolescent boys. The quantification of how much carbon dioxide is in a one liter bottle of a carbonated soft drink is calculated using a formula known as Henry's Law.

William Henry was an English physician and chemist who proposed what is now called Henry's law in 1803. The law states that at a constant temperature, the amount of a given gas dissolved in a liquid is directly proportional to the pressure of that gas. As the gas pressure increases, the solubility of the gas in the liquid increases. As the temperature increases, the solubility of gas in liquid decreases. The greater the pressure, the greater the quantity of a gas that can be absorbed by a liquid. Henry's Law explains why carbon dioxide in a pressurized container, such as in a can or bottle of a carbonated beverage remains in solution until it is opened. As soon as the container is opened the pressure is reduced causing the carbon dioxide gas to lose its solubility and escape in the form of bubbles or fizz.

The gas content in a one-liter bottle is a surprising two point eight liters. In other words, there is nearly three times the volume of the original container in excess gas under pressure hidden in those tiny bubbles. Do not forget another important law of the physics of gasses, Charles' Law. This law defines the activity of gasses expanding as the temperature increases. The cooler the liquid, the greater the amount of gas that it can absorb. As the temperature of liquid increases, the solubility of the gas decreases forming bubbles that allow it to escape. If you drink a cold carbonated beverage, and after swallowing it is warmed up to body temperature, it will exhibit another substantial increase in the volume of gasses released. The burping and belching that occurs after drinking a cold carbonated beverage may seem out of proportion to the small amount consumed. Just remember that whatever the volume of liquid carbonated beverage swallowed, there is nearly three times that volume of dissolved gas waiting to be released.

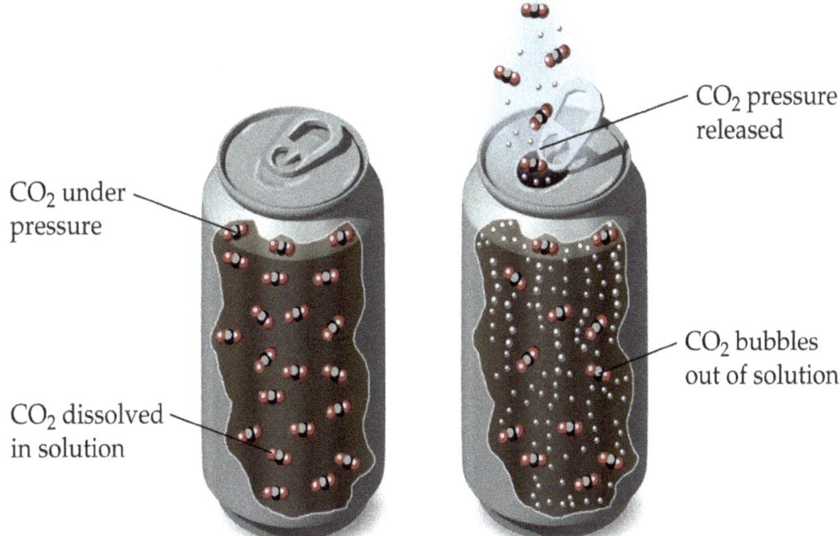

Creative Commons License

If you want further visual proof that Henry's Law is accurate take a look at the photographic evidence of another popular activity. The addition of a Mentos brand mint candy tablet to a liter bottle of a carbonated beverage, such as Diet Coke, sounds like such an innocent activity. This demonstration is repeated in countless elementary school science classes. The *Guinness Book of World Records* described one thousand three hundred and sixty students in the historic university town of Leuven, Belgium creating simultaneous Mentos with Diet Coke geysers.

The instantaneous foaming effect is a dramatic virtual geyser of carbonated foam shooting over twenty-eight feet into the air. This experiment is not without risk as the bottles will explode if not allowed to become a geyser. Scientific progress continues apace and Henry's Law was demonstrated with two thousand eight hundred and sixty-five simultaneous geysers demonstrated before a large crowd in a mall in Manila, Philippines, breaking the previous world record.

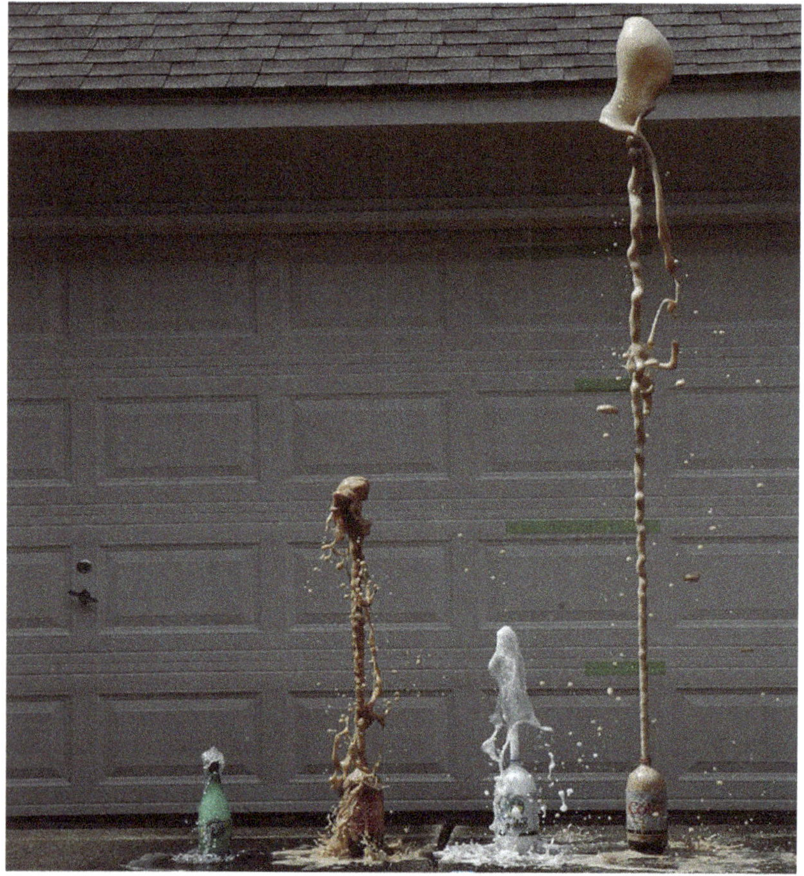

Mentos Geyser from carbonated beverages with the addition of Mentos. From left: carbonated water (Perrier), Classic Coke, Sprite and Diet Coke. The green marks in the background are at one half-meter increments. Photograph by K. Shimada Creative Commons License

Academic research physicist Tonya Coffey at Appalachian State University in Boone, North Carolina analyzed why the Diet Coke created the highest geyser. She determined that the aspartame in Diet Coke lowered the surface tension of the gas bubbles allowing the interaction between potassium benzoate with the gelatin and gum Arabic ingredients of the Mentos Mint. Surface tension is a physical property exhibited when certain liquids are in contact with a gas. It is particularly pronounced when liquid water is in contact with the gasses of the air.

Each water molecule contains two hydrogen atoms and one oxygen atom, giving rise to its familiar chemical shorthand of H_2O. Because of their atomic structure the negative charge of the electrons of the hydrogen atoms are attracted to the positive charge of the oxygen atom, creating was is known as a hydrogen bond. The electric charges also create an attractive force between water molecules, causing them to want to remain close together. These forces are balanced out when a water molecule is surrounded by other water molecules.

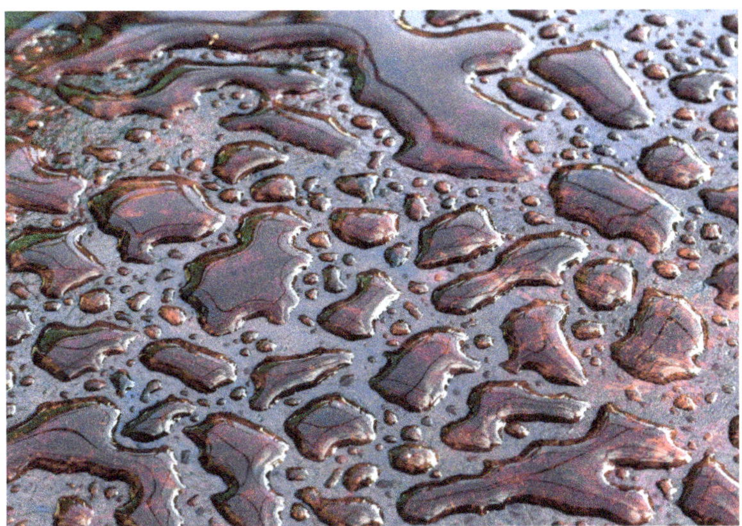

Surface tension is the physical principle, which creates islands of beaded water. Shutterstock/Kuruneko

When the water molecules on the surface are exposed to the gasses of the air above them they are no longer exposed to balanced charges. The water molecule on the surface exposed to the air is only subject to the electric charge pulling it down, keeping it in the liquid. This resistance to leaving its fellow water molecules behind gives it the property known as surface tension, a tension that prevents it from being separated from the remaining liquid. This surface tension is visible when you see water assume the shape of a droplet, or when you fill a glass to the brim and the fluid builds up above the lip of the glass before it begins to overflow.

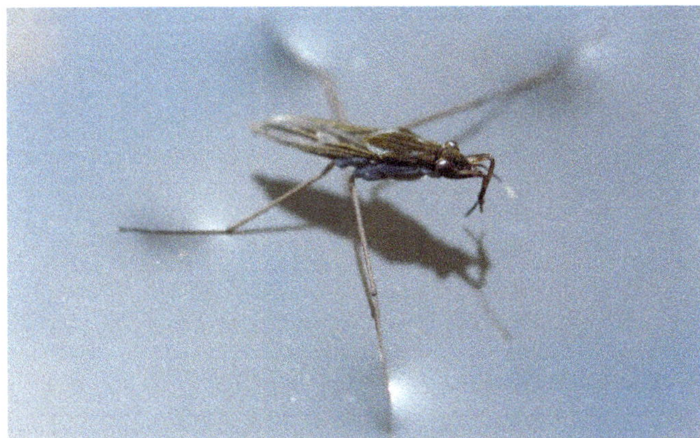

Pond skater using surface tension to walk on water Heteroptera suborder. Shutterstock/optimarc

It is also the principle that allows insects heavier than water, such as the water glider, to walk on water because the surface tension acts as a walkable surface.

Surface tension is the same force that allows the creation of bubbles. Surfactants are products that have the property of reducing surface tension and are used in detergents, as well as in anti-bubble and anti-gas products such as simethicone. Another principle of physics was also exhibited by the Mentos in Diet Coke geyser experiment. Because the mint has a microporous nature, the markedly increased surface area caused a rapid and vigorous foaming reaction. A single simple cube has a much smaller surface area for reactions to take place, than an identical volume cube that has been subdivided into many smaller cubes. The following illustration helps to visualize how the surface area can be dramatically increased with the same volume of material.

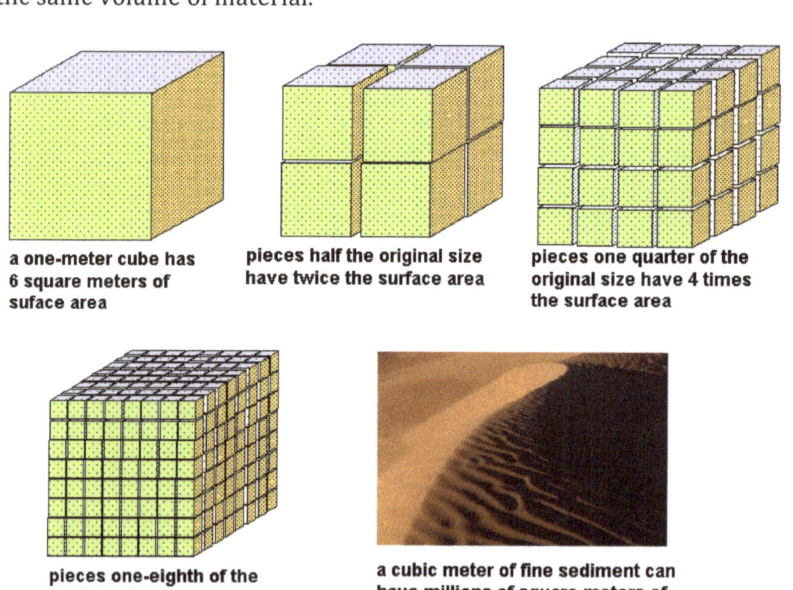

a one-meter cube has 6 square meters of suface area
pieces half the original size have twice the surface area
pieces one quarter of the original size have 4 times the surface area
pieces one-eighth of the original size have 8 times the surface area.
a cubic meter of fine sediment can have millions of square meters of surface area

Increase in surface area.. Phil Stoffer, Ph.D. Geology Cafe geologycafe.com Creative Commons License

The caffeine did not accelerate the reaction. Here is the reference for those who want to read all of the scientific details. Coffey, Tonya *"Diet Coke and Mentos: What is really behind this physical reaction?" American Journal of Physics* June 2008. 76 (6): 551–557. Competitions to see which beverage will create the highest geyser are very messy affairs that again seem to attract a disproportionate number of adolescent males in their middle years. As my spouse (who happens to be a reproductive endocrinologist, an expert on the subject) likes to remind me, there are five stages of the male life cycle: infancy, childhood, adolescence, adolescence, and adolescence!

In some beverages the carbon dioxide would interfere with the taste and flavor by reacting with the ingredients, giving it an acid taste from carbonic acid. An alternative is to use nitrogen as the gas of choice as it is a neutral gas and would not interact with the beverage. The most popular example is beer, which commonly uses nitrogen, or a combination of nitrogen and carbon dioxide, under pressure in kegs.

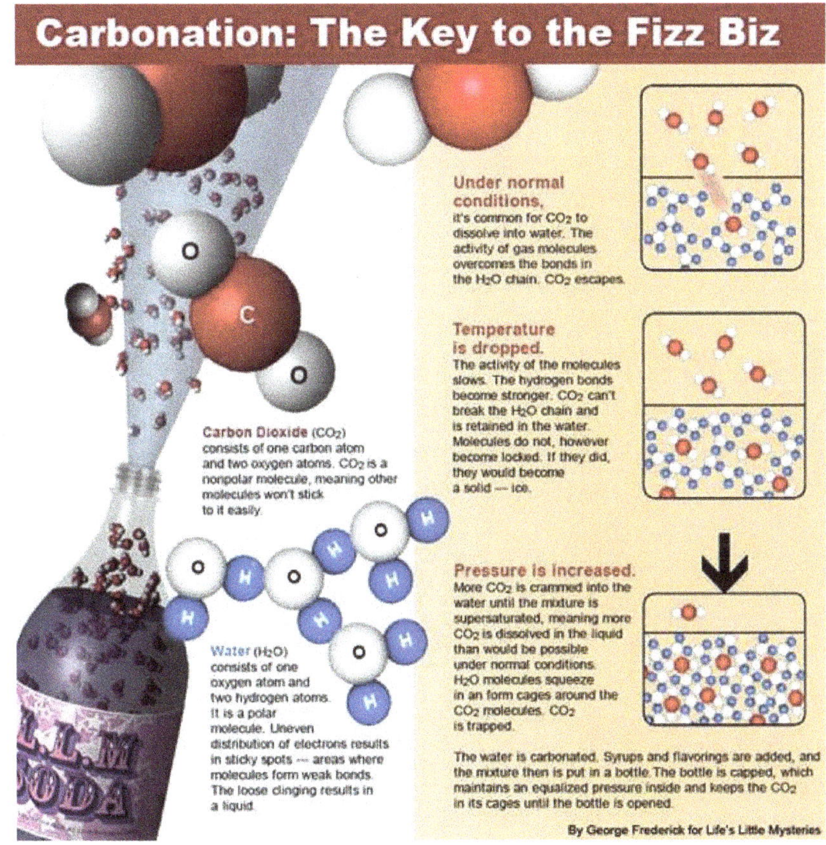
Carbonation: The Key to the Fizz Biz
Under normal conditions,
it's common for CO_2 to dissolve into water. The activity of gas molecules overcomes the bonds in the H_2O chain. CO_2 escapes.
Temperature is dropped.
The activity of the molecules slows. The hydrogen bonds become stronger. CO_2 can't break the H_2O chain and is retained in the water. Molecules do not, however become locked. If they did, they would become a solid — ice.
Carbon Dioxide (CO_2)
consists of one carbon atom and two oxygen atoms. CO_2 is a nonpolar molecule, meaning other molecules won't stick to it easily.
Pressure is increased.
More CO_2 is crammed into the water until the mixture is supersaturated, meaning more CO_2 is dissolved in the liquid than would be possible under normal conditions. H_2O molecules squeeze in an form cages around the CO_2 molecules. CO_2 is trapped.
Water (H_2O)
consists of one oxygen atom and two hydrogen atoms. It is a polar molecule. Uneven distribution of electrons results in sticky spots — areas where molecules form weak bonds. The loose clinging results in a liquid.
The water is carbonated. Syrups and flavorings are added, and the mixture then is put in a bottle. The bottle is capped, which maintains an equalized pressure inside and keeps the CO_2 in its cages until the bottle is opened.
By George Frederick for Life's Little Mysteries
i.livescience.com Creative Commons License

Carbon Dioxide (see Carbonation)

Carbon dioxide (CO_2) is a naturally occurring compound composed of two oxygen atoms bonded to a single carbon atom. It is a gas at standard temperature and pressure and exists in Earth's atmosphere as a trace gas at a concentration of 0.039 percent by volume. It is heavier than air, and when used as a fire extinguisher the dense ground-hugging layer of carbon dioxide prevents the flames from accessing oxygen.

As part of the carbon cycle, plants, algae, and cyanobacteria use light energy to photosynthesize carbohydrate from carbon dioxide and water, with oxygen produced as a waste product. However, photosynthesis cannot occur in darkness and at night some carbon dioxide is produced by plants during respiration. Carbon dioxide is exhaled in the breath of humans and land animals. It is also released from the fermentation of organic matter, volcanoes, hot springs, geysers and the combustion of hydrocarbons used as fuels. It contributes as a greenhouse gas to global warming. It is also a source of ocean acidification since it reacts with water to form carbonic acid.

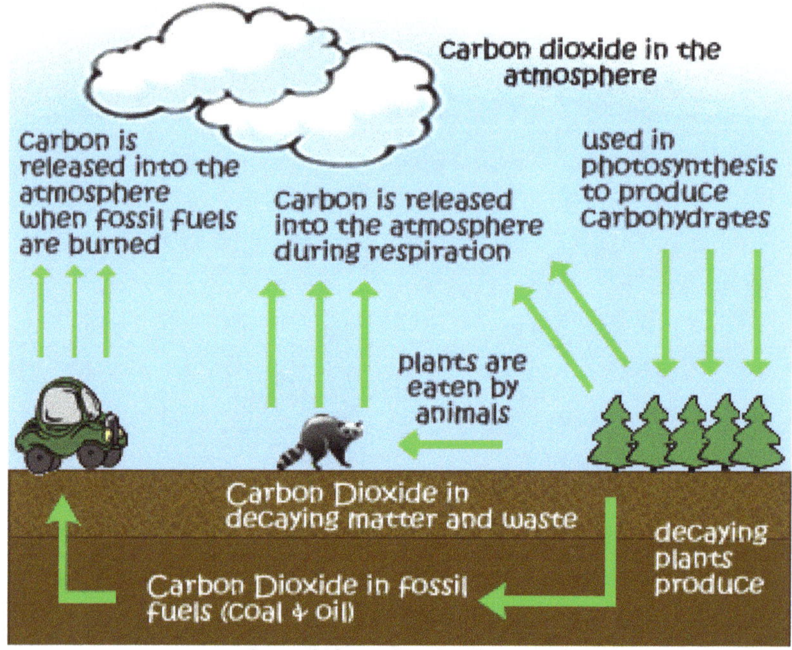

www.realtrees4kids.org Creative Commons License

A gas subsequently identified as carbon dioxide was identified by the Flemish chemist Jan Baptist van Helmont in the seventeenth century. In the 1750's Scottish physician, Joseph Black studied the gas more thoroughly. In 1772, English chemist Joseph Priestley published a paper entitled *Impregnating Water with Fixed Air*. The paper described how he forced carbon dioxide to dissolve in a bowl of agitating water, inventing what eventually became known as soda water. Soda water was the original product from which the major industry of carbonated beverages evolved.

Carbon dioxide is produced in large quantities in the digestive tract. The human stomach generates about one and one-half liters of very potent hydrochloric acid. With a pH of 1.5 it can make quick work of dissolving metal coins. The stomach lining is designed to handle the intense acidity, as well as the potent digestive enzymes released as zymogens and then activated as enzymes. The lining of the stomach is under constant attack and constant repair.

In fact, the turnover is so high that your entire stomach lining has been regenerated over the course of any three-day period. The gastric contents of food, acid, and enzymes transits through the pyloric channel and enters the duodenum. As it enters the duodenum it is in a brand new environment, and the digestive material is now known as chime. The material leaving the stomach requires prompt action from the duodenum to neutralize its high acid content. The duodenum neutralizes the acid by releasing sodium bicarbonate from its mucosal lining. It also receives a solution of pancreatic juices with a high concentration of alkaline sodium bicarbonate. The one and one-half liters of stomach acid is neutralized by one and one-half liters of sodium bicarbonate.

Do you remember from basic chemistry lessons what happens when you add an acid to an alkaline base? Did you ever perform or watch the school experiment of mixing baking soda (sodium bicarbonate) and vinegar (weak acetic acid) to create a fire extinguisher? In the demonstration a lit candle is placed on the bottom of a glass container. In a different glass pitcher the mixture of baking soda and vinegar were reacting with an impressive display of foaming and bubbling. They were reacting as expected from the mixing of an acid and a base, generating carbon dioxide as a free gas and neutral water.

Carbon dioxide is heavier than air so although it was invisible the rising level of carbon dioxide in the glass container was pushing the lighter air out and over the top. After just minutes of bubbling, the pitcher that was now full of heavier carbon dioxide was tilted over the glass containing the lit candle. Although it appeared that the tilted pitcher was not adding anything to the glass with the candle, the heavier but invisible carbon dioxide was pouring out of the pitcher and was now displacing the air around the candle with carbon dioxide. As soon as the invisible carbon dioxide reached the level of the flame the supply of oxygen was cut off, and the candle flame went out like magic.

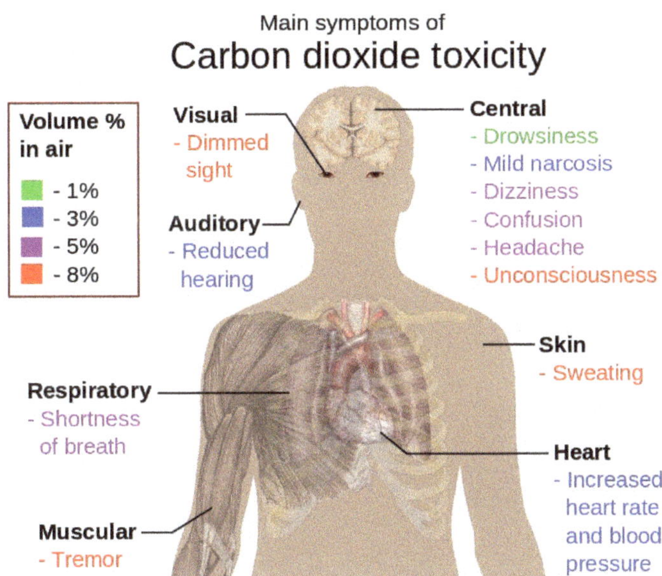

Main symptoms of carbon dioxide toxicity. Wikipedia. Mikael Häggström Creative Commons License

By the way there is another interesting fact about carbon dioxide and human respiration. It is the level of carbon dioxide in your blood, not the level of oxygen, that drives the respiratory center that controls breathing. The sensation of air hunger that arises when one is short of breath or suffocating is from carbon dioxide buildup, not from a lack of oxygen. That is why the trick of making your voice squeaky by breathing helium is actually very dangerous. If you breathe in and out pure helium your body continues to get rid of its carbon dioxide with each breath. It fools the body into thinking that everything is just fine, even though it is not obtaining any oxygen. The person breathing pure helium does not experience air hunger or suffocation because that sensation is only triggered by carbon dioxide which continues to be exhaled. Death occurs quickly and without warning, and because there is no sensation of air hunger it is supposedly very peaceful. As macabre as it may seem, advocates of capital punishment and euthanasia argue this would be a very humane, inexpensive, and simple way to end a life.

The one and one-half liters of potent hydrochloric acid and one and one-half liters of strongly alkaline sodium bicarbonate generate dozens of liters of carbon dioxide gas. The gas volume increases rapidly and dramatically and will lead to a bloated distended feeling within the small intestine. One may need to loosen a belt or tight clothing after a meal but fortunately the distended sensation is fairly short lived. The reason for this is that carbon dioxide gas in the intestines is rapidly absorbed and dissolved into the bloodstream. It travels to the lungs where the carbon dioxide is released via the alveoli into the airway and exhaled. The carbon dioxide present in intestinal gas is generated by colonic bacteria and other gut flora. It averages about ten percent of passed intestinal gas by volume. This figure can change significantly dependent on diet and the gastrointestinal microbiome.

Carminative

A carminative, also known as carminativum, is a herb or preparation that promotes the prevention or elimination of gas from the gastrointestinal tract. Many carminatives have been shown to work by releasing the air swallowed (aerophagia) by reducing the pressure of the lower esophageal sphincter to promote eructation (burp). This relaxation of the sphincter can also promote reflux, regurgitation and heartburn and can aggravate Gastroesophageal Reflux Disease (GERD), which may have atypical symptoms that are unrelated to heartburn.

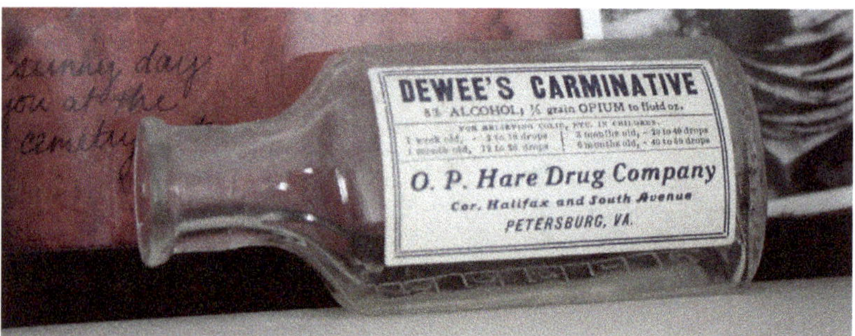

www.flickr.com Tess Shebaylo Dewee's Carminative Creative Commons License

Many folk medicines and remedies have a long tradition of being used as carminatives. They are often mixtures of herbs, spices, and essential oils. Many foods, social, and recreational products also relax the lower esophageal sphincter and encourage eructation, although one would not ingest them specifically for this carminative effect. This category includes onion, garlic, fried foods, fatty foods, chocolate, tobacco, alcohol, and marijuana.

In Western culture, the most common product that people see and use for its carminative property is mint, which relaxes the lower esophageal sphincter to encourage eructation. Chocolate can have a similar effect, so it is common to see the two combined as a traditional after dinner chocolate mint. Indian and Asian restaurants may offer other traditional carminative herbs and seeds usually found on the counter by the exit.

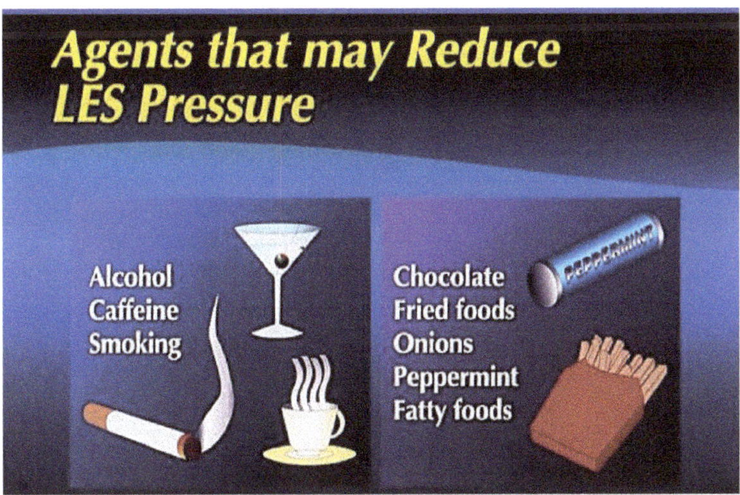
Agents that may Reduce LES Pressure
Alcohol
Caffeine
Smoking
Chocolate
Fried foods
Onions
Peppermint
Fatty foods
PEPPERMINT

Carminatives and other agents reduce the lower esophageal sphincter (LES) pressure, allowing the easier release of gasses and air from the stomach but at the same time make regurgitation and heartburn more likely. Restaurateurs want their customers to have enjoyed their meals, and they recognize that distension from the universal aerophagia of eating can cause discomfort. Most people have no idea that the air they swallowed, and not necessarily the meal, might be the cause of their distress. The carminative mint is offered to give prompt relief, but notice how it is offered on leaving the restaurant. The restaurant management does not want eructation to occur where others are dining in their refined accommodations. They prefer that the eructation occurs later to impress your 'significant other' or in the presence of your family and friends.

The following have all been described as having value as carminatives: Alcohol, Angelica, Anise, Asafetida, Basil, Black Pepper, Caffeine, Calamus, Capsaicin, Caraway, Cardamom, Chili (Cayenne) Pepper, Chocolate, Cinnamon (potency decreases with cooking), Cloves, Coriander, Cumin, Curcumin, Dill, Epazote,

Eucalyptus, fatty foods, Fennel, Garlic (potency increases with cooking), Ginger, Goldenrod, Hops, Lemon balm, liquorice (also spelled as licorice), Lovage, Marjoram, Mint, Motherwort, Muña, Mustard, Nigella, Nutmeg, Onion, Oregano, Parsley, Pepper, Pennyroyal, Peppermint, Rosemary, Saffron, Sage, Savory, Spearmint, Theobromine, Thyme, Tobacco, Turmeric, Valerian, Wintergreen, Winter Savory, Wormwood, and others.

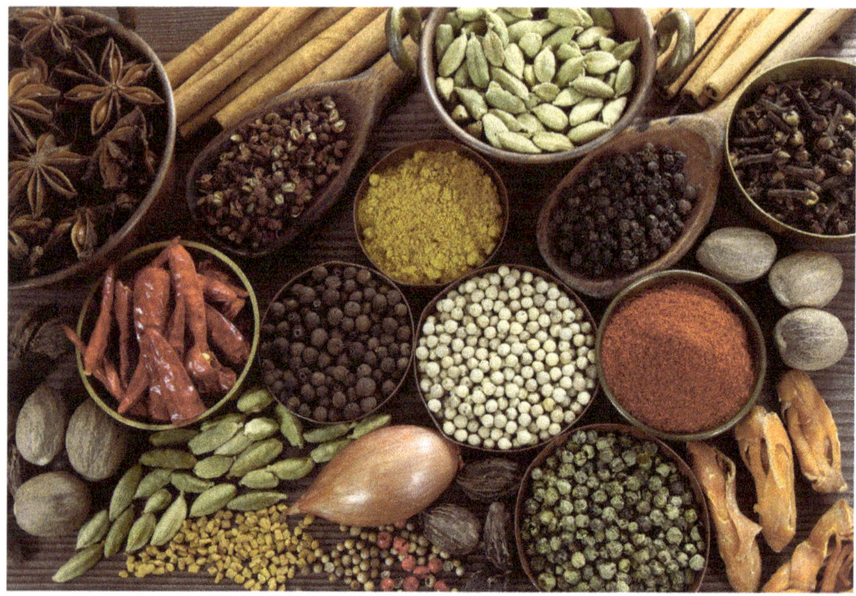

Herbs & Spices Shutterstock/KrzysztofSlusarczyk

As this exhaustive list confirms, a large number of herbs and spices have been described as having carminative benefits. The problem with anecdotes and folk traditions is that it is hard to separate true beneficial properties from those that do so as a result of a placebo effect. The business of selling spices and supplements is very lucrative, so there is a strong financial interest to keep the status quo and not investigate these herbs scientifically. Although many prescription drugs can affect the tone of the lower esophageal sphincter and promote eructation the carminative property is a side effect, and not an indication that the product should be used for that purpose. To encourage eructation avoid lying down after a meal. Sitting upright lets the air swallowed rise above the food in the stomach and when the lower esophageal sphincter relaxes air, rather than food, can then escape the stomach.

Carminatives relax the lower esophageal sphincter and can be used to allow burping or belching of swallowed air to give relief of gastric distension and bloat. Others drink a carbonated beverage or an effervescent product such as Alka-Seltzer to induce eructation by increasing the gas pressure within the stomach to overcome the resistance of the lower esophageal sphincter pressure. Fried foods, greasy, fatty foods, alcohol, onion, and tobacco can also act as carminatives as can a number of herbal preparations. A number of pharmacologic agents used in the treatment of a wide variety of medical disorders can also act as carminatives by relaxing the lower esophageal sphincter. Female hormones such as progesterone and estrogen are in this category. During natural periods of higher hormone levels, such as during a pregnancy, reflux is more common. One reason is that the hormones have an effect on the lowered esophageal sphincter, causing relaxation that may lead to reflux. A second reason is the increasing intra-abdominal pressure from a growing child and uterus.

Celiac Disease (see Gluten Sensitive Enteropathy, Sprue)

Chewing (Mastication)

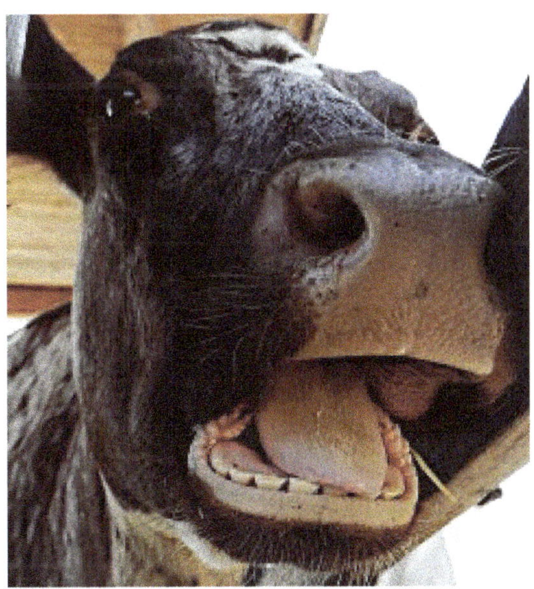

Chewing or mastication (Greek mastikhan-gnash the teeth) is the process of crushing and grinding food by the teeth. Mastication can be unconscious, or subconscious but can be modified by conscious control. This process increases the surface area of foods increasing the efficiency of enzymes and the absorption of nutrients. The bite pressure generated in the average human is one hundred and sixty-two pounds per square inch.

As impressive as the bite strength is, it is equally impressive how sensitive the chewing process is to recognizing when pressure should be released or withheld. It senses when a particle as small as a grain of sand is found in clam chowder, or a fragment of eggshell in an omelet. There is a very substantial amount of crushing and grinding power that macerates the food and disrupts the cellular structure of ingested plant and animal material. The disruption of cell structure often release enzymes within the cells themselves that assist in the degradation of cellular tissue and the process of digestion.

Chewing is obviously helpful in the digestive process. but it can inadvertently lead to excessive gas swallowing. With chewing the salivary glands are actively secreting more saliva. With the increased volume of saliva more swallows will take place. Each swallow allows the ingestion of excess air, on average three to five milliliters (about one teaspoon) per swallow. Chewing gum, ill-fitting dentures, drinking from a straw or bottle, tilting the head back while drinking, chewing tobacco, mouth candies and lozenges, etc. can contribute to excess aerophagia which may result in excess burping, bloating, and farting.

After chewing the food bolus is swallowed exiting the pharynx, transiting the esophagus via peristalsis, and entering the stomach. Chewing developed to handle the herbivorous diet, as carnivores generally engage in very little chewing activity and swallow their food whole or in large chunks. Cattle and other ruminants chew food more than once to allow further enzymatic digestion and bacterial fermentation to extract more nutrients. The regurgitated food bolus is called cud.

As a physician, I often ask if a patient has any difficulty chewing their food, such as from ill-fitting dentures. Chewing food well really helps the digestive process and can lead to less aerophagia, the swallowing of air, which can contribute to intestinal gaseousness. Medical words can be like a foreign language and easy to misinterpret. I always wondered what the response from some people would be if used the medical term for chewing and I encouraged them to masticate a lot with each meal. I imagine the response would be one of shock and indignation. What's the matter with you doctor, do you think I want to go blind!

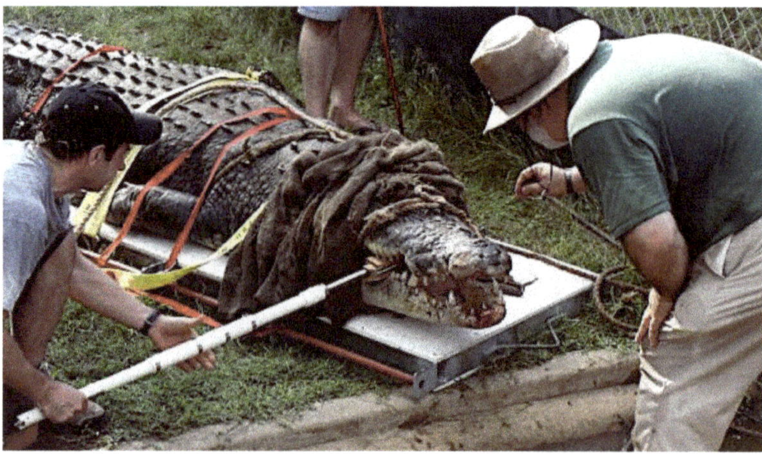

Greg Erickson, left, a paleobiologist on faculty at of Florida State University and Kent Vliet of the University of Florida measure the bite force of a saltwater crocodile in Australia. Contributed photo to St. Augustine Record, Florida

"The noise of the jaws coming together was like a gunshot. The power of the animal was astounding," said paleobiologist Greg M. Erickson of Florida State University. The crocodilians had a bite force of twenty-three thousand pounds per square inch, about double that of *Tyrannosaurus rex*, the scientist's estimate.

Dr. Brady Barr sponsored by the National Geographic Society measured comparative bite pressures of a sampling across the animal kingdom. Although humans have a very substantial bite pressure of one hundred and sixty-two pounds per square inch (psi), other species far exceed this amount of pressure generated.

Human: 162 psi
Dog: 310 psi
Lion: 600 psi
Shark: 600 psi
Hyena: 1000 psi
Turtle: 1000 psi
Crocodile: 2500 psi
Lion: 600 psi
Tiger: 1050 psi
Bear: 1200 psi
Gorilla: 1300 psi
Hippopotamus: 1821 psi
Jaguar: 2000 psi
Alligator: 2125 psi
Crocodile: 5000 psi

Chili Con Carne

Chili con carne is the Spanish name for a meal made as a stew that usually contains beans, chili peppers, tomato, and meat. Often other seasonings are added such as onions, garlic, and cumin. A wide variation of the ingredients and recipes often leads to competitions typically known as chili cook-off. It is often referred to by its abbreviated name chili in American English. It is the official culinary dish of the US State of Texas.

The high legume content has led to its recognition as a potent source of intestinal gas. The variety of spices, seasonings, and animal fat leads to an equally intense variety of subsequent farts and aromas, often of startling pungency. The use of chili as a staple of the diet of cowboys on the range has led to several comedic scenes. A famous example includes the infamous campfire scene in Mel Brook's movie *Blazing Saddles*.

Crepitation Contest

Attributed to the staff of the Canadian Broadcast Corporation in the 1940's, a recording called *The Crepitation Contest* was produced. Canadian Broadcast Corporation sportscaster Sidney S. Brown narrated it, with sound effects credited to his producer, Jules Lipton. The recording is a parody of a radio broadcast of a live sporting event with pre-game interviews of the contestants.

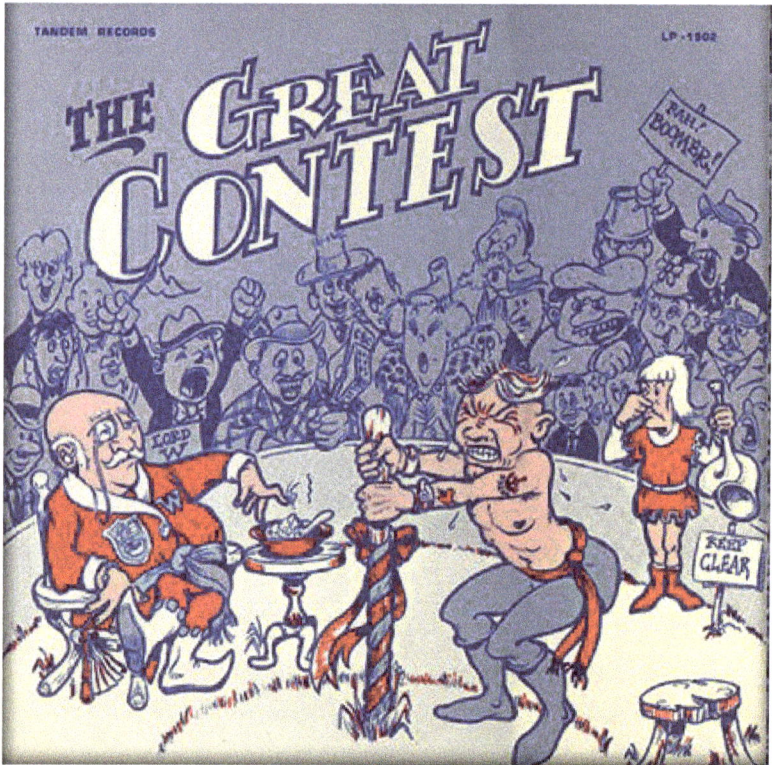

www.wfmu.org

The reigning champion is Lord Windesmear, and the challenger is Paul Boomer. The broadcast parody includes detailed descriptions of the competition including the rules, traditions, play-by-play reporting of the event and audience sounds and reactions. Reportedly the original recording was played at a New Year's Eve party in 1943 that was attended by an admiral of the United States Navy. He believed it would be a great morale booster for American serviceman. The original master recording at RCA Victor Studio in Toronto was obtained, and lacquer, and vinyl 78-rpm discs were pressed.

Diet

Diet obviously plays a major role in intestinal gas production. Certain types of vegetables and fruits contain carbohydrates with sugars and starches that may be poorly digested by people but happily fermented by bacteria comprising the gut flora. The starches, including potatoes, corn, noodles, and wheat are the source of the majority of gas generated by the gut microbial flora.

Rice is the one starch exception and rarely contributes to gas production. Wheat has the other 'distinction' of having the protein glutamate, which contains the nitrogen base product from which you generate ammonia-like aromatic compounds.

Common Foods that Cause Bloating and Gas

- Cabbage
- Cauliflower
- Beans
- Oats
- Apples
- Milk
- Fluffy wheat
- Broccoli
- Onions
- Corn
- Potatoes
- Pears
- Soft cheese
- Peaches

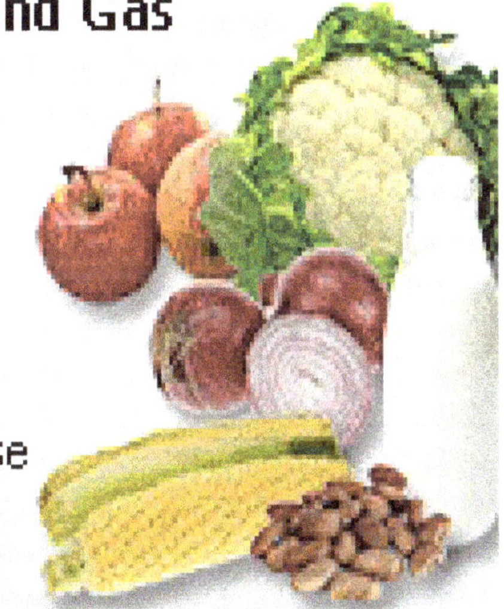

www.34-menopause-symptoms.com Creative Commons License

There are many specific enzymes required in the process of digestion, and deficiency in the quantity or activity of an enzyme can lead to food intolerance. The most common food intolerance is for the milk sugar lactose when an individual has decreased amounts and activity of the necessary enzyme for its digestion, lactase. The age of discovery is still in its infancy. Dozens of hormones, over one thousand and six hundred enzymes, over ten thousand species of gut microbes, and over one million genomes identified to date are just the beginning. Of the thousands of variables, we still have a clear understanding of only a few dozen. By the way, with so much remaining unknown and awaiting discovery, opportunity abounds if you have an interest in pursuing or supporting research activities.

If you are looking for a novel, practical, legitimate, and socially responsible way to avoid jury duty this may be your answer. A sincere desire to avoid inflicting your fart issues on fellow jurors may provide you with an excellent reason to be excused from jury duty. If you honestly believe you have excessive gas from an inherited enzyme deficiency you can bring the matter up with the clerk of the court and the presiding judge. If the court wants further clarification describe the scene of your intestinal gas leading the other jurors to flee the jury box complaining that it was a cruel and unusual exposure to a gas chamber. The judge just might have to declare a mistrial, stating that although justice is blind, she has not lost her sense of smell or hearing. A letter explaining the nature of your condition can go a long way to securing a permanent excuse from jury duty, and probably an invitation to use an absentee ballot to stay out of the voting booth on Election Day!

Chili con carne

Chili con carne is the Spanish name for a meal made as a stew that usually contains beans, chili peppers, tomato, and meat. Often other seasonings are added such as onions, garlic, and cumin. A wide variation of the ingredients and recipes often leads to competitions typically known as chili cook-off. It is often referred to by its abbreviated name chili in American English. It is the official culinary dish of the US State of Texas.

The high legume content has led to its recognition as a potent source of intestinal gas. The variety of spices, seasonings, and animal fat leads to an equally intense variety of subsequent farts and aromas, often of startling pungency. The use of chili as a staple of the diet of cowboys on the range has led to several comedic scenes. A famous example includes the infamous campfire scene in Mel Brook's movie Blazing Saddles.

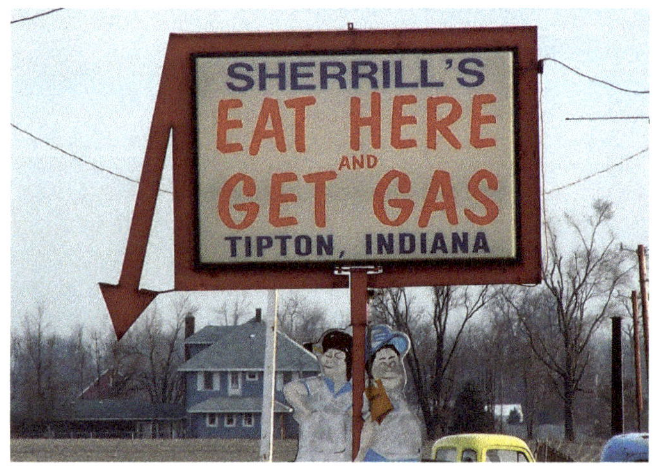

Refueling station and restaurant. Cindy Cornett Seigle www.flickr.com Creative Commons License

Legumes

"Beans, Beans, The Musical Fruit" is a schoolyard saying and children's song about the capacity for beans to contribute to flatulence.

Beans, beans, the musical fruit
The more you eat, the more you toot
The more you toot, the better you feel
So we have beans at every meal!
There are also several alternative versions, such as the one below:

Beans, beans, they're good for your heart
The more you eat, the more you fart
The more you fart, the happier/better you feel
So let's eat beans with every meal

Beans have a well-deserved reputation for contributing to intestinal gas production. Recent medical literature suggests that the degree of subjective complaints that legumes cause gas may be somewhat exaggerated. The bean is rich in the sugars raffinose, verbascose and stachyose. As humans do not produce the enzyme required for its degradation, alpha-galactosidase, these sugars undergo fermentation by the gut flora. The US Department of Agriculture is working on the development of a bean with lower levels of these sugars, and so far the Anasazi bean has been the leading candidate but no breakthrough yet. With genetically modified organisms (GMO) and foods being introduced in the marketplace, it is only a matter of time before products labeled as low-gas are promoted.

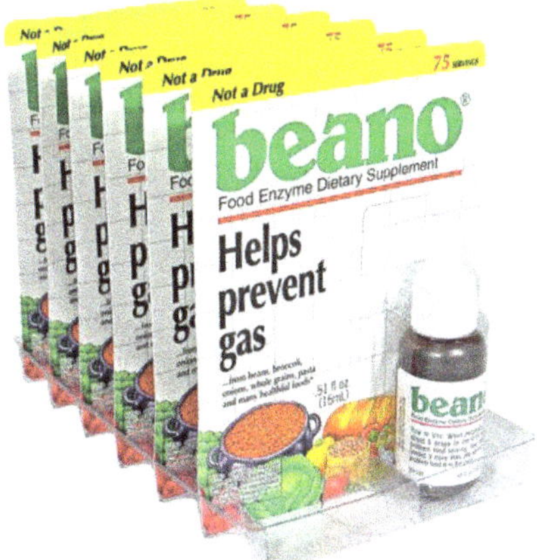

www.flickr.com Creative Commons License

Thankfully there are alpha-galactosidase enzyme supplements that can provide relief. The enzyme is not heat stable, so it will be inactivated by the heat of cooking. The enzyme should be added to the first bite of the beans consumed and if a large portion is ingested additional enzyme intake during the course of the bean meal is recommended. An alternative approach is to soak the beans for several hours, leeching out some of the sugars into the water, which is discarded. The best approach is to soak the beans until they begin to germinate. With germination the seed itself begins to release alpha-galactosidase to break down its complex sugar content for the nutritional use of the newly germinated bean plant. With germination approximately eighty percent of the complex sugars are digested.

A legume is a plant in the family Fabaceae (or Leguminosae) native to the Americas, grown agriculturally for their food grain seed, livestock forage and silage, and soil enhancement. Most legumes harbor the symbiotic bacteria Rhizobia in their root nodules, which convert nitrogen in the atmosphere into ammonia and ammonium. This source of nitrogen contributes to the plant's production of amino acids and high protein content. Legumes include alfalfa, clover, peas, beans, lentils, lupins, soybeans, and peanuts and a number of trees and shrubs. In farming crop rotation the growing of legumes near non-legumes is common. Legumes are sometimes referred to as 'green manure' because their symbiotic bacteria enrich the soil with nitrogenous products. A legume fruit is typically a pod that opens along a seam. They are an excellent source of protein but contain lower quantities of the essential amino acid methionine.

Like many legumes, the seemingly innocent lima bean should not be eaten raw, doing so can be lethal. Also known as butter beans, the legumes can contain a high level of cyanide, which is part of the plant's defense mechanism. In the United States there are restrictions about cyanide levels in commercially grown lima bean varieties, but not so in less developed countries, and many people can get sick from eating them. Even so, lima beans should be cooked thoroughly and uncovered to allow the poison to escape as gas. Also, drain and discard the cooking water to be on the safe side.

Many a granny came armed with a spoonful of castor oil to heal all ills, and studies show that it does indeed have health benefits to offer. Just be sure not to eat the beans from which the oil came. If castor beans are chewed and swallowed, they can release ricin, one of the most toxic poisons known to man. Eating just one or two castor beans can easily cause the demise of the eater. Ricin has been investigated as a warfare agent and has even been employed by secret agents and assassins.

Pumpernickel (Devil's Farts)

Pumpernickel (German Devil's Fart) is a heavy dark brown bread traditionally made with coarsely ground rye flour and whole rye berries and has been associated with the Westphalia region of Germany for over five hundred years. Like most rye breads, it is traditionally made with an acidic sourdough starter, which inhibits the rye amylase enzymes. The name is associated with the coarse bread-giving rise to flatulence. With its sourdough origins it can serve as a probiotic.

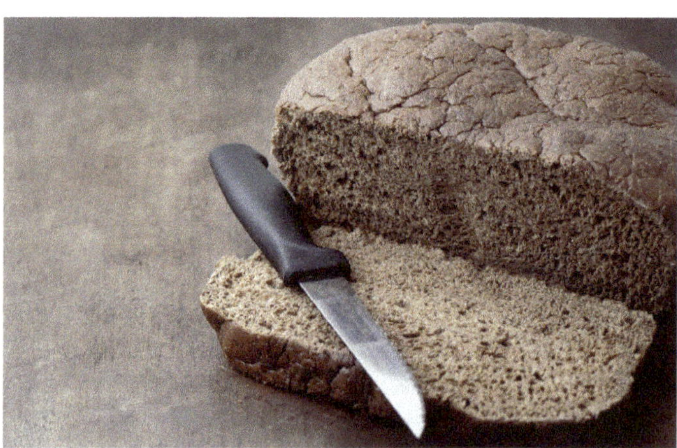

Shutterstock/eclipticblue

Pets de Nonne (Nun's Farts)

Pets de Nonne, also called Pets de Sœur, is translated as a nun's farts. They are a dessert puff pastry dating from medieval times and made from butter, milk, flour, sugar, eggs and sometimes honey is added. They are traditionally pan-fried in lard and then baked. Their lightness inspired their name in French, pets de nonne and Pets de Sœurs, suggesting that the farts of a nun were somewhat angelic.

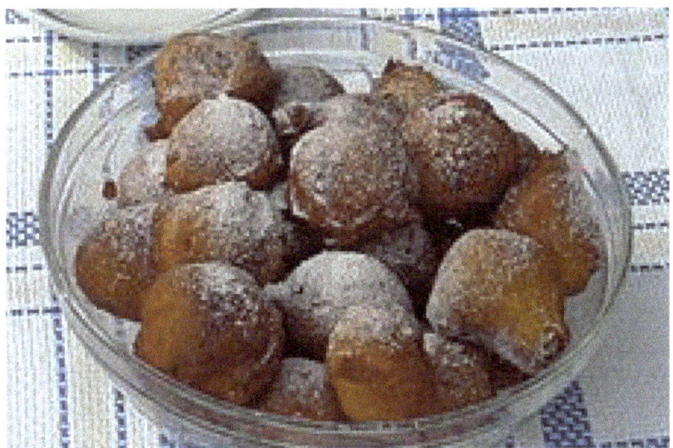

Pets de Nonne, also called Pets de Sœurs (Nun's Farts) French and Canadian Dessert Food photo by Ziga Creative Commons License

Digestion

The purpose of the digestive tract is to support life by providing the nutrition and energy we need for all of our body functions. Intestinal gas is simply a natural waste product and is rarely of consequence. Perhaps the analogy is not the best one, but think of the digestive tract as the reverse of the assembly line, a disassembly line. A factory has a goal to be efficient and profitable, and may not win too many awards for architectural beauty. So too with the digestive tract, the process has been refined over eons of evolution, yet still have its primitive origins and end products.

We begin our factory tour with a view much like you would get sitting in your car going through an automated car wash. Before you even go to the car wash, your brain has to make the conscious decision that this activity is what it wants to do. In the same manner, the mind begins the digestive process with the decision to satisfy its hunger call, or because an appetizing opportunity presents itself. When thinking about food and eating, the brain may activate the secretion of saliva and prime the digestive processes of the stomach and internal organs.

Much like the water hoses and spray that greet your vehicle as you enter the beginning of the car wash tunnel, the entrance of food to the mouth receives a similar welcome. Jets of saliva are secreted from the ducts of the salivary glands located strategically around the oral cavity of the mouth. Saliva that is in the resting mouth is viscous and coats and protects the teeth and the inner surface of the mouth. The secreted saliva with eating or drinking is of a thinner more watery consistency. It has digestive enzymes including amylase to digest carbohydrates and lipase to digest fats.

If your carwash is as sophisticated as your digestive tract, it will have a crew to make sure your side mirrors are tucked in. It will also provide a prewash scrub of your tires to remove residue that would otherwise be difficult for the machinery to reach. The teeth, jaws, and tongue work together in a remarkable and powerful dance with very few of the missteps which would be the dance equivalent of stepping on toes, the biting of the tongue.

The food has to be processed into smaller more manageable portions than that what is found on your plate. Your dining utensils of fork, knife, and spoon are just the preliminary, as the teeth do the real work in preparing food for the process of digestion. The teeth are subdivided into distinct categories that have unique functions. The incisors cut the food as you bite into an apple and the canines tear the food apart as you dig into your pastrami sandwich. The molars crush and grind the salad and crunchy vegetables that you have as a side dish. The grinding and crushing break the plant cell walls apart that would otherwise protect its internal nutritious content from our digestive enzymes. They also increase the surface area of the food increasing their exposure to digestive acid and enzymes.

The chewing process assures that the saliva and its active enzymes are well mixed with the increased surface area of the food. They begin the process of breaking down the carbohydrates and lipids into their essential components to ready them for further digestion and absorption. The saliva also moistens the food and lubricates it for the coordinated swallowing motion of the tongue, teeth, palate, and pharynx. These muscles and organs work together to roll it into an easy to swallow food bolus. The muscles of the swallowing process include those that protect the larynx and airway. The epiglottis closes off the passageway to the trachea, bronchi, and lungs, to prevent aspiration into the airways as the food and saliva swallow takes place.

The coordinated action is developed with age, which is why small children should avoid foods, such as nuts, grapes, larger oval or rounded candies. These foods, if inappropriately swallowed into the airway, can lead to fatal choking episodes. Tragically a number of children die because the oval or rounded shape can completely block the airway. An irregular shaped object, which can be life threatening, rarely completely obstructs the airway and usually allows some air to pass. The complicated swallowing neuromuscular coordination can also be affected by neurological disorders, stroke, surgery or other conditions, which may lead to the risk of aspiration. Once swallowed, the food bolus is propelled down the esophagus by coordinated snakelike muscular action, known as peristalsis. It is not recommended, but the swallowing mechanism is so efficient that you can swallow against gravity while standing on your head.

The muscular valve at the junction of the esophagus and stomach is called the lower esophageal sphincter. The lower esophageal sphincter is designed to allow food and fluid to enter the stomach, with the door closed behind them once they leave the esophagus. If the valve opens at the wrong time, gastric acid, digestive enzymes, and food can flow back into the esophagus. The reflux of stomach contents into the esophagus can lead to symptoms of heartburn or mucosal damage. If the refluxed material goes all the way into the airway hoarseness, sore throat, aspiration, choking, or pneumonia can develop. If it occurs frequently gastroesophageal reflux disease (GERD) can predispose to a change in the normal flat squamous epithelium cell tissue lining the esophagus. The growth of columnar epithelium, more of an intestinal type tissue, in place of the squamous epithelium gives rise to a condition called a Barrett esophagus. This type of cell lining is at a higher risk for abnormal atypical cell changes and a higher risk of cancer development. Individuals with Barrett esophagus are frequently treated for GERD and monitored carefully with surveillance endoscopy and biopsy for pre-malignant changes.

The stomach is a churning caldron of muscular mixing contractions, concentrated acid secretion, and potent digestive enzymes. The vagus nerve and gut hormones play a crucial role in the intricate balance of enzymes, acid, nutrients, and motility. When the conditions are right, the pyloric sphincter of the stomach opens to allow the acid, enzyme, and food mixture to exit. This digestive material is now called chyme as it enters the first portion of the small intestine, known as the duodenum. In Greek, this means the width equivalent to twelve fingers, which is what its small size would measure using your digits. For its small size, the duodenum plays an amazing and complex part.

The highly acid chyme would quickly damage the lining of the duodenum if it did not respond quickly with the pouring on, much like a fire extinguisher, of sodium bicarbonate. The sodium bicarbonate is produced in the duodenum as well as by the pancreas. The sodium bicarbonate produced in the pancreas is released through the pancreatic duct, which empties into the duodenum through the Ampulla of Vater. The fire extinguisher analogy shares another aspect of the story. Perhaps you made a fire extinguisher in a science class, or home experiment, by adding baking soda that contains sodium bicarbonate and vinegar that contains acetic acid. This neutralization of acid is the same type of reaction that takes place in the duodenum, when the hydrochloric acid of the stomach meets the sodium bicarbonate released to neutralize it. When the two react they produce water, sodium chloride (salt), and large quantities of carbon dioxide. The carbon dioxide is released as large volumes of gas that appears as bubbles arising from the reaction. The carbon dioxide is used as a fire extinguisher in the science experiment since it is heavier than air and cuts off the oxygen supply that the flame requires.

In the human duodenum, the carbon dioxide generated as a side product of acid neutralization only serves to bloat and distend the gut with gas. The body is pretty remarkable in getting rid of the bloat relatively quickly, in that it absorbs the carbon dioxide into the bloodstream where it travels to the lungs and is exhaled. The bile ducts from the liver join the duct from the pancreas bringing digestive enzymes and bicarbonate that enter the duodenum through the Ampulla of Vater. Within the ampulla lies the muscular sphincter of Oddi. The name sounds like a character from the story of *The Wizard of Oz*, and that would be an appropriate analogy. The coordinated release of hormones, enzymes, motility and vagal input is nothing short of wizardry.

Subconsciously, your body can sense what nutrients you have ingested. The body responds by releasing the correct recipe of enzymes, potent acid in the stomach, and bicarbonate in the duodenum, adjusting the pH as necessary. It adds just the right amount of bile to the mix, controls the timing and volume of stomach emptying, and controls the speed of transit and intensity of mixing contractions through the length of the intestinal tract. The majority of the sensing and control feedback takes place in a small confined space the width of twelve fingers, the duodenum.

The breakdown products of the digestive process are absorbed by a sea of finger-like projections called the villi. It looks like a field of waving wheat stalks; each upstanding villus is ready to use its enzymes and absorptive capacity to absorb nutrients. If you looked under the microscope, you would find that each villus has thousands of even smaller villi on its surface, given the appropriate name of microvilli.

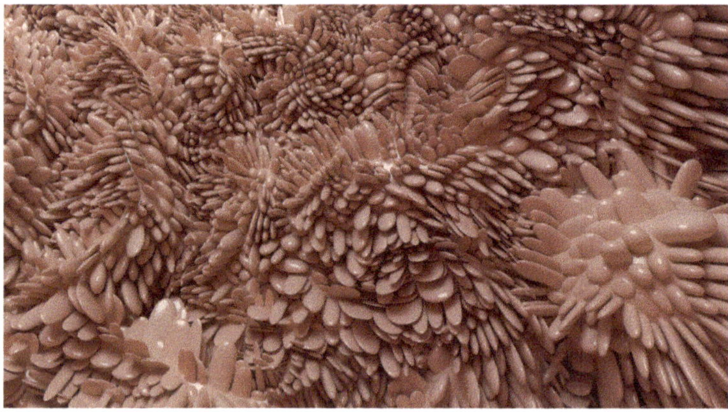

Villi Shutterstock/modella

All of these folds of absorptive tissue, if flattened out, would provide the equivalent absorptive capacity of a championship tennis court. A quote from Mark Twain also illustrates the concept of surface area: "If Switzerland were ironed flat it would be a very large country". The long intestinal tunnel of eagerly awaiting absorptive villi is about twenty feet long, and it is an amazingly efficient system of digestion and absorption. If injured, the ability of the small bowel to digest and absorb nutrients is compromised. A condition that temporarily damages the small intestine, such as a viral or bacterial gastroenteritis often called stomach flu, can cause a blunting or shortening of the villi. The villous blunting will also lead to the loss of digestive enzymes that reside on the villi.

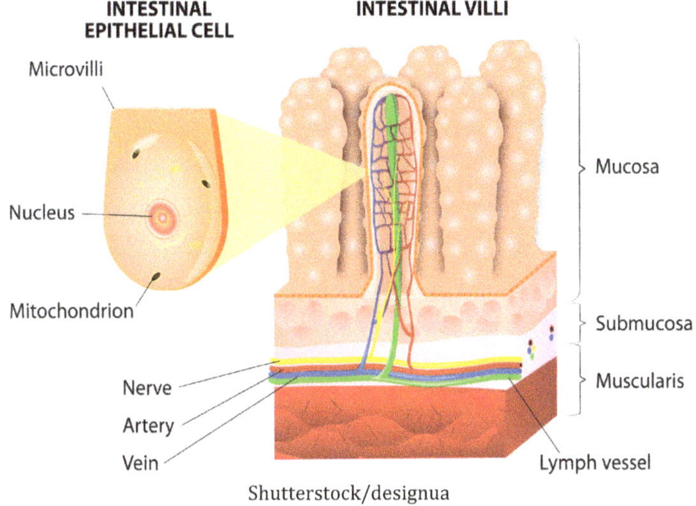

Shutterstock/designua

Without the ability to digest and absorb nutrients, the unabsorbed material can cause what is known as an osmotic diarrhea. People are often advised to avoid dairy products for a week or so after stomach flu to allow the villi and enzymes to recover. If you eat or drink lactose without waiting until the recovery is complete, you may end up with symptoms of temporary lactose intolerance such as gas and diarrhea. When the liquid chyme leaves the jejunum and ileum of the small intestine, it goes through the ileocecal valve to enter the colon. In the cecum of the colon lies the infamous appendix, which for thousands of years mystified science as to its purpose. It looks like its function has finally, and only very recently, been identified. It stores a reservoir of intestinal bacteria, representing the healthy gut microbiome, from which the gut flora can be replenished after a bout of intestinal dysentery.

The gut microbiome is much more important than most people realize. The microbes of the body far outnumber the number of human cells. In fact, if you just go by the number of cells and not their mass, they outnumber human cells by ten to one. In other words, you as a living system are only ten percent human and ninety percent microbes! The vast majority of the microbes living within and on us are commensals. The term commensal is used to describe a symbiotic relationship from which both parties benefit. They are able to process foods that would otherwise be indigestible, and convert them to absorbable nutrients and metabolites. It is not an understatement to say that they are a requirement for our health and well-being. The gut microbiome also plays a critical role in the gut-brain-microbiome-axis, which provides for the communication of information between the three. Many experts now include food as the fourth component of this important communication axis.

The colon, unlike the small intestine, is less involved in the digestion of foods and nutrients. It is primarily involved in the absorption of water and sodium, as well as some fat-soluble vitamins such as vitamin K. The colon removes the excess moisture from the watery chime solidifying the stool as it transits the gut. The ability to conserve water is necessary, and without this ability the risk of dehydration would be substantially increased. The fecal material of the stool is stored in the rectum, and sigmoid colon, awaiting the right opportunity to be eliminated through defecation. A process or illness that impairs the colon's absorption of water will lead to more fluid in the stool and diarrhea. The loss of water and electrolytes as a consequence of diarrhea, unfortunately, remains a life-threatening condition in many parts of the world, especially for infants and children.

If the elimination of the feces is delayed, the moisture continues to be absorbed, and the stools can become harder resulting in constipation. Constipation itself can be self-perpetuating as it aggravates the situation because the stools become harder and more difficult to pass the longer they remain in the colon. The more common treatments for constipation attempt to increase the moisture content of the stool. The feces excreted can provide information about bowel health. For most people going about their daily activities, the passage of the feces itself is the end of the story of digestion. The human digestive system, like that of other animals, does not remove all of the contained nutrients from food. For other organisms, including the common housefly, the feces are thus an available source of nutrition. For them, the elimination of feces is just the beginning of their story of digestion and can play an important role in the transmission of disease back to humans.

Farts are ubiquitous, all living creatures generate gas from the cellular respiration of metabolism, and humans are no exception. The bacteria in your colonic flora produce microscopic nanofarts and microfarts, which collect into larger bubbles of gas in the bowel. They are intermixed with the atmospheric air swallowed throughout the day and particularly at meals. The nature of the intestinal gas may provide clues to digestive health and disease.

Distension (see Bloat)

Distension and its synonymous term bloat are the familiar sensation that the abdomen is distended or overly full. There are many causes of bloating ranging from simple overeating and the regular production of intestinal gasses to abdominal ascites fluid buildup from an underlying tumor. Common causes of abdominal bloating include overeating, gastric distension, lactose intolerance, fructose intolerance and other food intolerances. Other causes include food allergy, aerophagia (air swallowing), irritable bowel syndrome, partial or complete bowel obstruction, and gastric dumping syndrome or rapid gastric emptying. The list continues with gas-producing foods, constipation, visceral fat, and obesity.

Less common causes include splenic flexure syndrome, menstruation, dysmenorrhea, premenstrual syndrome, polycystic ovary syndrome and ovarian cysts, and Alvarez' syndrome. The possibilities are an extensive list of ailments, infections, and disorders including intestinal parasites (e.g., *Ascaris lumbricoides*), diverticulosis, celiac disease, prescription medications such as phentermine, intra-abdominal tumors such as cancer of the ovary, liver, uterus, stomach, and colon. Temporary bloating is common after gastrointestinal endoscopic procedures. Rarely a megacolon, which is an abnormal dilation of the colon, can be caused by ulcerative colitis or Chagas disease caused by the parasite *Trypanosoma cruzi.* After surgical repair of a hiatal hernia or treatment for gastroesophageal reflux with a procedure known as a Nissen fundoplication, the ability to burp and belch is restricted resulting in uncomfortable bloating and distension.

A number of lifestyle and dietary factors can also affect the frequency and intensity of the sensation of bloating. Exercise stimulates the releases of hormones that encourage peristaltic activity in the bowels. In a similar fashion, caffeine containing beverages and food such as coffee, tea, cola, and chocolate also stimulate peristalsis and improve the transit time of food through the digestive tract. A rapid gastrointestinal transit gives the gut flora less time to ferment the material in the lumen of the bowel, with a resultant decrease in the total volume of gas produced by bacterial fermentation. Even a walk after a meal may help to move the contents along helping to ease the volume of gas produced. If nothing else, it at least allows you to release it outdoors!

Meals that are high in fat create the exact opposite effect as fat causes the release of hormones and slows down gut motility. As the food spends more time in the digestive tract continued bacterial fermentation produces increasing quantities of gas.' In addition, foods that are extremely hot or cold tend to be swallowed in smaller quantities resulting in more swallows being necessary to eat or drink the same volume at a moderate temperature. As each swallow contributes an additional quantity of air entering the esophagus and digestive tract, more swallows results in more air ingestion. Foods or snacks that require excess chewing with resultant excess swallowing of saliva, such as chewing or bubble gum, also contribute to excess air intake. Certain types of vegetables and fruits contain sugars and starches, which may be poorly digested by people but happily fermented by bacteria comprising the gut flora. The most common food intolerance is lactose intolerance.

The treatment is always directed at the underlying cause. Empiric trials of carminatives, probiotics, dietary restrictions, enzyme replacement therapy, simethicone, etcetera can be attempted. Alternative health approaches to treating bloating include acupuncture, homeopathy, and hypnosis. Sometimes the underlying bloat is not bloating from the air but from the increased body fat of obesity. Now that is a real challenge, but the benefits of eliminating that bloat can be profoundly beneficial to health and longevity. Another contributor to gastrointestinal bloat is reduced gut motility. With the reduction in peristaltic activity, the intestinal gasses accumulate and distend the bowel. Diabetes mellitus, neuropathy, various drugs including opiates, and other causes may lead to a reduction in peristaltic activity. Bowel obstruction leads to distension of proximal portions of the gastrointestinal tract because of accumulating gas, fluids, and undigested food residue.

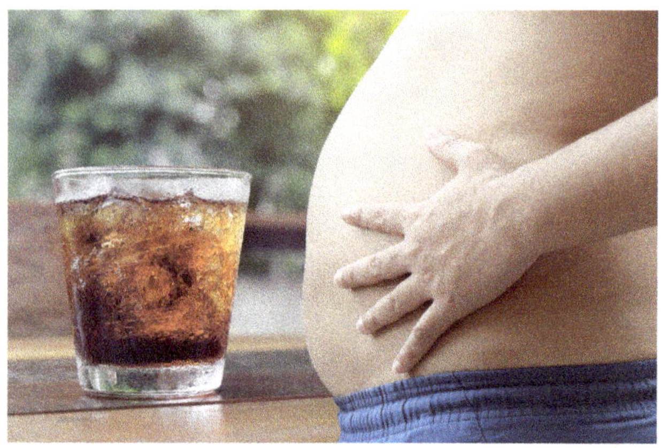

Shutterstock/sisacorn

Bloating and distension continue even after death. As there is no longer any gastrointestinal peristalsis or motility, the gasses rapidly accumulate. In the cases of victims of drowning the body, which initially descended deeper into the water, begins rise as the gasses accumulate. After a day or so enough gas has collected so that the body floats to the surface and remains there for a week or so. In cold water or colder climates the microbial metabolism is slowed so it takes longer for sufficient gas to be produced to float a body from submerged depths. In the San Francisco Bay area, the Golden Gate Bridge is a frequent location for tragic suicide leaps into the frigid waters below. The water is so cold it often takes a week for gasses to accumulate to allow retrieval of the body. The cold temperature also involves Charles Law, which dictates that the lower the temperature the smaller the volume the gas will occupy.

At some point the pressure of the gasses that are accumulating through the microbial metabolism and the decomposition process result in rupture of the body. This event can be explosive in nature and injury and death have occurred from proximity to decomposing bodies and animal remains. In most societies, early burial prevents exposure to the decomposition process. In Western and other cultures, a body may be displayed prior to burial. As the intestinal gas production does not cease with death, and indeed accelerates, gas may continue to escape as an audible fart. Part of the mortician practice is to perform a procedure that seals and secures the anus of the deceased so that the audible release of gas does not occur. Most people are not aware that the dead can fart, and when an uninformed person is exposed to a deceased person farting they are frightened, often believing that they are at least partly alive. Perhaps this has given rise to a belief in a zombie like state between life and death.

Diverticulosis

Diverticulosis is the presence of out pockets, called diverticula, of the colonic mucosa and submucosa through weaknesses of muscle layers in the colon wall. These are more common with advancing age and typically are most pronounced in the sigmoid colon. The incidence of ten percent of Americans having diverticulosis at age forty, to over fifty percent at age sixty is thought to be due to progressive weakening of the colon wall connective tissue. Diverticula are typically asymptomatic and the first sign of the condition may be painless lower intestinal bleeding. The bleeding can be brisk and life threatening or subtle presenting as an anemia of undetermined cause. The diverticula can also present as an infection called diverticulitis and if untreated abscesses, perforation, and life threatening peritonitis may develop. Diverticula can be visualized on colonoscopy and barium enema, but if an infection is suspect CAT scan or MRI is the preferred study to reduce the risk of perforation.

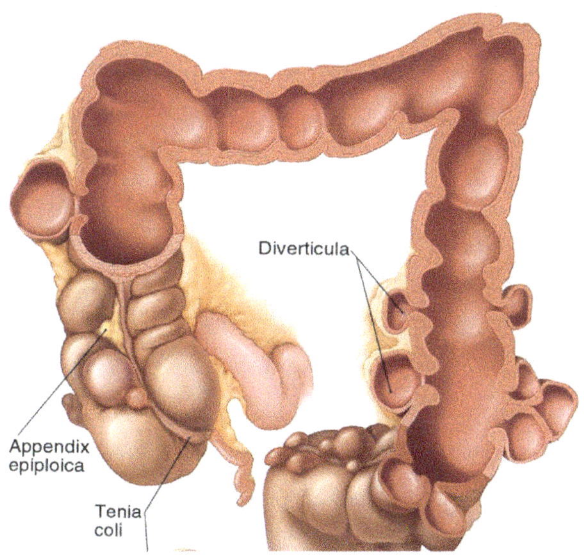

The passage of intestinal gas in African culture is basically a nonevent. It is considered part of the normal digestive process and not the cause of any embarrassment or suppression. It even came to be mentioned in a prestigious medical journal during a discussion of the cause of diverticular disease of the colon, discussed below. The development of diverticula has been ascribed to the high pressure generated within the bowel with the mass motion of feces. This is thought to cause herniation at the vulnerable location where blood vessels enter the colonic wall. Dr. Denis Burkitt, already famous for his identification of Burkitt Lymphoma a pediatric tumor seen in Africa, suggested an explanation for why diverticulosis is so common in Western society but rare in Africa. He theorized that because Africans eat a higher fiber diet than Westerners and use the natural squatting position for defecation, they pass soft bulky stools without straining. He wrote a book advocating his position and it became an international best seller

Another scientist challenged his theory with a letter to the editor published in the prestigious British medical journal, The Lancet. He theorized the reason Africans do not get diverticulosis was because they look upon farting as a perfectly normal activity and do so whenever the urge arises. In Western society, he argued, we sit in our office cubicles all day long holding on to internal gasses under very high pressure and only when we get into our cars at the end of the day do we allow ourselves to release the pent up high pressure gas and toot our way home. The fact that the incidence is identical in black and white Americans excluded a racial factor as a possible explanation.

An old theory ascribed diverticulitis to seeds ingested and lodged in the diverticula, because this was often seen in surgical specimens with the condition. More recent analysis concludes that these were just coincidental findings and those previous dietary restrictions of nuts, popcorn hulls, sunflower seeds, pumpkin seeds, caraway seeds, and sesame seeds were unnecessary. Although there is no scientific evidence showing statistical improvement, most scientists believe that a higher fiber diet may well be helpful in diverticulosis and has the added advantage that it may reduce cholesterol levels and the risk of colon cancer as well. Fiber is also an important prebiotic, and thus may be beneficial to improving the health of the gut microbiome.

Elevator (see Atmospheric Pressure, Fart Aroma, Fart, Diffusion)

Elevators are a source of frustration and humor when it comes to intestinal gas in confined small places. There is an underlying science as to why farts are more likely to occur when going up as opposed to coming down. Additional insights can be gathered by reading the entries on atmospheric pressure, altitude, ideal gas laws, fart aroma, and diffusion.

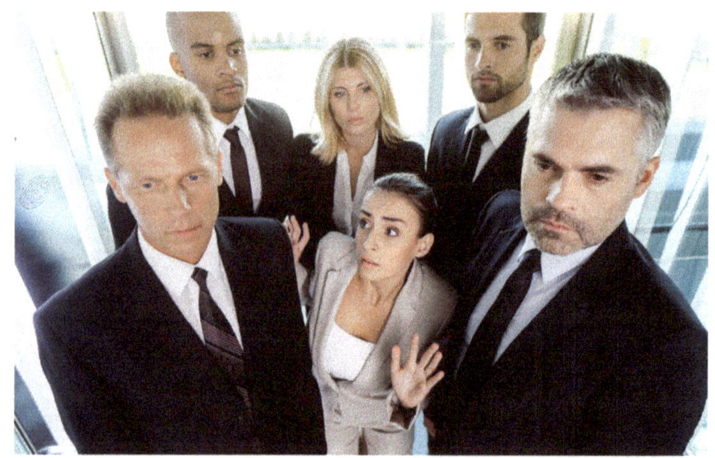

Shutterstock/g-stockstudio

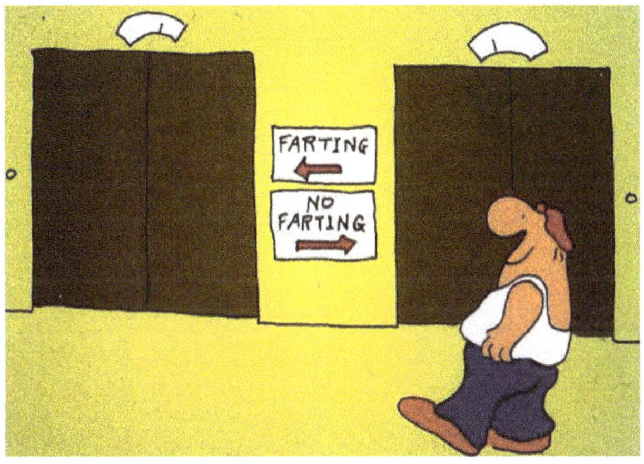

Enzyme

Enzyme deficiencies can lead to inadequate digestion of foods, which can result in excess material for the gut microbes to ferment with excess gas production. Enzymes are large molecules that are highly selective catalysts that greatly accelerate metabolic reactions. These range from the digestion of food to the synthesis of proteins and DNA. They are often described as being analogous to a lock and key. Most enzymes are proteins that have specific three-dimensional structure that acts like a key, with the substrate acting as a lock.

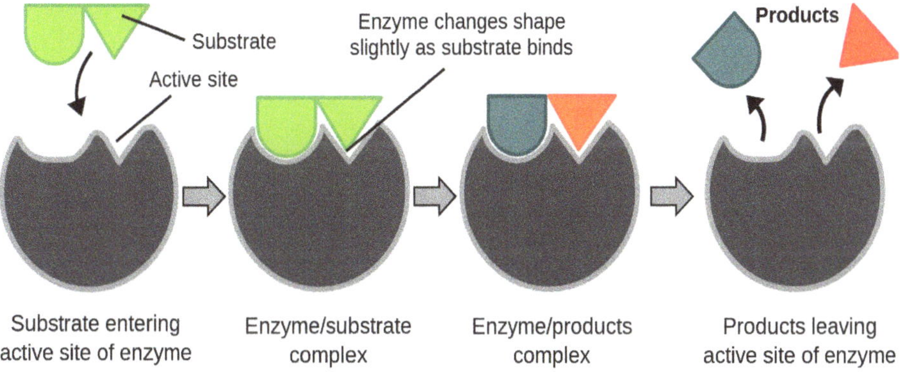

The molecules at the beginning of the process are called substrates, and are converted into different molecules called products. Most enzyme reaction rates are millions of times faster than reactions without the presence of the enzyme catalyst, and the enzymes are not consumed by the reactions and can be reused. Enzyme activity can be affected by other molecules such as inhibitors that decrease enzyme activity and activators that increase activity. Many pharmaceutical products, active ingredients from plants, and poisons are enzyme inhibitors or activators.

Five food Enzyme Families

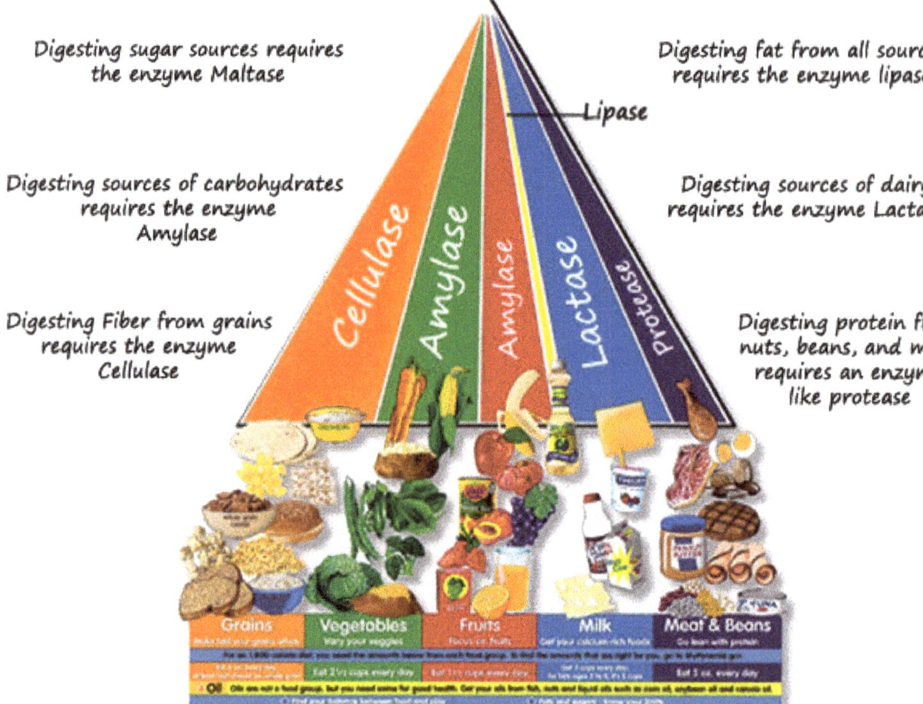
Digesting sugar sources requires the enzyme Maltase
Digesting fat from all sourc
requires the enzyme lipase
Lipase
Digesting sources of carbohydrates requires the enzyme Amylase
Digesting sources of dair
requires the enzyme Lacta
Digesting Fiber from grains requires the enzyme Cellulase
Digesting protein fr
nuts, beans, and m
requires an enzym
like protease
Cellulase
Amylase
Amylase
Lactase
Protease
Grains
Vegetables
Fruits
Milk
Meat & Beans

Many believe that raw food contains it's own specific enzymes to assist the body in breaking it down into nutrients for proper digestion.

PROTEIN DIGESTION

Substrate	Extracellular enzymes		Intestinal mucosal enzymes	End Products
Protein	*Pepsin* *Trypsin* *Chymotrypsin* *Elastases*	*Carboxypeptidase A* *Carboxypeptidase B*	*Aminopeptidase* *Tripeptidase* *Dipeptidase*	Amino Acids
Nucleoprotein	*Protein* *Hydrolysis*	*Ribonuclease* *Deoxyribonuclease*	*Oligonucleotidase* *5' Nucleotidase* *Alkaline Phosphatase* *Adenosine Deaminase*	Purine Bases Pyrimidine Bases Pentose-1-PO_4

CARBOHYDRATE DIGESTION

Substrate	Extracellular enzymes	Intestinal mucosal enzymes	End Products
Amylose Amylopectin Glycogen	*α Amylase*	*Maltase* *Isomaltase*	Glucose
Chitin	*Chitinase*	*Chitobiase*	Glucosamine
Sucrose		*Sucrase*	Glucose Fructose
Lactose		*Lactase*	Glucose Galactose
Trehalose		*Trehalase*	Glucose

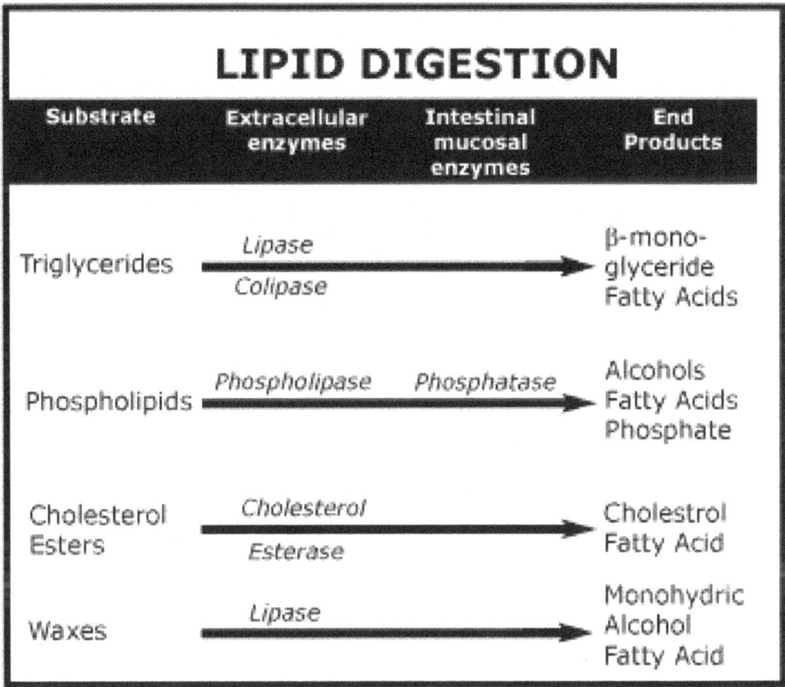

LIPID DIGESTION

Substrate	Extracellular enzymes	Intestinal mucosal enzymes	End Products
Triglycerides	*Lipase* *Colipase*		β-mono-glyceride Fatty Acids
Phospholipids	*Phospholipase*	*Phosphatase*	Alcohols Fatty Acids Phosphate
Cholesterol Esters	*Cholesterol* *Esterase*		Cholestrol Fatty Acid
Waxes	*Lipase*		Monohydric Alcohol Fatty Acid

Enzyme Type	Enzyme	Function
Carbohydrate-Specific Enzymes	Amylase, Alpha-Amylase	Converts complex starch in root vegetables and grains into maltose (a disaccharide), maltotriose (a trisaccharide), dextrins, and oligosaccharides
	Glucoamylase	Converts maltose, maltotriose, and oligosaccharides into glucose
Sugar-Specific (Disaccharide) Enzymes	Lactase	Converts lactose (milk sugar) into glucose and galactose
	Maltase	Digests maltose in malt, cereal grains, and processed foods into glucose
	Sucrase (Invertase)	Converts sucrose (table sugar) into glucose and fructose; forms sucrase-isomaltase complex in the intestinal lining that breaks down dextrins
	Pullulanase	Breaks down amylopectin starch molecules resistant to degradation that may otherwise remain trapped in the microvilli and contribute to inflammation
Vegetable/Fiber-Specific Enzymes	Cellulase, Hemicellulase	Liberates nutrients from fruits and vegetables, making them more bioavailable
	Alpha-Galactosidase	Breaks down hard-to-digest carbohydrates found in legumes and cruciferous vegetables
	Pectinase	Hydrolyzes pectin; reduces the bulking effect of some fibrous foods
	Phytase	Breaks down phytates in grains (wheat, oats, barley) and legumes
	Beta-Glucanase	Breaks down glucans in cereal grains and in yeast cell walls
	Galactomannase	Degrades hemicellulose, cellulose, and cell walls with mannose
Protein and Peptide-Specific Enzymes	Acid and Alkaline Protease	Breaks down plant, vegetable, and meat derived proteins
	Peptidase and Dipeptidyl Peptidase IV (DPP-IV)	Breaks down casein (dairy products) and gluten (wheat, barley, rye) and their exorphin peptides
Fat-Specific Enzymes	Lipase	Hydrolyzes fats in meat and dairy products, oils in nuts and seeds, and triglycerides
Specialty Enzymes	Lysozyme (highly purified from egg white)	Degrades polysaccharides found in the cell walls of many bacteria, yeast, and other pathogens
	Serratia Peptidase	Breaks down casein protein peptides; breaks down fibrin and protects sensitive GI tissues from irritation and inflammation

There are a wide variety of enzyme deficiencies and food intolerances that can be major contributors to gaseous distension and flatulence. Taking a Sherlock Holmes approach and trying an elimination diet is certainly reasonable. Enzyme supplements are commercially available and are another approach for an empiric trial if the suspect foods are not well defined. Medications can also interfere with enzyme activity and give rise to flatulence. Enzymes include proteases that digest proteins such as pepsin, pepsinogen, trypsin, trypsinogen, chymotrypsin, and chymotrypsinogen. Other enzymes include amylase, lipase, invertase, sucrose, maltase, lactase, and about one thousand six-hundred others!

It is important to take the appropriate enzyme with the appropriate food. The right enzyme for the wrong food, or the wrong enzyme for the right food, will not make a bit of difference in helping your digestion. The most common enzyme deficiency is lactase resulting in lactose intolerance. With over one thousand six-hundred known enzymes it is best to do your own Sherlock Holmes detective work with elimination diets or challenges to identify the foods you are best to avoid, or others will be avoiding you because of the intestinal gas that results.

All plants harbor the ability to generate digestive enzymes to break down the starch content of their own seeds and fruit. That is how the fertilized seed gets its nutrition for growth. In fact, we can take advantage of this property to ease our digestion of plants by letting them germinate before ingesting them. For some plants like sprouts and beans that is a very doable suggestion. For other fruits and plants by the time they germinate the starches have lost all culinary appeal to us. What may be surprising is the variety and diversity of enzymes the plants generate across various species. They number in the thousands and the vast majority have yet to be identified and analyzed. The development of plant genomics has accelerated our understanding of the vast diversity of enzymes we are exposed to. A number of plants also generate proteases to digest the plant storage proteins that a number of varieties have a rich storehouse of. For example, wheat has many endopeptidases. The plant world also uses proteolytic enzymes in defense against insect pests, to avoid being consumed by animals that do not assist them in their propagation.

Eructation (Burp, Belch) (see Aerophagia, Gastroesophageal Reflux Disease)

Commonly called a burp or belch the words are now synonymous with the medical term eructation. The English language, as all living languages, continues to evolve. Today the words are interchangeable but they were not always synonymous. In older times, a burp was considered an involuntary release of gas from the stomach. Encouraged and admired in infants and young children, tolerated in most cultures and societies if not in mixed company, and frowned upon by the female spouse, it was recognized as an involuntary act of nature. The belch however took on a more sinister demeanor being considered a voluntary and thus controllable outburst of gastric gasses. Although considered a talent worthy of development by adolescent males and those who remain in that mindset through their adult years, most of society frowns upon the activity.

Burping or belching may be a symptom of a hiatal hernia, GERD, or of lower esophageal sphincter dysfunction. The other dysfunction that is often associated with GERD and can lead to burping and belching is a motility disorder of the esophagus known as transient relaxation of the lower esophageal sphincter. As you can imagine, the lower esophageal sphincter (LES) isn't supposed to be tightly closed all of the time. The lower esophageal sphincter needs to relax every time you swallow to allow the material ingested to enter the stomach. It also needs to relax whenever you need to burp, belch, or vomit to allow for material to exit as well. The condition of transient relaxation of the LES is where the relaxation occurs for unknown reasons at an abnormal time, often without warning. It is much as if a security gate that is only supposed to open for authorized traffic opens on its own at random times. Many food products, herbs, pharmaceuticals, and social habits can contribute to relaxation of the lower esophageal sphincter by their carminative properties. The ability to identify and avoid these products may be the key to controlling gastroesophageal reflux disease without requiring expensive prescription therapy with potential side effects.

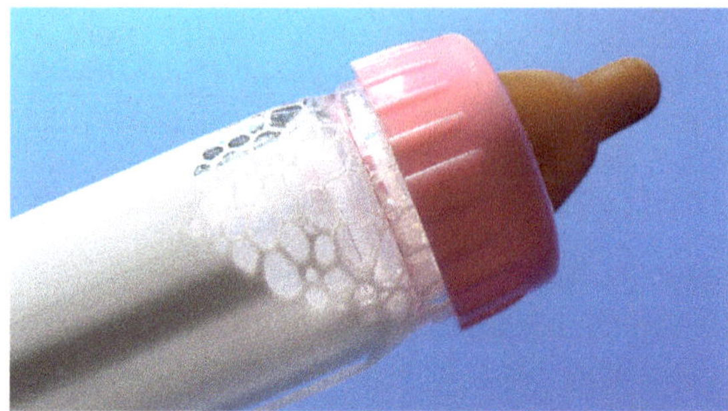

Baby bottles are a common source of aerophagia, air swallowing. Burping the baby after the feeding helps to release the swallowed air. Shutterstock/JohannaGoodyear

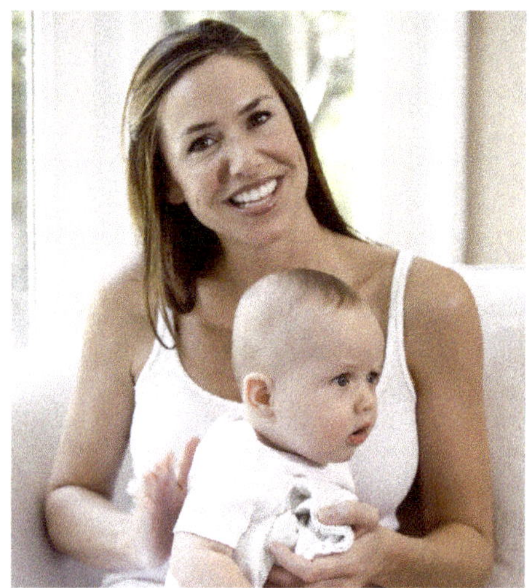

Burping the baby after the feeding helps to release the swallowed air. Shutterstock/GoldenPixels

Air swallowing is a universal event in humans and is also known as aerophagia. We do it with every one of the on average two thousand swallows we take every day, ingesting approximately five milliliters (one teaspoonful) of air with every swallow. Air is seventy-eight percent nitrogen, which is a poorly absorbed gas. If it is not released in a burp, it will contribute to bloating and distension. The volume of air swallowed is impressive, but is only a small percentage of what the digestive process can generate in terms of gas production.

Aerophagia is the swallowing of air, allowing it to enter the digestive tract, and it occurs naturally and without thinking in every individual. There is a variation of aerophagia in which the behavior becomes a purposeful, and at times obsessive-compulsive, behavior. More often, when excessive spontaneous aerophagia is occurring it is a subconscious or unconscious behavior, much like a nervous tic. The volume of air swallowed in these conditions can be impressive, and a plain x-ray of the abdomen may demonstrate that the entire digestive tract is filled with air from esophagus to rectum.

The important fact is that seventy-eight percent of air is nitrogen and the gastrointestinal tract poorly absorbs the nitrogen, unlike the oxygen and carbon dioxide. Once the nitrogen is swallowed it has only two ways to get out of the digestive tract. Coming up as a burp or belch is its closest exit, but it has to overcome the lower esophageal sphincter, the upper esophageal sphincter and the oncoming rush with peristalsis and gravity of more food, fluid, drink, saliva, and yes even more air being swallowed.

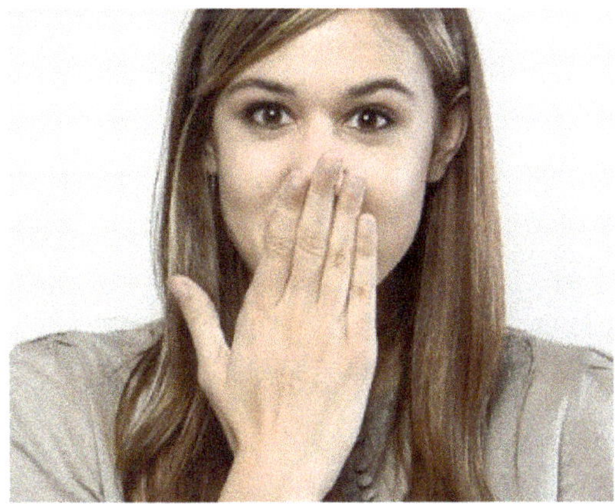

4.bp.blogspot.com Creative Commons License

Eructation is common after the ingestion of carbonated or nitrogenated (also called nitrogenized) beverages. The gas is kept in solution in the beverage while under the high pressure generated at the time of bottling or canning. Once the vessel pressure is released the release of gas is visible as bubbles arising in the beverage. When the beverage is ingested the bubbles of gas escape within the stomach. The common increase in temperature from a cold or room temperature beverage to higher internal temperature of the body also contributes to increasing the gas volume. The stomach will expand along with the gas accumulation until the intra-gastric pressure exceeds the pressure maintained by the lower esophageal sphincter. Once the sphincter pressure is exceeded the gas escapes as an eructation. The aroma of the gastric contents may escape with the eructation, so alcohol and the most recent meal ingested may discerned by those in near proximity.

A hidden source of swallowed air is the air content present within many foods. Many fruits contain a great deal more air than you would have imagined. If you take an apple and press all of the juice out you would have all of the air removed. When you add the volume of the juice and the pressed fruit together you will find that it was only sixty percent of the volume of the original fruit. In other words, of the entire fruit that you ate forty percent was air.

We have been in love with ice cream for thousands of years. All ice creams are not prepared in an identical manner. There is another important factor that leads to differences besides the ingredients such as cream or milk fat content, flavorings, sweeteners, stabilizers, emulsifiers, lactose, whey, casein, etcetera. It may be surprising to learn that the two largest ingredients in ice cream by volume are water (between fifty-five percent and sixty-four percent) and air (between three percent and fifty percent).

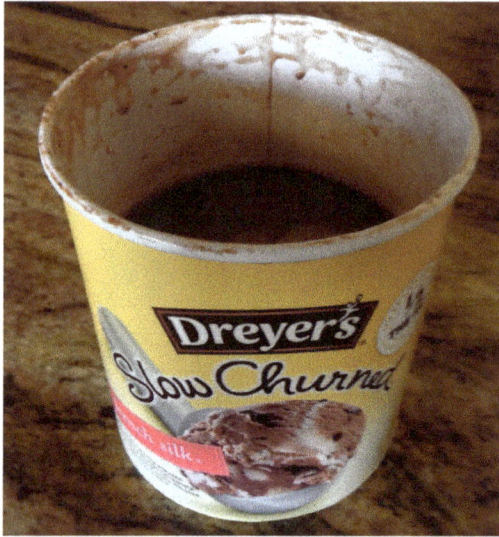

Overrun is the term used to describe air that is added into the finished food product to expand its volume as well as for texture. Air content of ice cream ranges from three percent to fifty percent and has a significant influence on texture, taste, and the value of the product purchased since ice cream is typically sold by volume, not weight. Photo by Lizabeth Weiss.

The same proposition is true for bread and most baked goods. The baking process often uses baking powder or yeast. When the dough rises you are seeing the additional volume of gasses such as carbon dioxide being produced by the yeast fermentation process. While we are on the subject of yeast, microbes of this type including *Candida albicans* are a normal constituent of the gut microbiome. Just like one sees with the rising of dough, the yeast organisms ferment carbohydrates and starches resulting in the release of gas. Excess yeast may lead to increase gaseousness. One of the thoughts as to why beer is known for producing intestinal gas are the residual yeast and carbohydrates, in addition to the nitrogen and carbon dioxide gasses already added to the beverage.

Many foods are whipped with air to increase their volume, which adds to the smoothness and creaminess of the product. It also adds to the bottom line of profitability to the manufacturer, as you are paying the commercial price for a product typically sold by volume, for extra air that virtually did not cost them anything. As long as they don't push it to the detriment of flavor and texture the more air added to a product increases its volume and profitability.

Carbonated beverages are very popular worldwide. In the United States sales of carbonated beverages exceed twenty billion dollars per year, four times the sales volume of dairy products. The majority consumed today already comes carbonated with large amounts of carbon dioxide forced into solution under high pressure. As the pressure seal of the can or bottle is released the carbon dioxide forms bubbles and comes out of the solution, giving a pleasant tickling sensation on the palate, and a full at times bloated feeling in the stomach and gut.

Nitrogen is poorly soluble in liquids, and the high density of bubbles contributes to a smooth creamy mouth feel. Most beers are saturated with a combination of thirty percent carbon dioxide and seventy percent nitrogen. The head serves both an aesthetic purpose, as well as accomplishing the dispersal of the beer aroma. You can get an idea of how high the nitrogen content is by looking at the size of the head created. A significant percentage of the volume of your drink is the head, and a friendly bartender will discard some of the head to give you more drink for your money, as well as to encourage a larger gratuity. Beer drinkers are famous for the burping and belching generated. The added nitrogen gives them an edge up in competitive burping and belching contests since it is not as rapidly absorbed and eliminated via the lungs as is carbon dioxide.

Yeast microbes including *Candida albicans* are a normal constituent of the gut microbiome. Just like one sees with the rising of dough, the yeast organisms ferment carbohydrates and starches resulting in the release of gas. Excess yeast may lead to increase gaseousness. One of the thoughts as to why beer is known for producing intestinal gas are the residual yeast and carbohydrates, in addition to the nitrogen and carbon dioxide gasses already added to the beverage. Nitrogen is also used in iced coffee beverages, providing a head of bubbles very similar to that of beer. Aerophagia is common with the use of chewing tobacco and even smoking tobacco whether as cigar, pipe, cigarette, or electronic smokeless cigarette. If you hold a conversation while you are eating it will cause even more air swallowing, as will drinking from a straw or tilting your head back to drink from a bottle or can. Rush through your meals and you swallow more air. See entry on aerophagia for more details

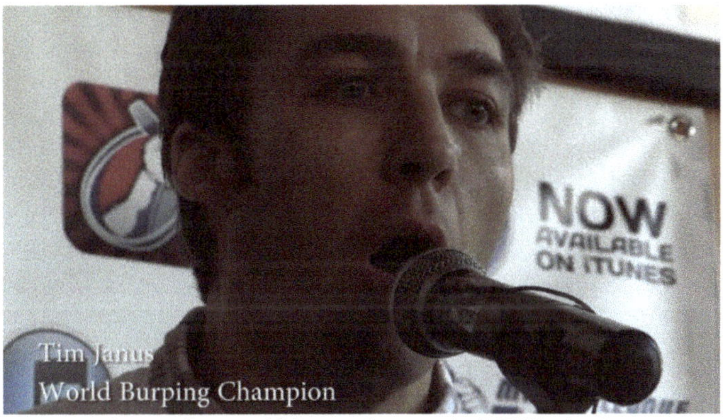

Longest burp at 18.1 seconds. youtu.be/gU3jBonhsrQ.

The World Burping Federation located in Geneva Switzerland holds the annual World Burping Championships. The *Guinness Book of World Records* has a listing for the loudest burp on record. The record holder is Paul Hunn of the United Kingdom. His burp was recorded with a car horn equivalent rating of nearly one hundred and ten decibels. The longest burp, by Tim Janus, has been recorded at over eighteen seconds. To achieve this record, he consumed approximately two gallons of Diet Coke and Mountain Dew. Imagine what would have happened if he swallowed a few Mentos tablets at the time of the competition.

Esophagus (Gullet, Foodpipe)

Esophagus (Greek oisophagos "entrance for eating.") (gullet) is a muscular passageway from the pharynx to the stomach. During swallowing, food passes from the mouth through the pharynx into the esophagus and travels via peristalsis to the stomach. There is an upper esophageal sphincter where it adjoins the pharynx and a lower esophageal sphincter where it joins the stomach, typically just below the diaphragm.

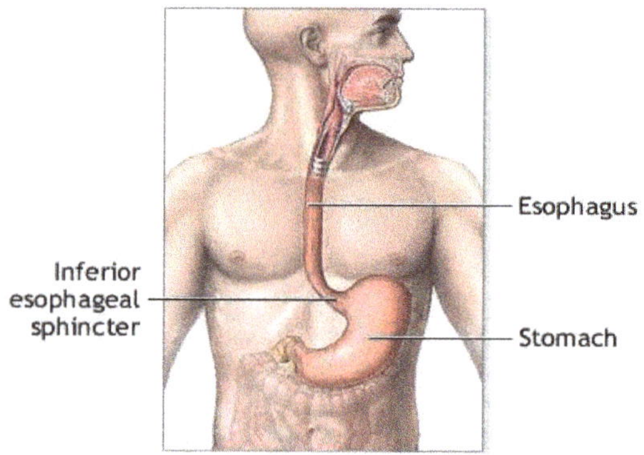

The lower esophageal sphincter is also referred to as the cardiac sphincter and gastroesophageal sphincter. It is a ring shaped area of high muscle tone at the distal esophagus typically just below the diaphragm that acts as a one valve to prevent gastroesophageal reflux except when vomiting is necessary. The lower esophageal sphincter is under involuntary control and is usually in a closed position. It relaxes during a swallow to allow the passage of the food bolus. In cases of gastroesophageal reflux disease, it may also relax inappropriately allowing acidic gastric contents back into the esophagus causing heartburn and mucosal damage. Lower esophageal sphincter pressure and relaxation are regulated by excitatory (e.g., acetylcholine, substance P) and inhibitory (e.g., nitric oxide, vasoactive intestinal peptide) neurotransmitters. Disorders of the lower esophageal sphincter can lead to the common disorder of gastroesophageal reflux disease (GERD) and its frequent symptom of heartburn. It also plays a major role in other conditions such as achalasia, nutcracker esophagus, and diffuse esophageal spasm.

The esophagus is normally lined by squamous epithelium similar to the mucous membrane lining the inside of the mouth. This epithelium is sensitive to acid and digestive enzymes and a competent lower esophageal sphincter is critical to protect it from reflux if gastric contents.

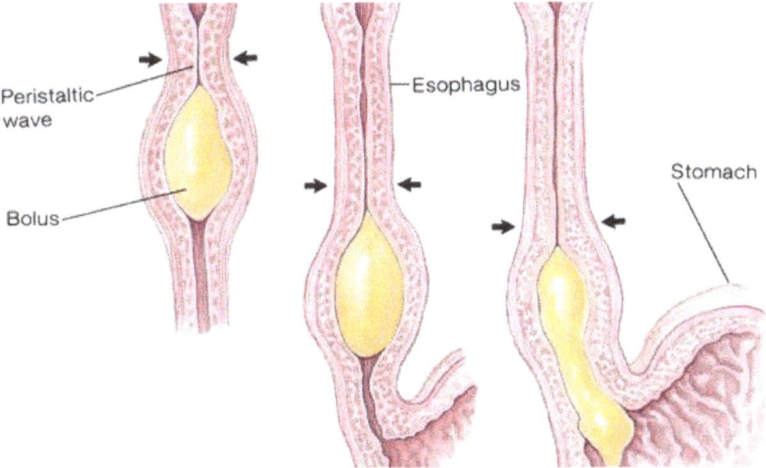

The symptom of heartburn is typically ascribed to the reflux or regurgitation of acidic stomach contents and may be a sign of gastro esophageal reflux disease (GERD). A number of esophageal disorders are associated with reflux and abnormalities of its motility. Unfortunately, cancer of the esophagus is not uncommon and its hallmark symptom of difficulty swallowing due to partial obstruction may make its first appearance when the disease is already incurable.

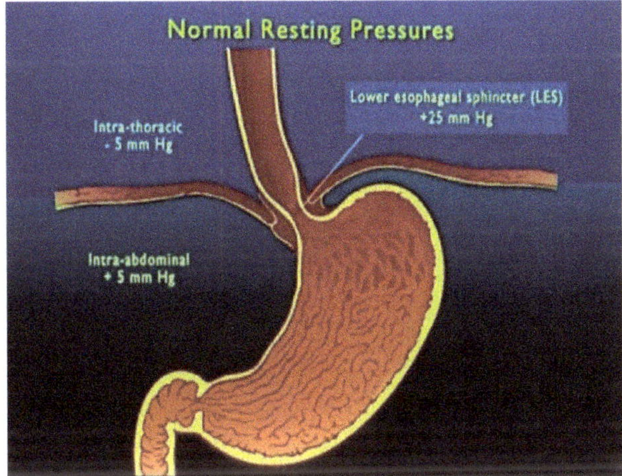

Pressure differential between intra-thoracic negative pressure of 5 mm of mercury vs. intra-abdominal positive pressure of 5 mmm of mercury, and lower esophageal sphincter (LES) pressure of positive 25 mm of mercury. Author presentation image.

Fart (Flatus)

The word fart is the correct word to use in the English language, and indeed is one of its oldest words. The alternative terms used, such as flatus and flatulence are not original English words as they have been borrowed from the Latin. There is controversy as to the derivation of the word fart. It is thought to have Indo-European roots in the Germanic language word farzen. One thought is that it originated as an onomatopoeia, a word that phonetically imitates the sound of the event it describes. Another thought is that it was related to the term for partridge, as the bird makes a similar sound when it is disturbed in its natural habitat and takes flight.

Farts are ubiquitous, all living creatures generate gas from the cellular respiration, and humans are no exception. The microorganisms in your intestinal flora produce microscopic nanofarts and microfarts, which collect into larger bubbles of gas in the bowel. They are intermixed with the atmospheric air swallowed throughout the day and particularly at meals, when chewing gum, when chewing tobacco, or when smoking tobacco or other recreational products.

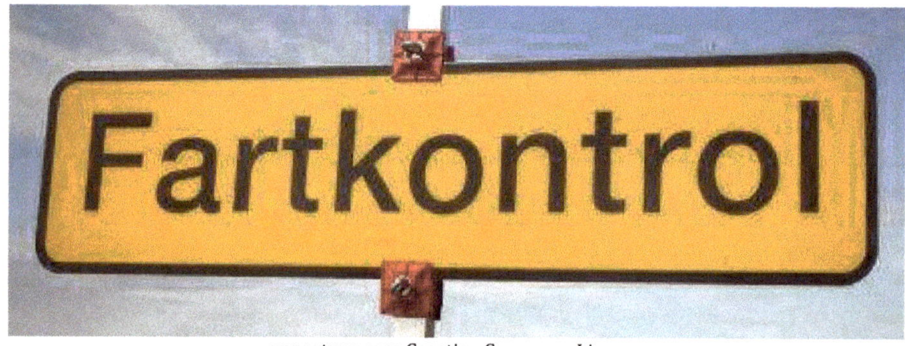

onpasture.com Creative Commons License

Aerophagia is universal, and we swallow on average three to five milliliters (one teaspoonful) of air with every swallow. Even when we are not eating or drinking, we regularly swallow the saliva we produce. The average human swallows over two thousand times a day. Chewing gum, hard candies, and use of chewing or smoking tobacco or other recreational products increase the volume of air swallowed. Drinking through a straw, directly from a can or bottle, or talking while eating, will also increase the amount of air swallowed.

Another common source of swallowed air is within the foods we eat. An apple is forty percent air by volume, and bread is over sixty percent air by volume. If you compress an apple or a loaf of bread, you will see that a sizeable portion of their total volume is air. Whipped foods, soufflés, and baked goods, all have high air content. Have you ever forgotten to put an ice cream container back in the freezer. Ice cream is typically forty percent air by volume and when it melts the air escapes, and the full container is no longer full. By the way, the ice cream industry knows that adding air, known in the industry as overage, enhances the mouth feel texture of the ice cream. They also know that it adds up to forty percent to the profit margin, because ice cream is sold by volume, not by weight.

Besides the swallowed air, additional gasses are produced during the enzymatic digestive processes, as well as the neutralization of gastric hydrochloric acid and pancreatic and duodenal bicarbonate. The result is that a large volume of gasses transit the bowel and a portion may be eliminated as a fart. Fortunately, the vast majority of the gasses produced are absorbed by the gut and then through diffusion into the bloodstream where it enters into solution. The gasses leave the blood when they arrive at the alveoli of the lungs where they are exhaled. The chemical component gasses have very different properties of diffusion through the bowel wall and into solution in the bloodstream.

Carbon dioxide readily diffuses and enters solution and is readily exhaled. It is the largest component of the volume of gas generated in the proximal intestinal tract. It is a major contributor to the temporary distension and discomfort that commonly occurs after a meal. Carbonation is also utilized as a common beverage enhancer and adds to the volume of carbon dioxide gas in the stomach. Carbon dioxide is the most rapidly absorbed component of intestinal gas and is the easiest to eliminate by simply exhaling it in the breath. As very little remains in the bowel, it is only a relatively minor component of a fart.

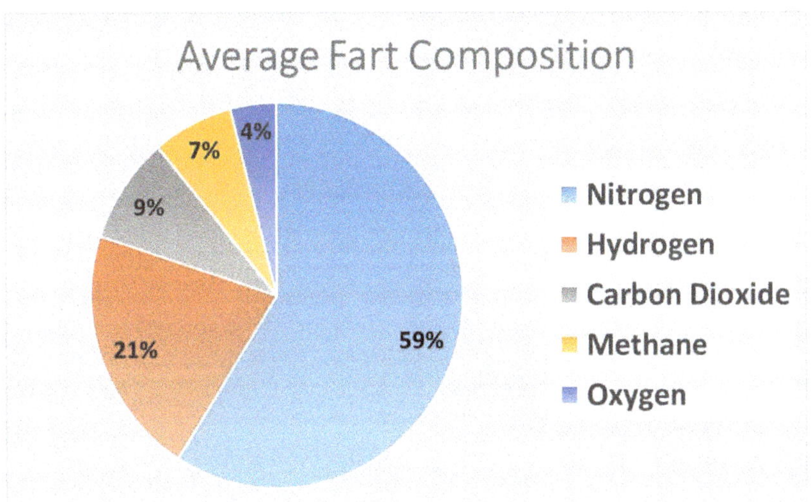

Creative Commons License

The volume of gasses in the gastrointestinal tract is dependent on many factors. The volume of gas produced is determined by the amount and nature of foods ingested, and the body's ability to synthesize and utilize specific enzymes for the various food types. The nature and quantity of the bacteria in the gut flora influences the nature of intestinal gas both by their active metabolism and by their ability to aid or hinder the digestive enzymes and processes.

One of the most common causes of excess gaseousness is the deficiency of the enzyme lactase. Lactase hydrolyses the complex disaccharide dairy sugar lactose into the readily absorbable monosaccharide sugars glucose and galactose. With insufficient lactase, the sugar molecule is not metabolized by the digestive system but is instead metabolized by the gut flora, also known as the microbiome. Lactase deficiency results in gas production and may also give rise to cramps and diarrhea. Another food sugar that can cause excess gaseousness is commonly seen in fruit and is thus known as fructose. The human digestive system can handle only a limited quantity of fructose at a time. If the fructose intake exceeds this capacity the gut flora ferment this sugar, with the release of gas, and often cramps and diarrhea.

That the microbes within our digestive tracts ferment foods that we have not fully digested is to our advantage, which is why the microbiome is considered essential to our good health. We can absorb some of the nutrients the microbes release in the fermentation process, including vitamins and bioactive molecules. We even use microbe fermentation in the preparation of many foods. When you add yeast to flour and watch the dough rise you are seeing the result of the release of gasses from the fermentation process. The spongy character of bread and cakes, and why they are sixty percent air by volume, is the result of the gas production of the yeast fungus. The characteristic holes in Swiss cheese are the result of microbial gas production. The entire production of wines, beer, and other alcohol beverages are based on microbial fermentation. In a very literal sense, we are ingesting the waste product of microbial fermentation.

Before you develop an opinion that a delicious baked good dependent on yeast farts loses some of its culinary appeals, recognize that this paradox was addressed hundreds of years ago. A French pastry delicacy is known as Pets de Nonne, also called Pets de Sœurs and translated as nun's farts. They are a dessert puff pastry dating from medieval times and made from butter, milk, flour, sugar, eggs and sometimes honey is added. They are traditionally pan-fried in lard and then baked. Their lightness inspired their name in French, pets de nonne and Pets de Sœurs. Another baked good named for its association with the fart is Pumpernickel (German: Devil's Fart) bread. It is a heavy dark brown bread traditionally made with coarsely ground rye flour and whole rye berries. It has been long associated with the Westphalia region of Germany for over five hundred years. Like most rye breads, it is traditionally made with an acidic sourdough starter, which inhibits the rye amylase enzymes. The name is associated with the coarse bread-giving rise to flatulence.

Beans are known as the musical fruit because of the gas they produce in all humans. The reason for this is that legumes contain complex sugars known as raffinose, verbascose, and stachyose. Humans and other animals lack the enzyme, called alpha-galactosidase, needed to metabolize these complex sugars into absorbable simple sugars. Without the enzyme, the complex sugars are fermented by the gut microbiome producing gas. Alpha-galactosidase is now commercially available as a dietary enzyme supplement to reduce the gas production associated with particular foods such as legumes. Another enzyme that humans do not possess is cellulase, without which we cannot digest the cellulose found in most plants and grasses. Herbivorous animals do have those enzymes, which is why they can subsist on grazing of grasses and forage.

Another factor in gas production is the speed of gastrointestinal transit. Drugs, hormones, food products, and illness may influence this. The absorptive capacity and health of the mucosal lining, and the physical length of the individual's gastrointestinal tract also play a role. The often-quoted figure of twelve farts per day is a reasonable approximation of the average number of farts passed, but there is a very wide range of what is considered normal. Besides the numerical quantity of farts passed per day is the question of what is considered an average volume of gas passed. If you are familiar with physics, a series of natural laws were defined that express the relationship between temperature, pressure, and volume. The relationship between temperature and pressure is direct, i.e. the higher the temperature, the larger the volume of space a gas would occupy.

The expansion to a larger volume of occupied space may result in intestinal bloating, discomfort, and increased burping and farting. The relationship with pressure is inverse, i.e. the greater the pressure, the smaller the volume.
We experience a change in intestinal gas volume based on temperature when we drink a cold carbonated or nitrogenated beverage. As the temperature of the gas increases from refrigerated to body temperature the gas volume increases dramatically. We will also often experience significant changes in volume due to pressure changes, as beverages from highly pressurized containers are exposed to the much lower pressures found within the intestinal tract they expand dramatically. Increases in pressure reduce the volume of gas, which is not a problem when it comes to the gut and our symptoms of gas if atmospheric pressure is increasing, such as with scuba diving or going down a mine shaft. It can become a major problem when the pressure decreases and the gas volume increases such as upon ascent from a dive or a mine, or going higher in altitude such as air travel or mountain climbing.

The atmospheric pressure changes as we go higher or lower from sea level. The effects on intestinal gas are seen in scuba divers, pilots, airplane passengers, mountain climbers, living at higher elevations, and even taking an elevator to the top of a skyscraper. When the pressure change is rapid, for example, a scuba diver returning to the surface, or an astronaut on the ascent to orbit, the consequences can be dramatic and life threatening and are known as barotrauma. Most gasses that are commercially available (oxygen, helium, air, etc.) are compressed and contained in hardened metal canisters that can withstand very high pressure. Compression of the gas allows for significant savings of space, for example allowing scuba divers to have the equivalent of a roomful of air within a single tank. The intestinal tract is flexible and expandable to a degree, more like a balloon than a metal container. As such changes in the surrounding atmospheric pressure can result in significant volume changes, which in the extreme of barotrauma may lead to perforation and rupture.

The fart would not be as notorious as it is if it were not for its aroma. Over ninety-nine percent of the gasses in a fart are odorless. While a number of individuals may have methane present in their farts, methane is odorless. If you smell a natural gas (methane) leak, it is not the methane you smell, but an odorant gas added by the gas company as a safety precaution to give notice of danger. The majority of the aroma from a fart comes from hydrogen sulfide, skatole, indole, and aromatic fatty acids, the majority coming from the digestion of animal fats. While vegetarians may fart more than carnivores, the aroma is not nearly as pungent or offensive.

Aerophagia is universal, and we swallow on average three to five milliliters (one teaspoonful) of air with every swallow. Added into the mixture are the gasses produced during the enzymatic digestive processes as well as the neutralization of gastric hydrochloric acid and pancreatic and duodenal bicarbonate. The result is a large volume of gasses transiting the bowel that may be eliminated as a fart. Fortunately the vast majority of the gasses produced are absorbed by the gut, then into the bloodstream through diffusion dissolving into solution. They are finally released when they reach the alveoli of the lungs and are exhaled. The component gasses have very different properties of diffusion through the bowel wall and into the bloodstream.

Carbon dioxide readily diffuses, enters solution, and is readily exhaled. It is the largest volume of gas generated and is the major contributor to distension and postprandial (after meal) discomfort. The good news is it is the easiest to eliminate from the bowel because of its rapid diffusion into the bloodstream. Carbon dioxide is only a minor contributor to flatulence. The volume of gasses in the gastrointestinal tract is dependent on the quantity and nature of foods ingested, and the body's ability to synthesize and utilize specific enzymes for the various food types.

The nature and number of microorganisms in the gut flora also play a major role. It may also be affected by the speed of gastrointestinal transit, which likewise may be influenced by drugs, hormones, food product, illness, absorptive capacity, and the physical length of the individual's gastrointestinal tract. The often-quoted figure of eleven and one-half farts per day is a reasonable approximation of the average number of farts passed, but there is a very wide range of what is considered normal. There are so many variables that what is reasonable for an individual can only be determined over a longer period than a single day.

Fart, Art

The fart has been the subject of numerous works of art over the ages. It has been represented in virtually all of the artistic media including literature, music, paintings, sculpture, cinema, photography, etcetera. It has been the material for live and stage performances for thousands of years, and of course is notorious for personal and up-close entertainment. The following images are just a few of the visual representations over the years. A thorough review of the fart through the arts is found in the unique companion volume to this book, entitled *Artsy Fartsy, Cultural History of the Fart.*

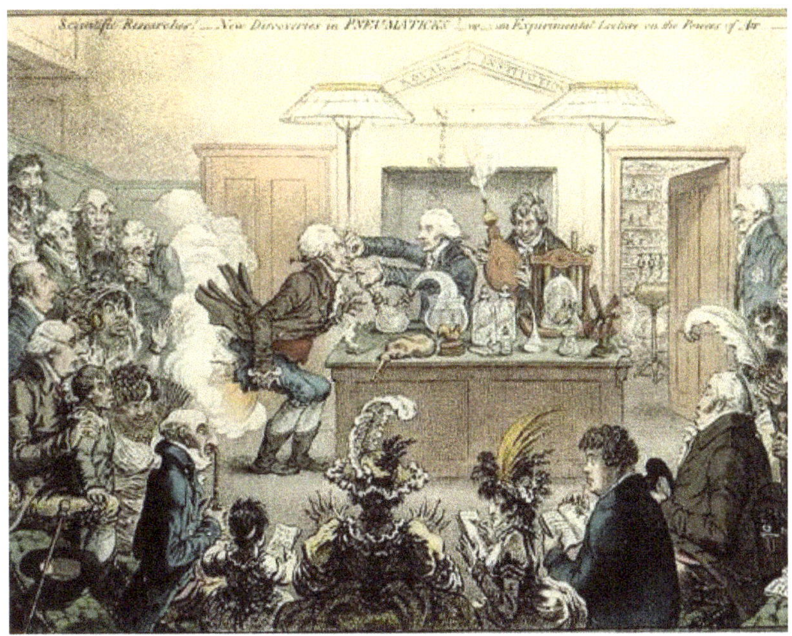

James Gillray, *Scientific Researches! New Discoveries in PNEUMATICKS! or an Experimental Lecture on the Powers of Air.* Public Domain

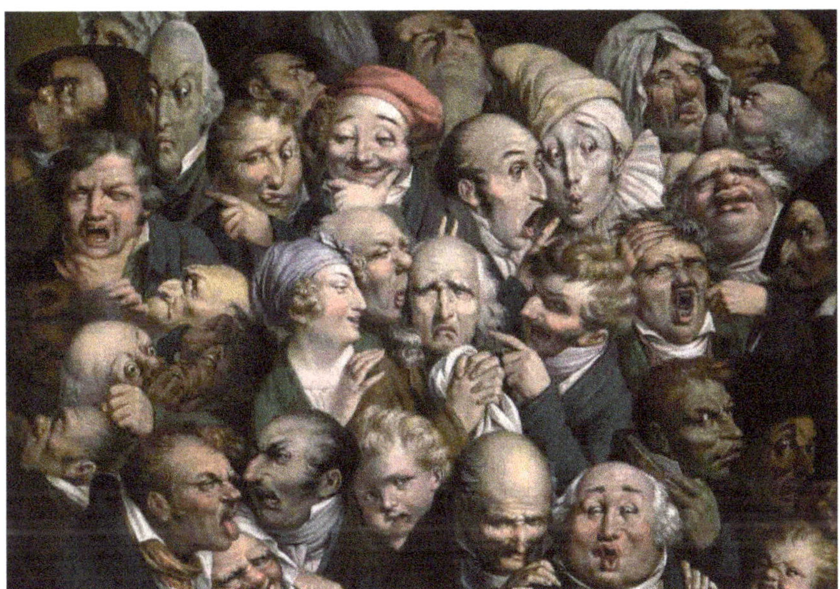

Louis-Léopold Boilly *Thirty-Six Faces of Expression.* Public Domain

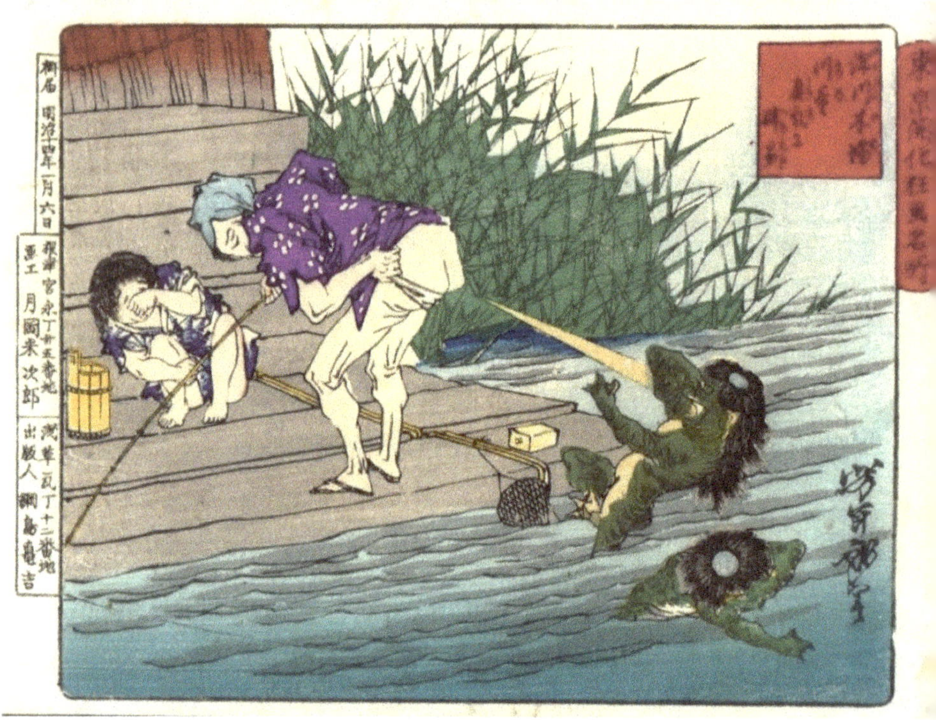

Public Domain

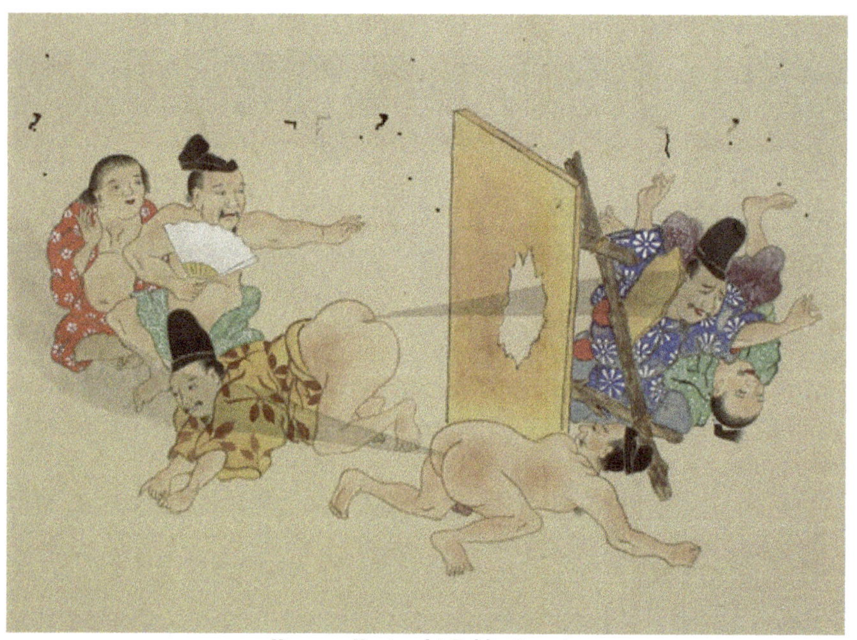

Utagawa Kuniyoshi, Public Domain

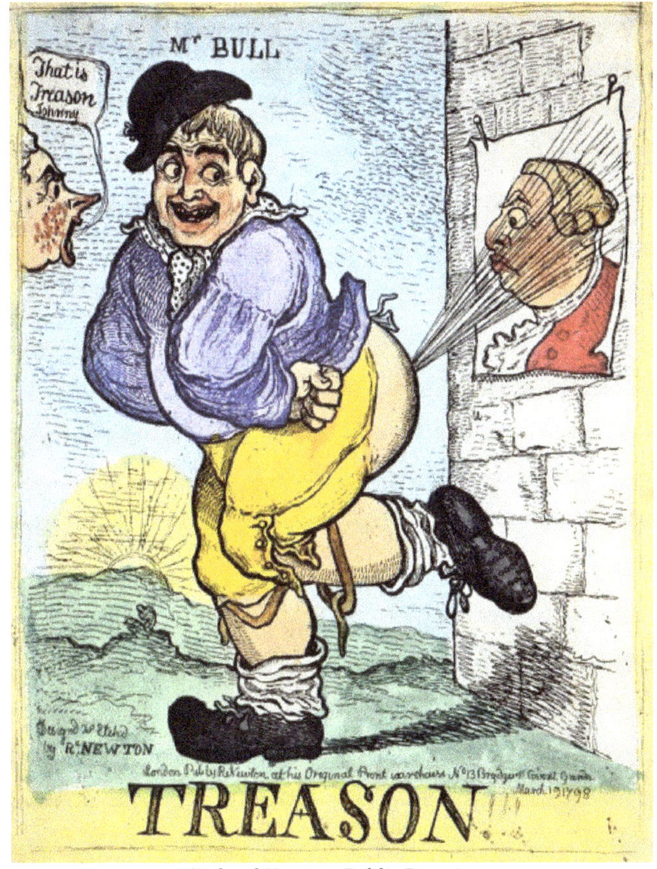

Richard Newton, Public Domain

Fart, Diffusion

The word Fart in northern European languages including German and the Scandinavian languages means speed. In you go by a school or hospital you may go by a no farting zone. Or you might receive a police citation for exceeding the fart limit! The sense of smell requires that molecules from the source material travel to the nasopharynx and touch the olfactory nerve receptors. The detection of a fart by odor requires the direct contact of the odorant molecule and the cilia of the nerve cell. Most people do not realize that a fart actually contains odorants as well as transmissible microbes, so although not as well recognized as a source of communicable disease like a sneeze or a cough, a fart could reasonably be considered a public health hazard, as well as a nuisance.

It is possible to become ill and acquire a pathogenic infection from a fart, similar to what can occur with a cough or sneeze. Coughing and sneezing release a large plume of aerosolized droplets impregnated with microbial pathogens. A single sneeze can disperse up to forty thousand aerosol droplets, which can transmit pathogens and disease. The sneeze is a much more effective dispersant of infectious material than a cough, speaking, or squeaking a fart. On the other hand, the farts plume of microbes is of fecal origin, giving rise to an entirely different microbial exposure, consistent with the fecal oral contamination route of many communicable diseases.

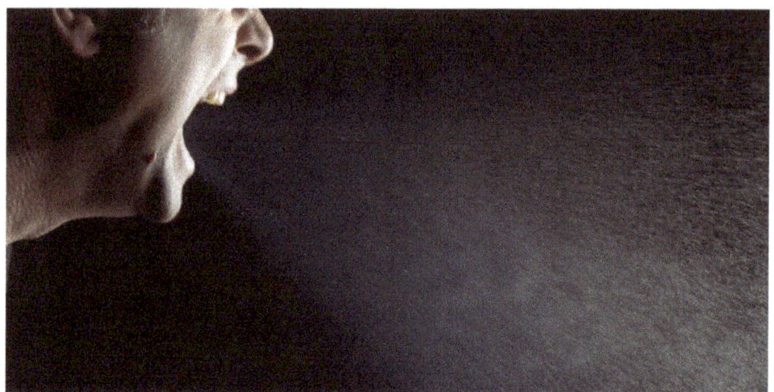

Shutterstock/JamesKlotz

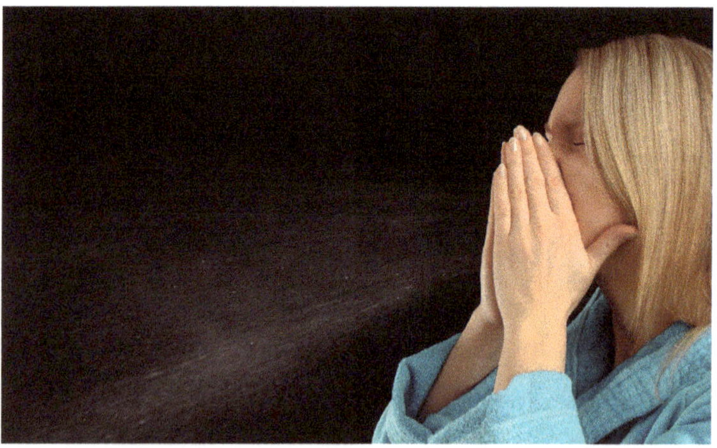

Sneezes reach a velocity of up to five hundred miles per hour (eight hundred kilometers per hour) Some sneezes are so loud the volume may give the impression that they have broken the sound barrier! Shutterstock/RioPatuca

A sneeze, or sternutation, is a powerful rapid expulsion of air from the lungs through the nose and mouth. The average velocity of a sneeze is forty-two meters per second), equivalent to approximately ninety-five miles per hour. The average speed of a cough is fifteen meters per second and the average velocity of the breath of ordinary speech is four meters per second. The sneeze and cough can quickly reach a velocity of over one hundred miles per hour (one hundred and fifty kilometers per hour) and has been recorded at speeds up to five hundred miles per hour (nine hundred and fifty kilometers per hour). These discharges will spread contaminants throughout a large size room. The flushing of a toilet will aerosolize fecal microbes that would cover a room with dimensions of twenty feet by twenty feet in a matter of seconds.

The mechanism of increasing intra-abdominal pressure for a fart is similar to generating intra-thoracic pressure for a sneeze. The size of the exit orifice is a major determinant of velocity. No one has voluntarily gotten close enough to a fart blast to measure its ejection velocity or count the vapor droplets. The brave soul who does so may not get a Nobel Prize, but would certainly be worthy of nomination for an IgNobel Prize.

Farts have been recorded with the speed of aroma travel at a conservative ten miles per hour. It was not clear if this was from an individual wearing clothing at the time. Science or a dedicated researcher somewhere will one day answer the question about fart speed. Perhaps a luxury watch company will sponsor a competition for the *Guinness Book of World Records* which has a number of fart categories already entered into the competitive arena, but somehow missed out on the exciting competition of fart speed!

Back in the 1946 a spoof recording of the International Crepitation Contest was created, and it is still commercially available today. It was produced by recording engineers for the Canadian Broadcasting Corporation and was supposedly held on February 31, 1946 as the World Championship Crepitation Contest. The fictitious location of the Maple Leaf Auditorium at Thunderblow, Canada between competitors Paul Boomer and Lord Windesmear completed the scene for the blow-by-blow description of the announcer.

Fart, Etymology

English is the richest language on the planet, with more words by far in its vocabulary than any other. This richness is due to the significant influence of its history of occupation by foreigners, especially during the days of the Roman Empire. Unlike other conquerors, the Romans did not impose their own language, in this case Latin, on the inhabitants of the British Isles. The population adapted their native tongue to include words borrowed from the occupiers and foreign influences. This led to the rapid expansion of the English vocabulary, including many different words that are synonyms.

The word fart is the correct word to use in the English language, and indeed is one of its oldest words. The alternative terms used, such as flatus and flatulence are not originally English words as they have been borrowed from the Latin. In Latin these words have the general meaning of a wind or a blowing.

There is controversy as to the derivation of the word fart. It is thought to have Indo-European roots in the Germanic language word farzen. The word fart may have originated as an onomatopoeia, a word that phonetically imitates the sound of the event it describes. Another thought is that it was related to the term for partridge, as the bird makes a similar sound when it is disturbed in its natural habitat and takes flight. How it made that transition may be an enlightening example of the evolution of words and language.

The Indo-European word *perd* means fart, and this led to the Latin word *pedere* the verb form of fart, and *peditum* the noun form of fart. The Indo-European *perd* led to the Greek word for fart πέρδομαι *perdomai*. It is also cognate with Sanskrit *pardate*, Avestan *pərəδaiti*, Italian *fare un peto*, French "péter", Russian пердеть (perdet') and Polish "pierd". The related Greek word *perdix* referred to a type of bird that made an explosive fart-like sound when it was flushed from the brush when startled. While being incorporated from Greek to Old French it became *perdriz*, then Middle English *partrich*, and finally Modern English *partridge*. The final step that has yet to be taken would be to complete the circuitous history and modify the name of the partridge to *fartridge*!

The word fart is also found in other languages, but there it often has a different and unrelated meaning. In the Scandinavian languages, it usually denotes speed or motion. In Danish and Norwegian, it is often used in combination with other words that obscures the meaning even more. For example in Danish a *fartcertifikate* means a trade certificate. In Norwegian, a *fart plan* means a schedule. The Norwegian phrase *stå på fartin* pronounced as stop-a–fartin means ready to leave. Likewise, the phrase *farts måler* pronounced as fart smeller refers to a speedometer. In Swedish, a speed bump is called a *farthinder*. *Fartlek* is speed training for athletes by running at alternate intervals of fast and slow paces.

Likewise if you travel on a Scandinavian marine vessel, you may see the control of engine speed labeled as *half fart* and *full fart* for half speed and full speed respectively. Fart kontrol zones are speed zones. In Germany, a similar word *fahrt* means a journey, trip, tour, or passage. It is often seen in signs that say e*infahrt* (sounds like in-fart) and *ausfahrt* (sounds like out-fart) denoting entrance and exit respectively.

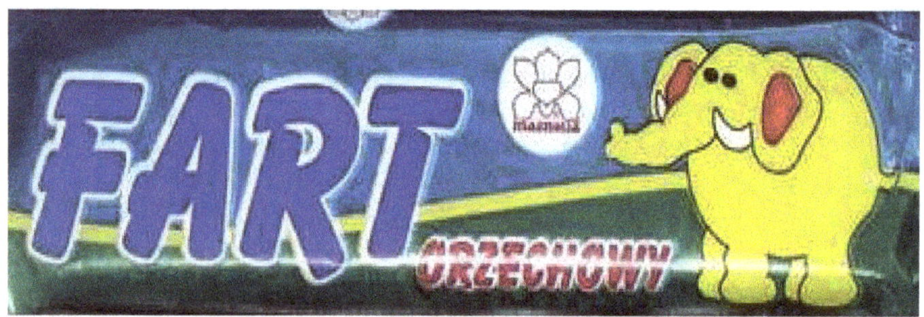

In Spanish and Portuguese *fart* means an excess of anything, especially food. One of the richest desserts they offer is called a *farte*, which means a fruit tarte in Spain, and usually a sugar almond or cream cake in Portugal. In Italy, the word *farto* means mattress. In Hungary, *fartaj* means buttocks. In Poland, if you want to buy a local favorite candy bar with a name that that means lucky, you will be looking for a *Fart* bar.

Several languages have a number of different words for variations on a theme for which there is only one word in English. The word snow is one example where we have a singular word, but the Inuit, Eskimo, Aleut, Sami and other languages of the native people of the Arctic and northern latitudes may have hundreds of words. When it comes to the word fart, the English language is very limited with just the singular word. I will not leap to the conclusion that the language that has the most words for fart needed to do so for necessity. Their population may or may not have the world's highest rate of fart production, but they certainly have the most descriptive fart words.

The Russian words for fart include *perdyozh* (first act of breaking wind), *perdun* (perpetrator and outcome), *perdil'nik* (place from where it comes), *Perun* (ancient God of wind), *bzdun* (silent fart), *bzdyukha* (silent fart as well as a stupid jerk). Some of the Russian verbs for the action of farting are particularly colorful. *Perdet'* (to fart with or without sound), *bzdet'* (to fart silently), *pereperdet* (to fart repeatedly), and my favorite word *nabzdet'sya* (to fart silently to one's complete and utter satisfaction!).

The word fart is one of the oldest words in the English language. One of the most influential dictionaries in the long history of the language is Samuel Johnson's *A Dictionary of the English Language* published in 1755. An important innovation in his dictionary was the use of quotations from literature to illustrate the usage of the word defined.

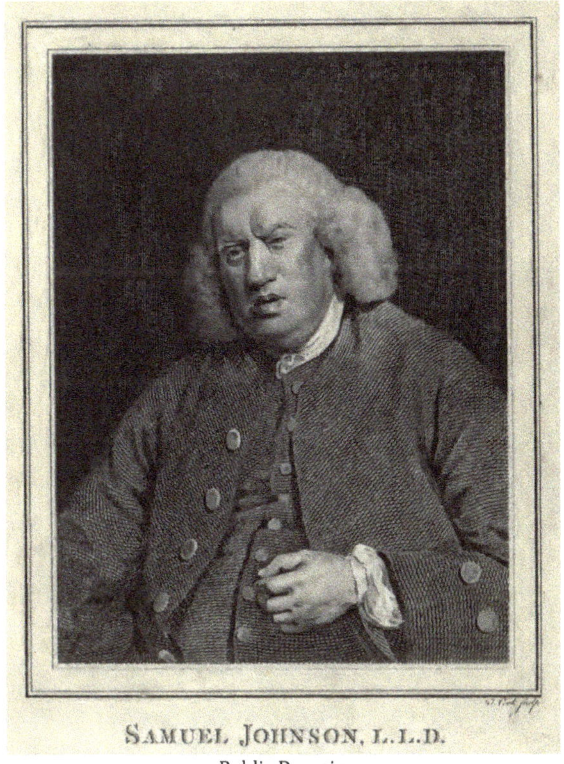

Public Domain

The word fart is proper English and was in use for hundreds of years before relatively recent polite and civil society considered it taboo. Without an alternative term, euphemisms were created and used. The number of terms that were synonymous with fart numbers in the many hundreds.

FART. *n. ſ.* [ꝼeꞃꞇ, Saxon.] Wind from behind.

Love is the *fart*
Of every heart;
It pains a man when 'tis kept cloſe;
And others doth offend, when 'tis let looſe. *Suckling.*

To FART. *v. a.* [from the noun.] To break wind behind.

As when we a a gun diſcharge,
Although the bore be ne'er ſo large,
Before the flame from muzzle burſt,
Juſt at the breech it flaſhes firſt;
So from my lord his paſſion broke,
He *farted* firſt and then he ſpoke. *Swift.*

Public Domain

The origins of these phrases and their acceptance into the cultural lexicon, are often obscured. Sometimes new words are added directly by an author creatively using a newly invented word in a literary work. I am fond of a new word coined by David Gilmour, an entrepreneur, and philanthropist. He described a word that combines the sense of anticipation and subsequent disappointment, when the experience is not as satisfying as expected. The word he created 'anticipointment' is a portmanteau that should stand the test of time.

I am tempted to add to new words in the lexicon as well. I am using the author's prerogative to place the word in print below, and although I have not heard them elsewhere before, someone may well have created them before me. The word is fartigenic, or its alternative, fartogenic. Fartigenic is a portmanteau combining the word fart, with the Latin root suffix -genic of Genesis and creation fame. The term describes a substance, which induces the creation of a fart. Refried beans and chili con carne would be good examples of fartigenic foods.

The colloquialisms, idioms, and synonyms that for better or for worse, are part of the lexicon can be found in a number of resources including the unique companion volume to this book *Artsy Fartsy, Cultural History of the Fart.* This volume provides an informative and entertaining overview of the fart through human history and culture, including works of literature, music, and the arts.

Fart, Flammable (see Methane, Hydrogen, Oxygen)

The individual gasses that make intestinal gas flammable (inflammable and flammable are synonyms and interchangeable words, their antonym nonflammable means the exact opposite) and explosive are hydrogen, methane, and oxygen. Hydrogen is a chemical element which has the symbol H and atomic number one. It is the lightest element and in its single atom form it is by far the most abundant element in the universe, comprising approximately seventy-five percent of its total identifiable mass. In the earth's atmosphere as the diatomic H_2 molecule, it is a colorless, odorless, tasteless, non-toxic, highly explosive gas. Most of the hydrogen on Earth is in molecules such as water and organic compounds because hydrogen readily forms covalent bonds.

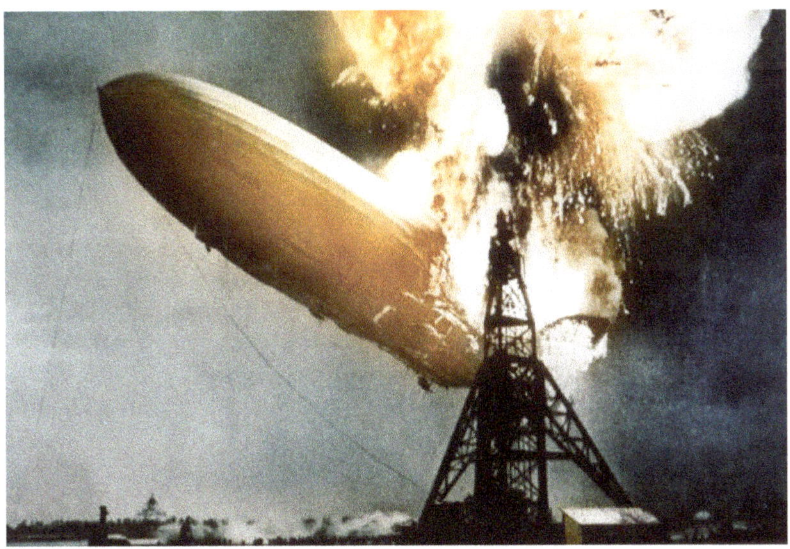

Public Domain

Hydrogen is lighter than air and lighter than helium. Unfortunately, it is also explosively flammable. Hydrogen fires are less destructive to immediate surroundings because of the buoyancy of H_2, which causes the heat of combustion to be released upwards as it ascends in the atmosphere. On May 6, 1937, the hydrogen-filled German airship Hindenburg burst into flames while attempting to land at Lakehurst, New Jersey. In little more than thirty seconds, the largest object ever to soar through the air was incinerated with a tragic great loss of life.

In 1766, Henry Cavendish was the first to identify hydrogen gas. In 1783 Antoine Lavoisier gave the element the name hydrogen (Greek ὕδρω hydro water and γενῆς genes creator) when he and Laplace confirmed Cavendish's finding that water is produced when hydrogen is burned. Methane is produced in the human intestinal tract by microbial organisms. Methanogens are microorganisms of the Kingdom Archaea, not bacteria as previously thought. They produce methane as a metabolic byproduct in anaerobic conditions when oxygen is not present.

Methanogens have been found in a variety of extreme environments, and can thrive and reproduce in boiling water as well as in ice cores taken miles down in arctic glaciers. They are common in wetlands, where they produce marsh gas, and in the digestive tracts of animals and humans where they generate the methane content of flatulence as well as the ruminant belch. It was discovered by Carl Scheele Sweden in 1773, but his publisher delayed publication for two years. The delay in publication inadvertently allowed British clergyman Joseph Priestley, who independently discovered it a year later, to be given priority as its discoverer because his work was published first.

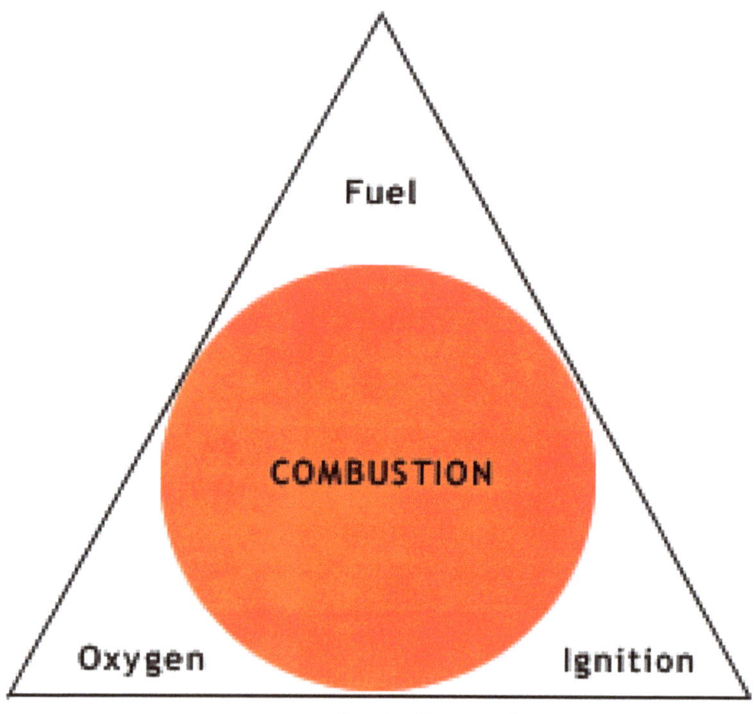

www.omega.com Creative Commons License

Oxygen is a chemical element with symbol O and atomic number eight that forms dioxygen a colorless odorless and tasteless gas. It was mistakenly named Oxygen (the Greek ὀξύς (oxys) "acid", and γόνος (gonos) "producer"), by Antoine Lavoisier because he incorrectly thought that all acids required oxygen. Acids actually require the element hydrogen, not oxygen.

Oxygen is a highly reactive element that forms compounds with most elements except the noble gases. Oxygen is a strong oxidizing agent, and only fluorine has greater electronegativity. Oxygen is the third most abundant element in the universe, after hydrogen and helium. On the surface of the Earth, it is the most abundant element making up half of the earth's crust and nearly twenty-one percent of the air.

Intestinal gas that contains hydrogen or methane, in addition to oxygen, is potentially combustible. Electrical cautery devices used during routine colon and intestinal surgery can potentially ignite these gasses. With the advent of colonoscopy electro-cautery loop snares to remove colon polyps was developed. A few cases of fatal colonic explosions occurred before the danger of explosive intestinal gas was recognized as a risk of the procedure. The bowel preparation solution was found to increase hydrogen and methane gasses and raised the risk of explosion. The bowel preparation has been changed, and carbon dioxide is often used to inflate the colon to reduce the risk of explosion even further.

hydrogen and methane are combustible gasses and in the presence of oxygen and an ignition source, you have a potent flammable commodity. When methane burns, it has a characteristic blue flame that you may see in a pilot light if you have a gas stove or furnace. Adolescent males and those who remain as adolescents intellectually have a fondness for demonstrating their dragon like ability to be human flamethrowers by igniting their farts. The lighting of farts is not a recommended activity, and severe injury has resulted from the successful ignition of flammable gasses near exposed sensitive anatomy.

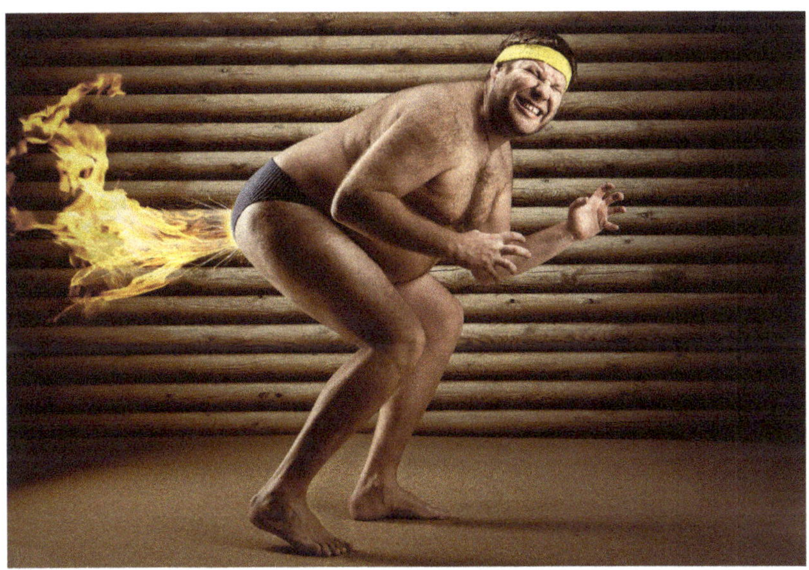

Shutterstock/Nomad_Soul

One of the more unusual injuries from a lit fart was second and third degree burns on the buttocks and a broken arm. The stout gentlemen was sitting on the toilet defecating and farting extensively for some time. Being overweight his buttocks formed a firm seal around the toilet seat, retaining all of the gasses in the enclosed space of the toilet bowl. He was smoking at the time and made a little space under his cheeks to innocently toss the lit cigarette into the toilet bowl. It promptly ignited blowing him off the seat, shattering the porcelain toilet bowl, and causing extensive burn injuries to his buttocks. His wife called the paramedics, and as he was being carried down the stairwell to the waiting ambulance he told them what caused the explosion. They laughed so hard they dropped the gurney thus breaking his arm.

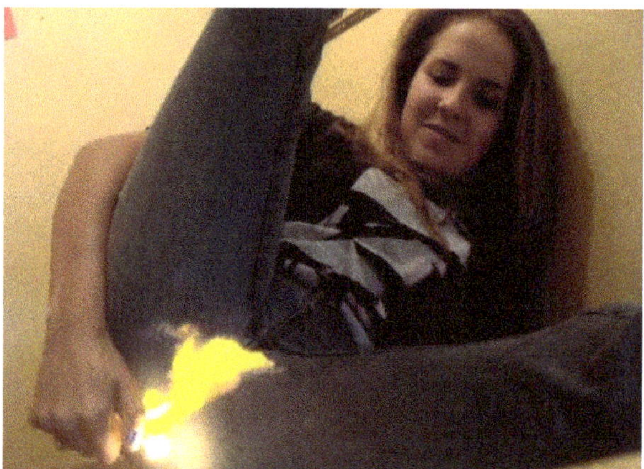

Moment of ignition of a fart, video is at youtu.be/Zt9rvaijpPY

Hydrogen and methane are the two flammable gasses that may be found in a fart making them flammable. Lighting a fart to see if one produces these gasses is a dangerous activity. Significant burns to the anogenital area have occurred, especially when ignited without a clothing barrier. The popular television show *Mythbusters* filmed an episode confirming that many farts are indeed flammable. It appears that the network found the episode too provocative and, perhaps for liability concerns that children watching might attempt their own demonstrations, decided to not 'air' the episode.

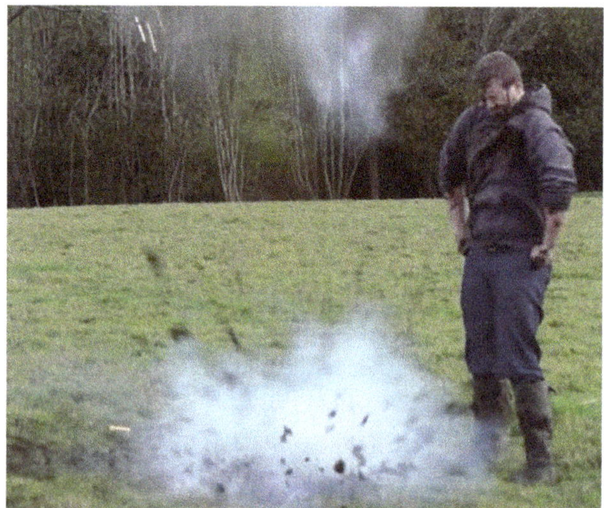

Lighting a match to a pile of cow dung is not a sign of higher intelligence. The methane and hydrogen generated by the microbes active in the manure pile may accumulate to explosive levels. youtu.be/bZI1eeV88lQ

On occasion dung and excrement can be more than just flammable, it can be explosive. The microorganisms that produce hydrogen and methane that lead to ignitable farts continue their activity while sitting in a pile of manure. For those foolish enough to light a match in a pile of cow dung to see what happens up close and personal the link to the video above should be convincing.

Now that you know intestinal gasses are flammable see if the numbers from the following Internet survey surprise you with how many people already knew this from personal experiments.

Women: Have you ever considered lighting one of your pass intestinal gas?

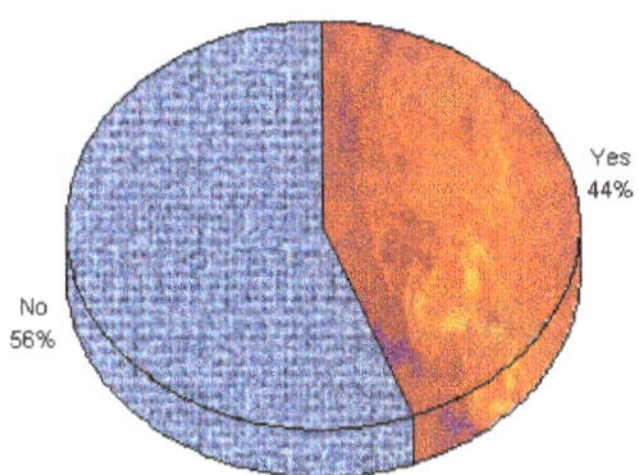

Almost half of the women surveyed indicate that they have considered an attempt to ignite their release of intestinal gas. They may not have done it or tried it, but they have thought about it.

Women: Have you ever attempted lighting one of your passages of intestinal gas?

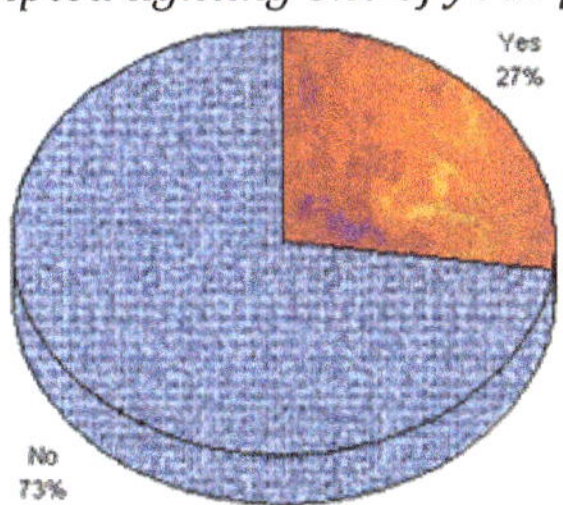

About a quarter of the women surveyed have attempted to ignited their passed intestinal gas.

Women: When you attempted to light your passed intestinal gas, did it ignite?

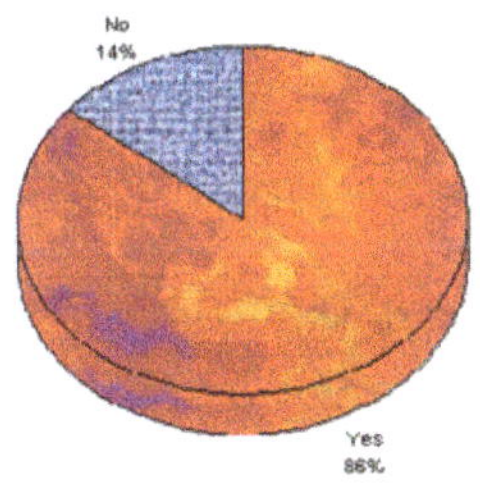

The large majority of women that have made the attempt were successful in confirming that the gas was flammable. The other fourteen percent may not have tried to ignite enough gas, or their diet and gut flora did not generate a flammable mixture of gasses. It appears that most women in the survey passed intestinal gas that burned with a blue flame due to the methane. Those who produced hydrogen had intestinal gas that burned with a yellow flame. Yellow flame was the second most common flame color.

Women: If you have lit your pass intestinal gas have you ever gotten burned?

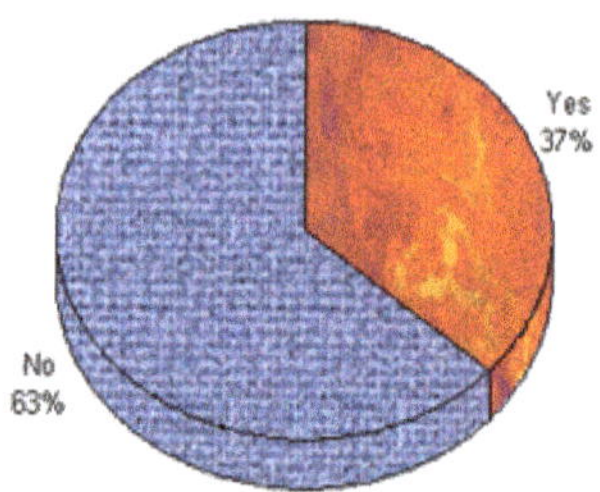

Women: If you lit your own pass intestinal gas and been burned was the of burn of your body, hair, or pants:

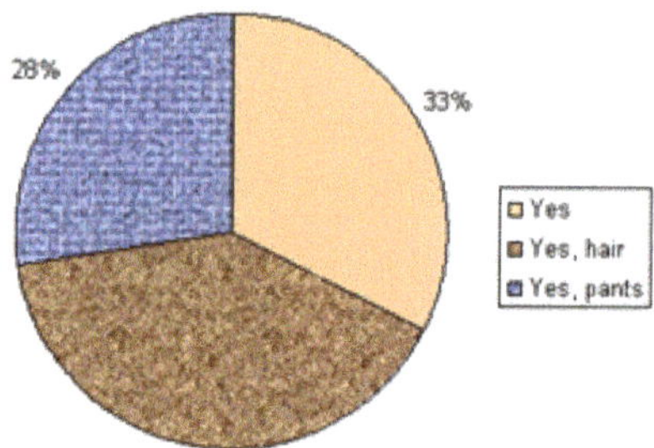

Lighting passed intestinal gas can be very dangerous. About a third of the women that admit lighting their intestinal gas ended up getting some type of burn. About half of these burns consisted of just the singeing of hair. Twenty-eight percent of these burns consist of burning a hole in one's underwear, and thirty-three percent are unfortunate enough to burn their skin.

Women: Have you ever lit another person's intestinal gas?

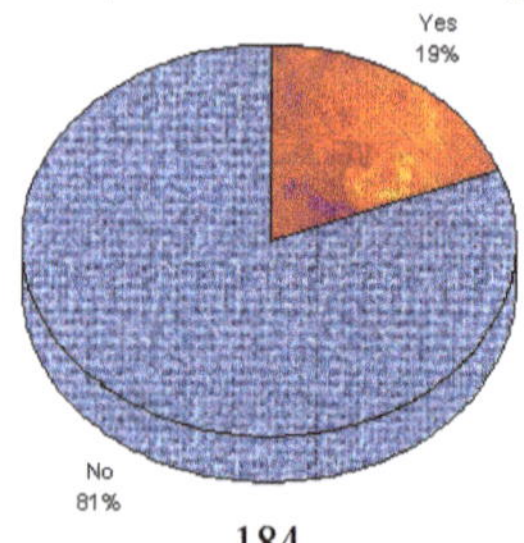

About one-fifth of the women surveyed were brave or foolish enough to light another person's intestinal gas. Most of these experiences were with friends or spouses. About half of the women surveyed admit seeing someone light a fart.

Spontaneous Human Combustion

As explosive and flammable farts are a well-recognized phenomenon, a theory has developed that they may also be responsible for spontaneous human combustion. A rare and bizarre event, spontaneous human combustion has been a proposed explanation of cases where a human body is consumed by flame without an external source of ignition. Typically the body is incinerated but the surrounding area has not been damaged by fire. Once a body begins to burn the tissue can continue to fuel the flames with a wick effect drawing on melted fat and other tissues.

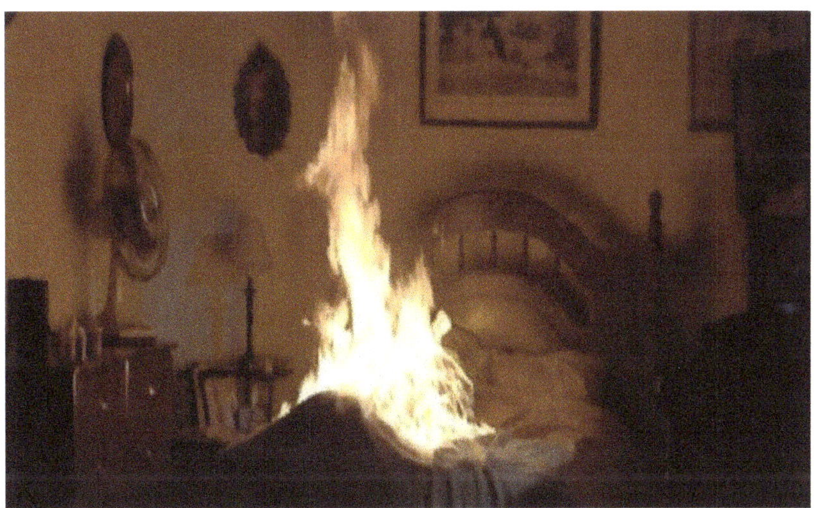

img.gawkerassets.com

Although the external source could not be identified, there are several potential explanations. Combustible fuel is undoubtedly present, perhaps as the gases methane and hydrogen, flammable clothing and alcohol, as well as body fat. Human fat is similar to the animal fats that were used in tallow candles. The external ignition source may have been a cigarette or spark of static electricity. Curious rural phenomena with similar spontaneous combustion effects include swamp gas, St. Elmo's fire, ball lightning, gamma ray discharges, and others.

Static electricity is an imbalance of electric charges between objects. As the imbalance is discharged with the transfer of electrons between the objects, most people can feel, see, and hear the spark of the static shock. Lightning is a static discharge, different only in its intensity. A spark, which is responsible for the majority of industrial fires and explosions, occurs between objects at different electric potentials.

The energy released in a static electricity discharge may vary over a wide range and the charge buildup increases as the humidity decreases. As little as 0.2 millijoules is the ignition energy required for methane, and a miniscule 0.017 mJ is the ignition energy for hydrogen. The low spark energy is often below the threshold of auditory, visual, or sensory perception of humans and may the source of the ignition that appears to be spontaneous.

The ignition of the flammable gasses of hydrogen and methane often present in a fart may thus appear to be a spontaneous occurrence. Of course, there may have been a more obvious source such as a lit cigarette that was consumed in the event, never to be found. There is a saying in medicine that is used as analogy for the search for a disease that will explain the symptoms. When you hear hoof beats, look for a horse, but be prepared for a zebra.

In spontaneous human combustion, the most likely explanation is an accidental fire from a cigarette. The cigarette may ignite the clothing and then the wicking effect continues to burn fueled by human tissue and fat until the body fire has exhausted itself. To be a bit more creative one can imagine a large fart with hydrogen and methane attracted the pet dog to come over and investigate the noise and smell. Close contact of the pet may have released a static spark and the rest is history. When in doubt, the standard excuse is to simply blame the poor dog.

Fart, Frequency

The fact is that all living creatures create gas from the cellular respiration, which is ubiquitous through a variety of life forms. The bacteria in your intestinal flora generate microscopic nanofarts and microfarts, which collect into larger bubbles of gas in the bowel. They are intermixed with the atmospheric air swallowed throughout the day and particularly at meals, when chewing gum, chewing tobacco, or smoking tobacco or other recreational products.

Aerophagia is universal, and we swallow on average three to five milliliters (one teaspoonful) of air with every swallow. Now add into the mixture the gasses produced during the enzymatic digestive processes as well as the neutralization of gastric hydrochloric acid and pancreatic and duodenal bicarbonate. You now have a virtual windstorm of voluminous gasses transiting the bowel.

Fortunately, the vast majority of the gasses produced are absorbed by the gut. They then enter into the bloodstream through diffusion, finally being exhaled when they reach the alveoli of the lungs. The component gasses have very different properties of diffusion through the bowel wall and into the bloodstream. Carbon dioxide readily diffuses and enters solution and is exhaled. Carbon dioxide is the largest volume of gas generated, and is a major contributor to distension and postprandial (after meal) discomfort. It is also the gas most readily absorbed and eliminated from the bowel. Carbon dioxide is thus only a relatively minor contributor to flatulence.

Nitrogen is the largest volume component of atmospheric air, and as would be expected, represents an identically high proportion of the gasses swallowed through aerophagia. Once in the body the carbon dioxide of the air is absorbed and eliminated as discussed above. The nitrogen however, is a very poorly absorbed gas, and will either come back up as a burp or come out the other end as a fart.

The oxygen in the air, representing nearly twenty-one percent of the air gasses swallowed during aerophagia, is absorbed slowly, as the gut is not nearly as efficient at oxygen absorption as the lungs are for respiration. As the carbon dioxide and oxygen are absorbed the percent of the gastrointestinal tract air that is nitrogen increases. As soon as the digestive process begins, the hydrochloric acid of the stomach is neutralized by bicarbonate of the duodenum and pancreas. Large volumes of carbon dioxide gas are generated, as are smaller quantities of hydrogen, methane, and other aromatic gasses.

The amount of gas in the gastrointestinal tract is dependent on the quantity and nature of foods ingested, and the body's ability to synthesize and utilize specific enzymes for the various food types. It is also dependent on the nature and number of the microorganisms in the gut flora, and the speed of gastrointestinal transit. Gastrointestinal transit may be influenced by drugs, hormones, food product, illness, the absorptive capacity of the mucosal lining, and the physical length of the individual's gastrointestinal tract.

The question of what is the average number of farts per day is similar to the question if what is an average price for a typical used car. To answer that question you would need more information, such as which year, make, model, condition, diesel or gas or electric or hybrid, mileage, etcetera. The quoted figure for fart production of eleven and one-half farts per day is a reasonable approximation. It came from a very small sample size of male medical students, but how one defines normal is subject to a very wide range depending on the variables. The female medical students were too smart to participate in the study, so as far as science knows, women do not fart.

Later suggestions that they fart, but less than the guys, is just as suspect. The differences in the physical attributes of the male and female of a species represent their sexual dimorphism. The theory of sexual selection advanced by Charles Darwin in 1871 is closely associated with sexual dimorphism. On average, adult humans males are four percent taller and eight percent heavier than females. In a number of other species, it is the female that is larger, occasionally dramatically so. The triple wart sea devil, an anglerfish, exhibits extreme sexual dimorphism. The male becomes little more than a stunted sperm-producing body permanently attached to the female. It lives a parasitic existence off of the females hard work and effort in providing livelihood and producing the next generation of offspring. Some human males appear to have evolved their behavioral patterns from the anglerfish modus operandi.

In most mammals, humans included, the males are larger in size, mass, and caloric intake. In most species is the female that is diminutive in size, sometimes dramatically so. It would only make sense that males would generate more gas, but how do the two compare if the caloric intake and composition were identical. Since there are no identically comparable cases studies, one would have to study averages from large populations of each gender and minimize the variables as much as possible.

As curious as we may be to know the answer to this question vital to gender politics and security, no studies are planned or anticipated. There have been reports of extreme flatulence in the medical literature of what may be considered the upper limits of the normal range, up to one hundred and fifty farts in a twenty-four hour period. There are probably more accurate reports of what is the upper limit of spousal tolerance in divorce court proceedings and depositions.

For general health we talk about achieving our target heart rate during exercise. Is there an equivalent for a target fart rate? For harmonious relationships, ideal would be below the quoted figure of eleven and one-half farts per day, that way you could reasonably suggest that you fart less than average. You could also argue that the twenty-three farts you passed were each only a half-fart so you still are within the normal range.

As we age, we produce less digestive enzymes, and there is an argument to be made that there should be an adjustment and tolerance allowed for 'old farts'. The sheer number of variables allow many explanations for why you fart much less than expected for your given circumstances. But perhaps the best excuse is that you did not do anything, it is the billions of nanofarting and microfarting microorganisms that are to blame. If you are told to pick on someone closer to your own size, you could blame the dog and claim it is a talented ventrilo-farter.

Trying to arrive at a definition of what constitutes a discrete individual fart is a challenge worthy of drafting and getting unanimous approval of a United Nations resolution. Is a staccato stutter, often very small farts completed in rapid succession, to count as one single fart or as ten? Is one large long loud fart the equivalent of four small farts over thirty seconds. Should a loud eardrum shattering tuba blast count the same as a faint and dainty toot? Perhaps the nebulous definition should allow the creator of the uniquely individual fart poetic license.

Fart, Global Warming

Global warming due to greenhouse gas production from human activity is mainly due to deforestation, the combustion of fossil fuels, livestock enteric fermentation and manure management, and landfill emissions. In terms of biomass, bacteria would be the main contributors to global warming by their methane production. A ruminant (Latin *ruminare* - to chew over again) is a mammal that digests plants in a multi compartment stomach through bacterial fermentation. It regurgitates the semi-digested mass, called cud, and chews it again and repeats the swallow.

The process of re-chewing the cud is called "ruminating". There are about one hundred and fifty species of ruminants, which include both domestic and wild species. Ruminating mammals include cattle, goats, sheep, giraffes, yaks, deer, camels, llamas, and antelope.

Other contenders nominated have been termites, which have over two thousand species and are prolific methane producers (initial reports suggested that they produce forty percent of global methane), livestock such as cows, sheep, and pigs, and lastly dinosaurs, which are no longer around to defend their reputations.

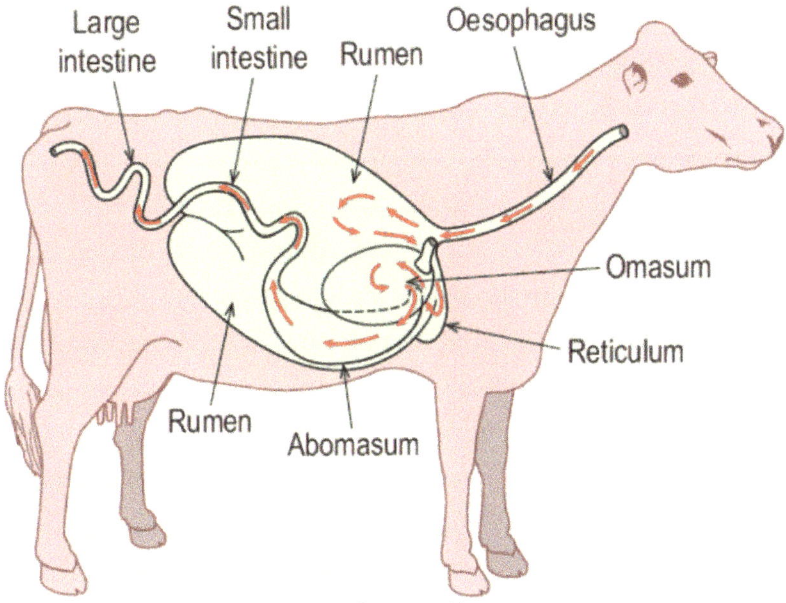

Creative Commons License

Ruminant bacterial fermentation is a significant contributor to global methane production, which is over twenty times as potent a greenhouse gas compared to carbon dioxide. To incentivize efforts to reduce livestock methane production a number of countries have proposed taxes on the release of greenhouse gasses. University of Alberta, Canada, Professor Stephen Moore is examining the genes from ruminant stomachs with the goal of developing a cow breed which burps less to reduce methane in the greenhouse gases responsible for global warming. A different approach is being undertaken by Professor of Animal Nutrition Winfried Drochner at the University of Hohenheim, Stuttgart, Germany. A fist-sized plant-based pill bolus combined with a special diet and strict feeding times reduces the methane produced by cows. "Our aim is to increase the wellbeing of the cow, to reduce the greenhouse gases produced and to increase agricultural production all at once. It is an effective way of fighting global warming. We could use the energy to boost the cow's metabolism, the fist-sized tablets mean that microbiotic substances can slowly dissolve in the cow's stomach over several months," said Professor Drochner.

Another method being used to reduce methane emissions is reducing the grass and low efficiency foods the livestock are receiving that require excessive fermentation. Replacing the feed with a diet higher in energy and rich in edible oils can reduce methane production by up to twenty-five percent. New Hampshire-based Stonyfield Farm reduced emissions from their cows an average of twelve percent by adding alfalfa, flax, or hemp to livestock feed. "If every U.S. dairy farmer reduced emissions by twelve per cent it would be equal to about half a million cars being taken off the road," said Nancy Hirshberg, Vice-President of Stonyfield's Natural Resources department. It took extensive scientific experimentation to collect the intestinal gasses of herds of cattle before it was discovered that the methane production was coming from the other end of the cows and other ruminants. It is the burps and belches from the multi compartment ruminant stomach that is the primary source of methane.

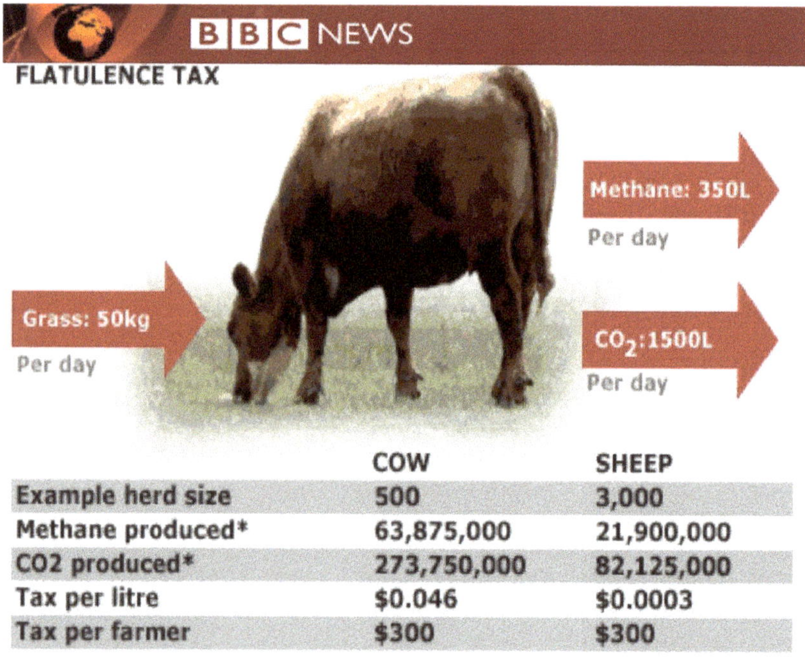

	COW	SHEEP
Example herd size	500	3,000
Methane produced*	63,875,000	21,900,000
CO2 produced*	273,750,000	82,125,000
Tax per litre	$0.046	$0.0003
Tax per farmer	$300	$300

*- Litres per year

In spite of it being labeled as a flatulence tax, the predominant source of global warming from ruminants comes from fermentation in their multi compartment stomachs. It should really be called a burping and belching tax, but that is not as newsworthy.

Kangaroos are herbivores and as marsupial their burps and farts contain little or no methane, a potent greenhouse gas. It appears that the reduced methane emissions are due to the microbes in the kangaroos' gut flora. Australian researchers hope that introducing a similar gut flora to other methane producing herbivores such as cattle and sheep will contribute to a reduction in greenhouse gasses and the resultant global warming. Methane can cause about twenty times as much atmospheric warming as an equivalent volume of carbon dioxide.

Kangaroos, like cattle and sheep, are ruminants that re-chew their cud with the assistance of the gut flora to digest and metabolize their cellulose based grazing diet. In the foregut the meal is broken down by fermentation with carbon dioxide and hydrogen released. In cows and other ruminants, microbes called methanogens transform these gases into methane. But in the kangaroos' guts the same hydrogen and carbon dioxide may be utilized by bacteria called acetogens to produce acetate, a volatile fatty acid.

These microbes compete with methanogens to use the carbon dioxide and hydrogen, so the more acetogens the less methane production. The odds are in generally in favor of methanogens, since the process of methane production is generally more energy efficient than producing acetate. One of the acetogen microbes, *Blautia coccoides,* is in the gut flora of cows as well as in kangaroos. Further research is being undertaken to understand why the organism is more successful in competing with the methanogens in kangaroos than in other herbivores.

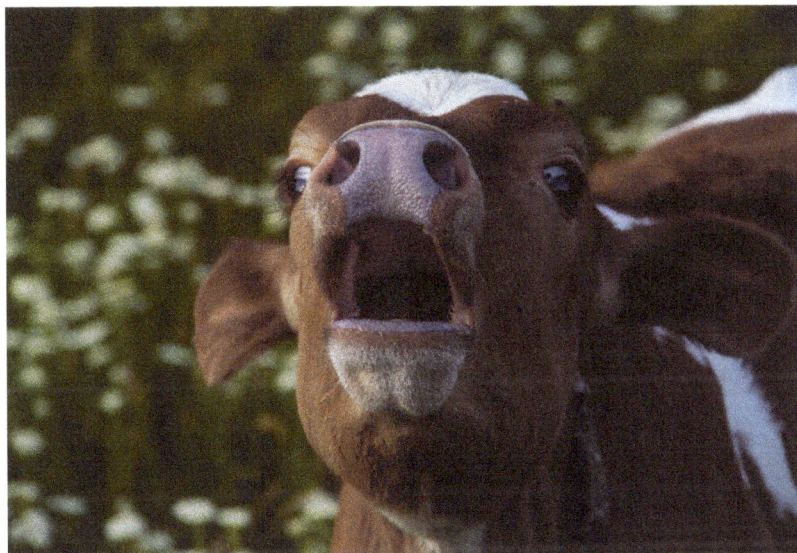

It is the burps and belches from the multi compartment ruminant stomach that is the primary source of methane. Shutterstock/AlisaBurkova

Carbon dioxide, methane, nitrous oxide (N_2O), and three groups of fluorinated gases (sulfur hexafluoride (SF_6), hydro fluorocarbons (HFCs), and per fluorocarbons (PFCs) are the major greenhouse gases impacted by human activity. These are regulated under the Kyoto Protocol, an international treaty that was adopted in 2005. Nitrogen dioxide (NO_2) warms the atmosphere three hundred and ten times more than carbon dioxide and methane twenty-one times more than carbon dioxide. Although CFCs are greenhouse gases, regulations were initiated because CFCs' cause ozone depletion, not because of their contribution to global warming. Ozone depletion itself has a relatively minor effect on greenhouse warming.

Dinosaurs are no longer around to defend themselves and have been accused of contributing to global warming. We do not know if they were ruminants and contributed by belching up gasses as well, but there should be no doubt that they were big time farters. Their nickname "thunder lizards" may have more to do with their farts than their footsteps. For more information about fart contributions to global warming see entries on methane and carbon dioxide.

Fart, History & Culture (Art, Music, Literature)

Artsy Fartsy: Cultural History of the Fart is a fascinating and factually correct review of the common fart through human culture and history. The cough, sneeze, hiccup, stomach rumble, burp, belch, and other bodily sounds simply cannot compete with the notoriety of the fart. Whether encountered live and in person or through the medium of literature, television, film, art, or music it may leave a powerful and lingering memory.

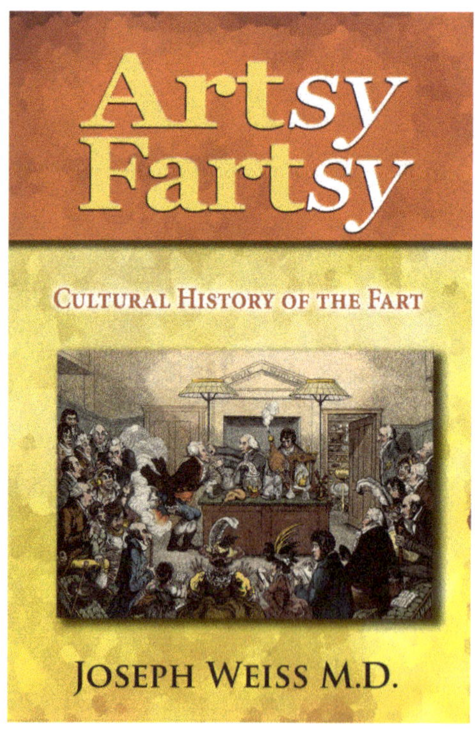

The history of the fart in culture and society is a seldom told but fascinating tale. The very same fart that has triggered wars and the deaths of thousands of innocents (see entry on Flavius Josephus) has also led to the laughter and entertainment of millions worldwide (see entry on Joseph Pujol and Cinematic

Arts). Even today the response to a fart can reach from the extremes of triggering violence to inducing spasms of uncontrollable laughter.

The intent of *Artsy Fartsy: Cultural History of the Fart* is to demonstrate that the ubiquitous fart has a more illustrious story to share than just lowbrow humor. The societal standards and cultural acceptance of this normal physiologic event have evolved over the years, and it is currently popular as a point of humor even in sophisticated circles. *Artsy Fartsy*, is a chronological survey of some of the high and low points in the cultural history of this ubiquitous but inherently controversial activity. Rather than an exhaustive and long-winded discourse, this volume is meant to introduce the reader to the colorful and extremely varied response to the fart over the course of human history.

The book provides an entertaining overview of the fart in human culture and history, not an extensively referenced academic treatise. The number of references to farts in the arts, especially over the recent years, is so numerous that a complete list is not practical or possible. The good news for those wanting more in depth information about any author, artist, or topic of interest is the powerful reference resource of the Internet. I expect that many will be surprised that the fart was a subject near to the hearts and minds of many illustrious and enlightened notables over the course of thousands of years of human history. The cultural mores of Western society have evolved and the fart has become a normal physiological event that has become more tolerated, although not yet universally accepted.

Fart Non-Human

Blue Whale

The Blue Whale is the largest animal on Earth, up to one hundred feet (thirty meters) long and three hundred and forty thousand pounds (154,545 Kilograms or one hundred and seventy tons). The blue whale is a mammal that ingests and digests up to sixteen thousand pounds (7,272 kilograms or eight tons) of plankton per day. The whale digestive tract generates large quantities of gas and when the blue whale releases a fart the bubble expands as it rises to the surface. The decreasing atmospheric pressure as it continues to rise contributes to its expansion as described in physics by Boyle's Law. When it just reaches the surface of the ocean the fart bubble is so huge it could easily enclose and asphyxiate a large horse. The smell is just as powerful as its size would predict.

Cat

Cats fart just like dogs, but they are wiser and more discreet. Because they are generally more diminutive in size than dogs they are not as easily identified or innocently blamed as the source of the fart. The alpha-galactosidase enzyme has also been marketed as a veterinary product with the brand name Curtail. It has been offered as a solution for dogs and cats that have farted one time too many. Although that particular product is no longer actively being marketed, the active ingredient is alpha-galactosidase. That is the same enzyme found in other products marketed for human consumption to reduce intestinal gas production.

Cow, Sheep, & Ruminant

A ruminant (Latin *ruminare* - to chew over again) is a mammal that digests plants in a multi compartment stomach through bacterial fermentation. It regurgitates the semi-digested mass, called cud, and chews it again and repeats the swallow. The process of re-chewing the cud is called "ruminating". There are about one hundred and fifty species of ruminants, which include both domestic and wild species. Ruminating mammals include cattle, goats, sheep, giraffes, yaks, deer, camels, llamas, and antelope. Ruminant bacterial fermentation is a significant contributor to global methane production, which is over twenty times as potent greenhouse gas. Please see the entries on Global Warming and Methane for more details about ruminant gas production.

Dinosaur

Dinosaurs are no longer around to defend themselves and have been accused of contributing to global warming. We do not know if they were ruminants and contributed by belching up gasses as well, but there should be no doubt that they were big time farters. Their nickname "thunder lizards" may have more to do with their farts than their footsteps.

The hulking sauropods were widespread about one hundred and fifty million years ago, and methane-producing microbes aided the sauropods' digestion by fermenting their plant food. Dave Wilkinson of Liverpool John Moores University, Graeme Ruxton from the University of St Andrews, and methane expert Euan Nisbet at the University of London studied the implications. Wilkinson, Ruxton, and Nisbet calculated global methane emissions from sauropods to have been approximately five hundred and twenty million tons per year. By comparison modern livestock ruminant animals produce methane emission of up to one hundred million tons per year.

There is a common public misperception that petroleum is predominantly derived from the organic remains of the great dinosaurs. Rather than the enormous dinosaurs, it was microscopic bacteria that produced the petroleum reserves of our time period. Single-celled bacteria evolved in the earth's oceans about three billion years ago, and were the dominant life form on the planet until about six hundred million years ago. In fact, if dominant is qualified as largest by biomass, bacteria retain that distinction today.

As microscopic as the individual bacteria may be, the bacterial colonies known as "mats" were of enormous proportions. They had masses of millions of tons compared to the hundred tons for the largest dinosaur, the sauropods. As these massive colonies died off and decayed they subsided to the bottom of the sea and were covered by layers of accumulating sediments. Over millions of years these layers of sediment thousands of feet underground were compressed under tremendous pressure and temperature, and developed into the liquid hydrocarbons we recognize as petroleum.

The vast majority of the world's coal deposits date back to the Carboniferous period, about three hundred million years ago. The first dinosaurs would not make their grand entrance in the evolutionary timetable until seventy-five million years later. During the Carboniferous period the earth was heavily forested. With the death and decomposition of these trees and plant life buried under great pressure and temperature under heavy layers of sediment, they were transformed into solid coal rather than liquid petroleum. As the search for petroleum and coal preserves often entails drilling and excavation of deep layers of sediment, it is not uncommon for fossils of dinosaurs and other prehistoric forms of life to be uncovered. The discovery of a theropod dinosaur during fossil fuel exploration in China has been given the appropriate name Gasosaurus. It looks as though Dino's story may have come full circle.

Dog

Dogs are just like any other organism, they do fart. Some breeds fart more than others especially the short snouted English bulldog and similar breeds that are serious air swallowers and farters. Several hundred years ago lap dogs were specifically bred to be small enough for a lady to keep with her at all times and if intestinal gas ruffled her undergarments it would not ruffle her composure as she would simply excuse her dog for the emission

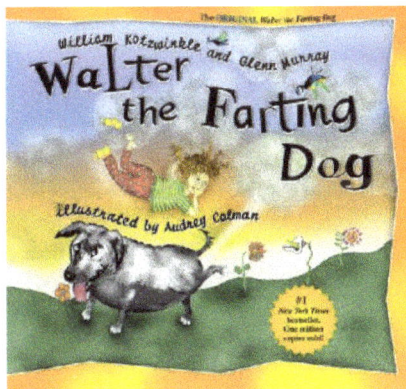

Walter the Farting Dog by William Kotzwinkle & Glenn Murray.

Hippopotamus

The hippopotamus (Greek hippos-horse and potamus-river) is considered by many experts to be the most dangerous animal in Africa (excluding the malaria carrying mosquito) having killed many more people than lions have. The hippo is extremely aggressive with its huge canine teeth and sharp incisors, unpredictable and fearless of humans. Most deaths occur when the victim gets between the hippo and deep water or between a mother and her calf.

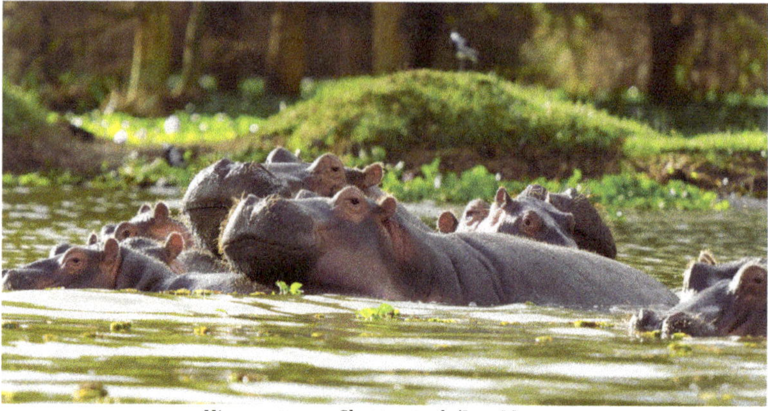

Hippopotamus Shutterstock/IvanMateev

Hippos weigh up to eight thousand pounds, gallop at eighteen miles per hour (twenty-nine miles per hour), sleep or lounge around on riverbanks and in the water most of the day, and graze on the grasslands at night. Their skin secretes a sticky pinkish oil that helps protect them from the sun. They defecate generous amounts of excrement into the rivers and ponds in which they wallow all day, punctuated by voluminous farts. They also participate in marking territory by what the hippo experts refer to as "dung showering." They blow feces mixed with urine over a large area around their watering hole, twirling their relatively short tails like fans to distribute the aromatic spray.

Horse

The well-known phenomenon of horse farts have been exploited on television with an episode of the comedy series *Seinfeld* entitled *The Rye*. Cramer feeds the horse a beef and pasta meal pulling a hansom carriage in Central Park in New York City. It makes the horse so extremely flatulent that Cramer and the passengers in the carriage cannot bear the gas exposure.

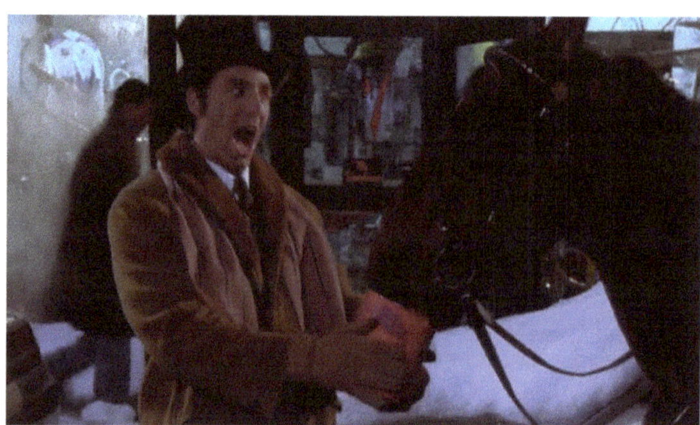

mapsaboutnothing.wordpress.com

A similar equine theme took place in a prime and extremely expensive American football Super Bowl advertisement for Budweiser beer. A man and a young woman are in a romantic horse drawn carriage. He presents her with a lit candle and reaches down to pull up some bottles of Budweiser beer. As he is out of the way getting the beer the horses tail lifts, releases a fart, and the candle explodes in a ball of flame singeing her features. When he resurfaces he smells smoke and asks if she smells a barbeque.

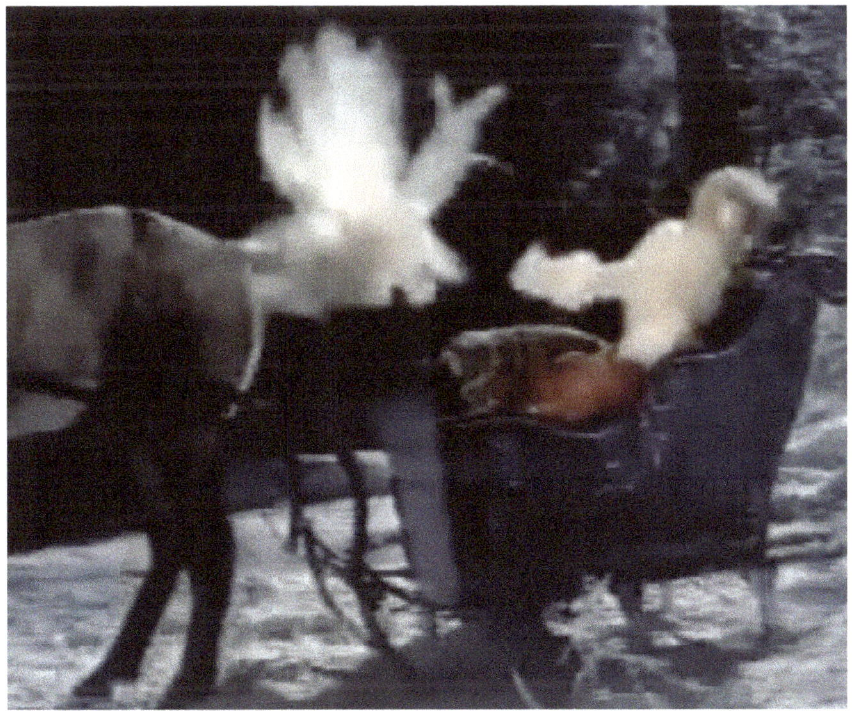

critbritlit.blogspot.com Creative Commons License

Ronald Wilson Reagan (1911–2004) was the fortieth President of the United Sates. I heard an apocryphal story from a normally reliable source that served in a high position in the administration of former president Ronald Reagan. Then again the source was a politician, which should automatically double the suspicion that this story was just the continued passage of excessive hot air. Her Majesty, Queen Elizabeth II was visiting the presidential ranch, Rancho Cielo, in the Santa Ynez Mountains of California. The ranch is at a high elevation (Rancho Cielo is Spanish for Sky Ranch) and as both the president and queen are horse aficionados they went for a ride on the ranch trails. At higher altitude, as you may recall from Boyle's Law of the physics of gasses, the atmospheric pressure is less than at sea level and the volume of gasses expands. The horse's intestinal tract likewise experienced expanding gasses and being natural animals they release it at will, even if they are in the presence of a Royal Queen and President.

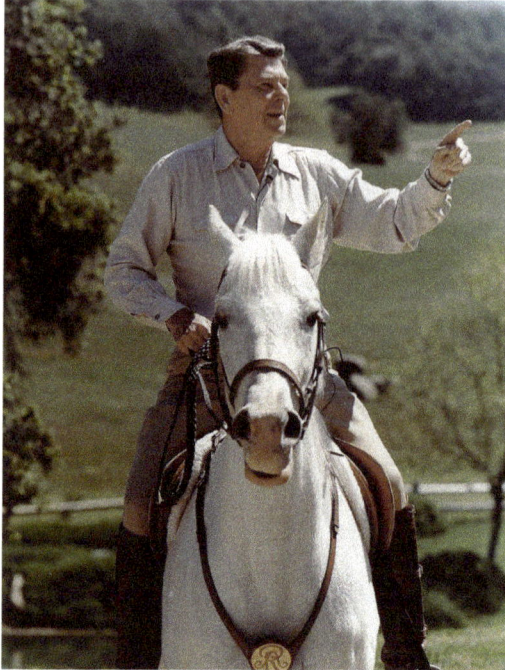

US President Ronald Reagan riding a white horse. 2004 Pete Souza official White House photographer Public Domain

Along the trail the Queen's horse in particular became increasingly flatulent with noisy and pungent emissions. At one point the aroma became particularly strong and the Queen said to Mr. Reagan. "Mr. President I really must apologize for the terrible aroma." Some observers thought that perhaps President Reagans Alzheimer Disease was beginning to take hold, but much more likely it was his quick wit that rose to the occasion. Mr. Regan responded, "Your Majesty, you needn't have apologized at all. In fact, if you hadn't said anything, I would have thought it was the horses!"

<u>Kangaroo</u>

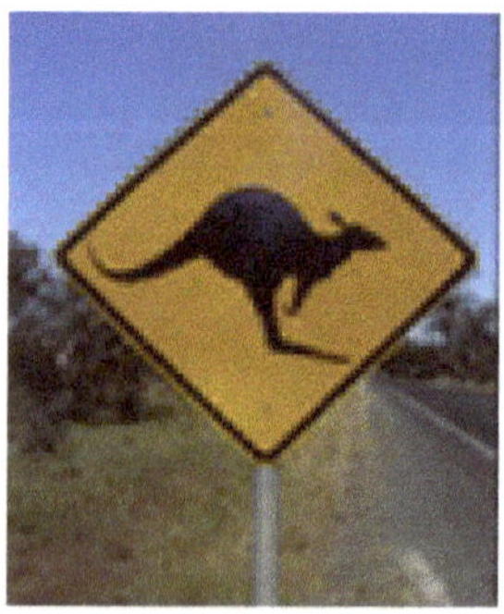

Kangaroo Farts Could Help Curb Warming

Secret to methane-free gas could be transferred to cattle and sheep

img1-azcdn.newser.com Creative Commons License

Kangaroos are herbivores and as marsupials their burps and farts contain little or no methane, a potent greenhouse gas. It appears that the reduced methane emissions are due to the microbes in the kangaroos' gut flora. Australian researchers hope that introducing a similar gut flora to other methane producing herbivores such as cattle and sheep will contribute to a reduction in greenhouse gasses and the resultant global warming. Methane can cause about twenty times as much atmospheric warming as an equivalent volume of carbon dioxide.

Kangaroos, like cattle and sheep, are ruminants that re-chew their cud with the assistance of the gut flora to digest the and metabolize their cellulose based grazing diet. In the foregut the meal is broken down by fermentation with carbon dioxide and hydrogen released. In cows and other ruminants, microbes called methanogens transform these gases into methane. But in the kangaroos' guts the same hydrogen and carbon dioxide may be utilized by bacteria called acetogens to produce acetate, a volatile fatty acid.

These microbes compete with methanogens to use the carbon dioxide and hydrogen, so the more acetogens the less methane production. The odds are in generally in favor of methanogens, since the process of methane production is generally more energy efficient than producing acetate. One of the acetogen microbes, *Blautia coccoides,* is in the gut flora of cows as well as in kangaroos. Further research is being undertaken to understand why the organism is more successful in competing with the methanogens in kangaroos than in other herbivores.

Microbe

Microbes including bacteria, Archaea, fungi, viruses, protist, and parasites are a major component of the gastrointestinal tract flora, also known as the gut microbiome. These organisms play a major role in the metabolism of the diet, and thus play a direct role in intestinal gas production. Although the organism's microfarts may seem to be inconsequential, the trillions of their numbers make them major contributors to the intestinal gasses of all larger organisms. The methane production that used to be blamed on bacteria is actually generated by the non-bacterial microbes from the Kingdom Archaea.

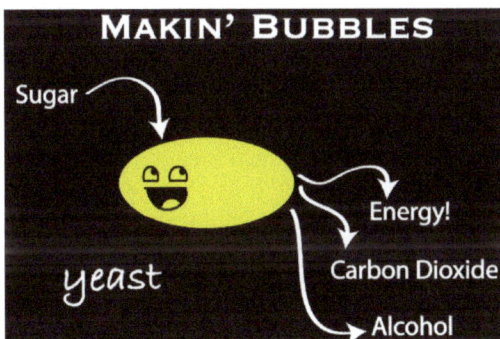

domesticlabrat.files.wordpress.com Creative Commons License

The gastrointestinal tract flora, is influenced by many environmental factors. These include diet, water purity, antibiotic exposure, chemicals, pesticides, and exposure to the microbiome of others. The gastrointestinal tract of the newborn is sterile at birth, but rapidly becomes colonized by microbes that are swallowed. Infants born via a normal vaginal delivery have a markedly different microbiome than those delivered by Cesarean section. Those born by Cesarean section have a higher incidence of allergies, asthma, and immune disorders. Many experts now suggest swathing the infect in its mother's vaginal secretions to expose it to the microbiome it would have been naturally exposed to.

Plant

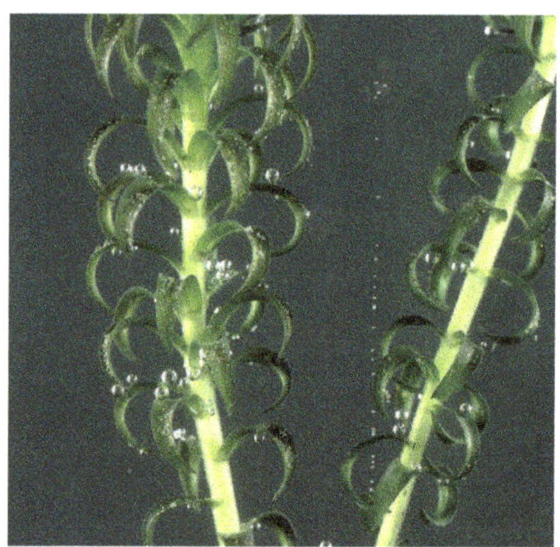

Plant placed underwater to demonstrate the production and release of oxygen gas bubbles
www.pinterest.com Creative Commons License

Plant life also contributes to gas production, but one of the most important gasses they produce as far as humans are concerned is oxygen. Although not described as a fart, the plant release of gas is analogous to a fart, as it is a gas waste product of their metabolism. It just so happens that their waste product of oxygen is one humans and other animals require for life. Plants are also critically important in taking carbon dioxide out of the atmosphere as well as fixing nitrogen into products that the other life forms can access and utilize. With plant death the decay of decomposing organic matter adds gasses that can contribute to global warming.

Stinkbug

The stinkbug is an agricultural pest which has caused significant losses of fruit and vegetable crops in numerous countries including the United States. They invade human domestic dwellings during cold winter months. When they find a comfortable habitat they release an aggregation pheromone to attract other stinkbugs, which huddle closely together. The pheromone does have an aroma which most find unpleasant. They lay about four hundred eggs which hatch in less than a week, which can lead to large populations of stinkbugs in a home. One home was found to be harboring over twenty-six thousand stinkbugs. They do not damage the house structure and they do not bite humans. The stink glands are located on the underside of the thorax, between the first and second pair of legs, and on the dorsal surface of the abdomen. Although the stink glands are associated with the insect's abdomen they are not an intestinal gas, although some incorrectly believe this is the source of odor.

The odor from the stink gland is due to its release of chemicals including the aldehydes trans-2-decenal and trans-2-Octenal, both of which have a pungent odor similar to cilantro and coriander. Most people find the aroma offensive but others do not, perhaps due to a genetic basis. Some species also release a cyanide compounds with a rancid almond scent. The odor is a defense mechanism and the insect can control the quantity ejected as well as whether just one or both glands are activated. Stinkbugs are commonly eaten in Laos, where the extremely strong odors are believed to enhance the flavor. The insects are crushed and mixed with seasoning including chilies and herbs creating a paste known as cheo.

Termite

Termites are major producers of methane, and because of the enormous size of the termite population and biomass they are thought to be significant contributors to global warming, producing over twenty-five percent of the world total methane production. Of interest, termites trapped in the sap of a tree have often been found frozen in time as the sap turns to amber over the ages. The tiny bubble of gas at the tail end of the termite entrapped in amber has been analyzed and is indeed methane produced thousands of years ago from the bacterial fermentation of the wood termites ingest. The termite gut microbiome flora generates tiny bacterial nanofarts, which coalesce into the termite microfarts that have been captured in amber eons ago.

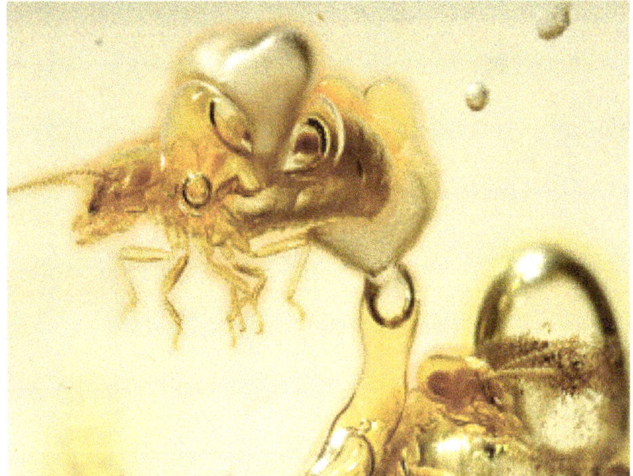

Termite farts trapped in amber have been analyzed for gas composition and indeed it is methane.
1.bp.blogspot.com Creative Commons License

Fart, Smell (Aroma, Olfaction)

Olfaction, also known as olfactics, is the scientific term for the sense of smell. Olfaction occurs when odorant molecules bind to specific sites known as the olfactory receptors. The olfactory receptors are specialized sensory cells in the nasal cavity of vertebrates. Invertebrates, such as insects, typically house their olfactory sense organ on their antennae. In the snake the olfactants are acquired by the tongue, which taking advantage of its forked anatomy deposits them on the olfactory cells on the respective sides of the nasal cavity. The difference in concentration of the olfactants on each side of the nasal cavity allows the receptors to discriminate and localize the source of the scent, much like binocular vision allows depth perception. Because humans and other animals have two nostrils, each with separate inputs to the brain, it is possible for them to have perceptual rivalry in the olfactory sense akin to binocular vision.

Many vertebrates, including most mammals and reptiles, have two distinct olfactory systems. The main olfactory system identifies general odorants while the accessory olfactory system is used mainly to detect pheromones. For air-breathing animals the main olfactory system detects volatile aerosolized chemicals, and the accessory olfactory system detects chemicals usually in the fluid phase. Olfaction, along with taste, is a form of chemoreception. Although taste and smell are separate sensory systems in land animals, water-dwelling organisms often have one combined chemical sense.

Odors are also commonly called scents, and these terms can refer to both pleasant and unpleasant stimuli. The terms fragrance and aroma are used primarily by the food and cosmetic industry to describe a pleasant odor, often referred to as a perfume or bouquet. In contrast malodor, stench, reek, and stink are used specifically to describe an unpleasant odor. The sense of smell gives rise to the perception of odors, mediated by the olfactory nerve. The olfactory receptor cells are neurons present in the olfactory epithelium, a small patch of tissue in back of the nasal cavity. There are millions of olfactory receptor neurons, each neuron has hair-like projections known as cilia. The cilia has receptor proteins that are in direct contact with air and bind directly with the odorant chemicals and molecules initiating a neuron mediated electric signal. Volatile small molecule odorants, non-volatile proteins, and non-volatile hydrocarbons may all produce olfactory responses and sensations. Much like some animal species are able to visualize ultraviolet or infrared beyond the spectrum visible to humans, a number of species can smell carbon dioxide and other odorants that are not detectable and thus considered odorless based on human sensitivity.

Olfaction, taste, and trigeminal receptors with a property known as chemesthesis together contribute to flavor. The human tongue is able to distinguish five distinct qualities of taste, salt, sweet, acidic, bitter, and umami. The nose and olfactory sense of smell has a much greater sense of discrimination and can distinguish among hundreds of substances, even in extremely minute quantities. The olfactory sense of smell takes place during inhalation, while the olfactory contribution to flavor occurs during exhalation. The olfactory system is unique among the human senses in that the neural pathway bypasses the thalamus and provides neural input directly to the forebrain. In human females the sense of olfaction is strongest around the time of ovulation, significantly stronger than during other phases of the menstrual cycle and stronger than the sense in males. The association of heightened olfactory sensitivity in association with ovulation has raised speculation about pheromone activity in humans but it has yet to be scientifically confirmed.

Scent hounds as a group can smell one to ten-million times more acutely than a human. Bloodhounds, which have the keenest sense of smell of any dogs, have noses ten to one-hundred-million times more sensitive than a human's. They were bred for the specific purpose of tracking humans, and can detect a scent trail a few days old. The second most- sensitive nose is possessed by the Basset Hound, which was bred to track and hunt rabbits and other small animals. The silvertip grizzly bear found in parts of North America, has a sense of smell seven times stronger than that of the bloodhound. This keen sense of smell is essential for its skill in locating food underground. Bears can detect the scent of food from up to eighteen miles away.

Olfaction, the sense of smell, is a form of chemoreception that in humans occurs when odorant molecules bind to olfactory receptors. The stimulation of olfactory and taste receptors is through a process known as chemesthesis. Cloning of olfactory receptor proteins and identifying that odor molecules bind to specific receptors led to the 2004 Nobel Prize award to Linda B. Buck and Richard Axel.

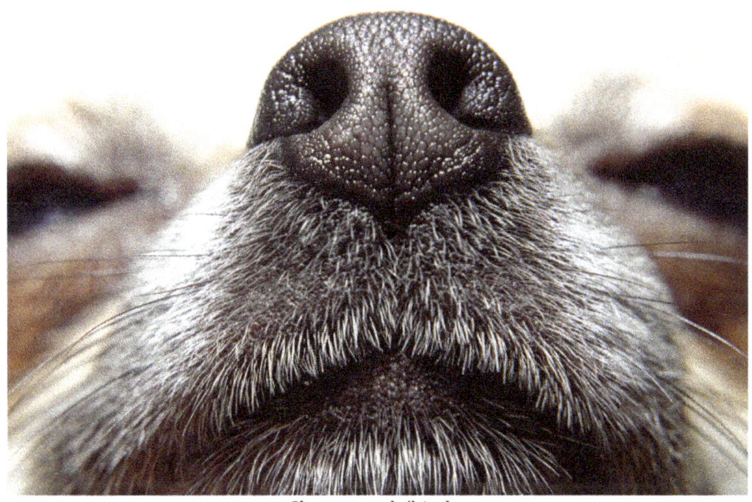

Shutterstock/bimka

Females have greater olfactory sensitivity than males, particularly at the time of ovulation. More than pheromones is involved and females can detect by olfaction potential mates that have a genetic diversity that would be beneficial for their offspring. Odor information is retained in long-term memory and the olfactory system is anatomically associated with the regions of the brain associated with emotion. It has been long recognized that odors can trigger memories and emotions from remote times.

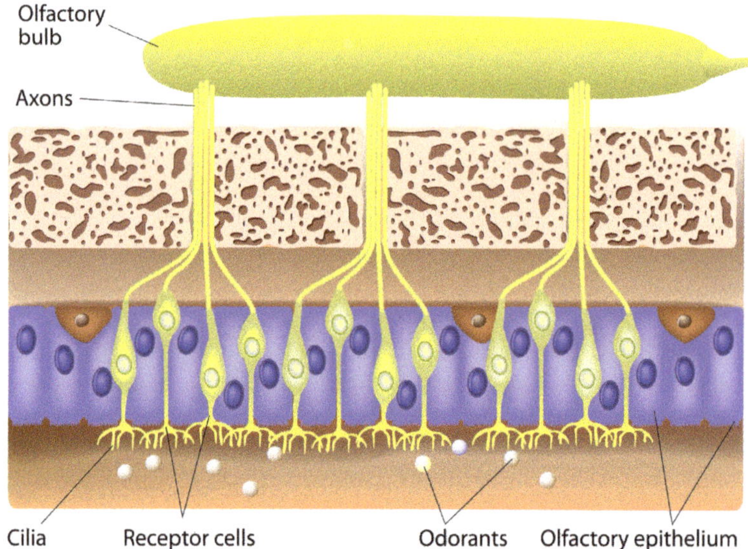

Illustration of olfactory bulb, dendrites with cilia, and odorants traveling across the olfactory epithelium. Shutterstock/Ollyy

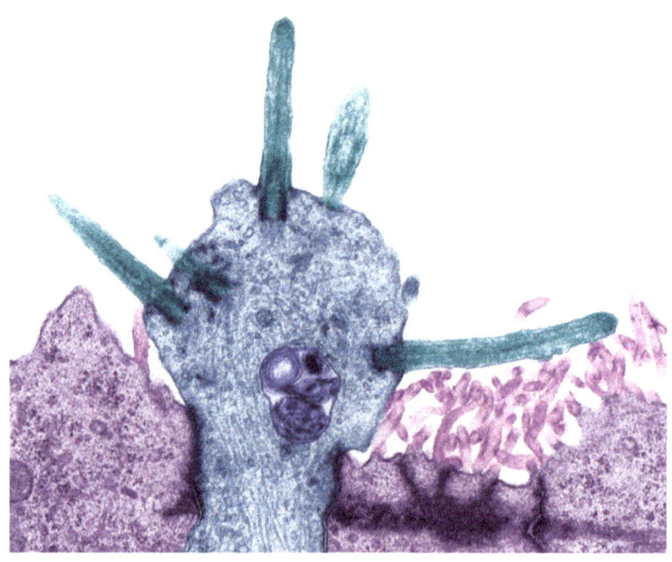

The sense of olfaction is the most sensitive of all human senses. The nose can identify the single scented molecule hiding amongst two billion unscented ones. To use a visual analogy, paint one single square sheet of a toilet paper roll the

color red. Now wrap that unlimited length roll of toilet paper around the twenty-five thousand mile long equator of the planet earth, and go around a second time, a third, a fourth, and a full fifth time.

Your nose can instantaneously identify the single red square of a one hundred and twenty-five thousand mile roll of toilet paper. Are you impressed with our sense of smell? Just like wealth and beauty there is always someone who has more to keep us from being number one. Human's olfactory epithelium is less than ten percent of the surface area of a dog's olfactory epithelium, which also has one hundred times more receptors per square centimeter. Bloodhounds have olfactory receptors up to one hundred million times the sensitivities of humans, and are trained to track a human trail several days old. North American grizzly bears have the keenest sense of smell seven times greater than the bloodhound. Salmon utilize their keen sense of smell in ocean waters to locate the stream from which they hatchlings years earlier to return to spawn. A mosquito smelling the "odorless" carbon dioxide that mammals exhale to locate their next blood meal illustrates the specialized olfactory sensitivity located on their antennae.

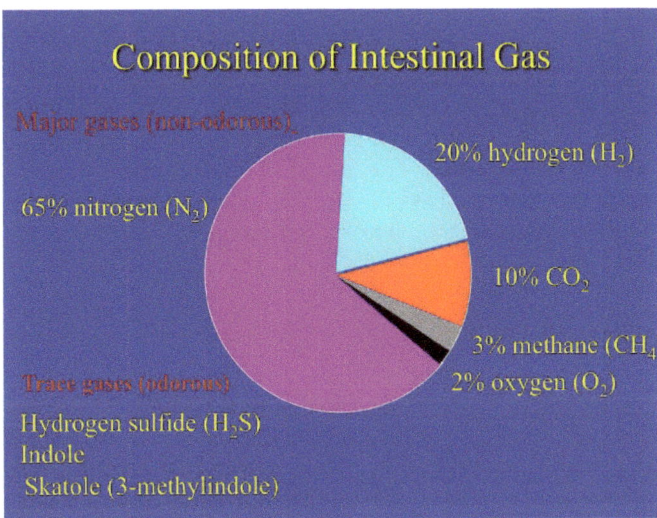

The vast majority of the gasses in intestinal farts including nitrogen, hydrogen, carbon dioxide, methane, and oxygen contributing 99.9% by volume are odorless. So what on earth is in that other tiny but overwhelming fraction of less than one percent? Indole skatole, thiol, sulfhydryl, mercaptan, and aromatic fatty acids are the major culprits. The aromas generated by farts are normally considered unattractive or offensive. There is a surprising percentage of the presumably normal population (predominantly males) who profess enjoyment and pleasure with the olfactory stimulation generated by their own farts, but not those of others. The utility of specific odors to diagnose a limited number of diseases has been a part of the diagnostic medical armamentarium for thousands of years. When it comes to farts, particularly offensive aroma has been associated with fat malabsorption and inflammatory bowel conditions.

Indole

Indole is an organic compound known as an aromatic heterocyclic because it consists of a six-membered benzene ring fused to a five-membered nitrogen-containing pyrrole ring. Indole is often used as a component of fragrances and is used in the production of a number of pharmaceutical products. The amino acid tryptophan is the precursor of the neurotransmitter serotonin and is an example of an indole derivative. Tryptophan is one of the twenty-two amino acids, and is also considered an essential amino acid. Essential amino acids are those amino acids that cannot be synthesized by humans, and therefore must be obtained through the diet. Because of its importance as an essential amino acid, tryptophan is a common constituent of most protein foods and supplements. A diet rich in tryptophan can contribute to the fecal aroma of intestinal gas.

Indole occurs naturally in human feces and contributes to the characteristic fecal odor. Surprisingly, at very low concentrations it has a flowery smell and is a constituent of many perfumes. The name indole was created from the words indigo and oleum. Indole was first isolated by the dye industry in treatment of the deep blue indigo dye with oleum. Jasmine is a climbing shrub native to northern India and China that has a delicate night blossoming white star like flower that is highly prized for its fragrance. It is harvested only at night and an experienced picker can collect ten thousand blossoms a night. It takes three and one-half million jasmine blossoms to make one pound (half a kilogram) of natural jasmine oil, which is less than three percent indole. It is priced at over one thousand times as much as synthetic jasmine, which takes advantage of the commercial production of indole.

Skatole

Skatole (from the Greek το σχατος = feces), or methylindole, is a mildly toxic organic compound belonging to the indole family. It is the primary source of the odor of feces and is produced from the breakdown of the important amino acid tryptophan, the precursor of the neurotransmitter serotonin. Surprisingly, in low concentrations skatole has a very pleasant flowery smell and is found in orange blossoms, jasmine, and other flowers and essential oils. It is used as a fragrance in many perfumes. Skatole is attractive to males of various species of bees, who gather the chemical to synthesize pheromones. It is also an attractant to gravid (pregnant) mosquitos. The U. S. military has used skatole as a non-lethal malodorant weapon. The German physician Ludwig Brieger, who also identified cadaverine and putrescence, discovered skatole in 1877. His neighbors were probably not pleased with the smell coming from his laboratory as the names he gave his discoveries were derived from their source material.

Skatole also plays a major role in the aroma of pork obtained from mature male pigs (boars). After puberty, under the influence of the male hormone androstenone, the gut microbiome of the male pig generates skatole. This odorant is deposited in the fat and muscle giving it an offensive smell and taste known as taint. Because it cannot be sold at market, male pigs are typically castrated at a young age or slaughtered before puberty. The male of the human species, under similar hormonal influence is also a large producer of skatole contributing to the enhanced offensive potency of male farts after puberty.

Of particular interest to some scientists is that androstenone, and its effect on skatole, appear to have a pheromone like effect on the human female. Much like color-blindness, there appear to be some odors that cannot be smelled by all people. Initial studies suggested that about thirty percent of human females could not sense androstenone. Further studies revealed that the majority of the non-scenters could be trained to identify it, yet there remained a small proportion of less than five percent who could not perceive the scent. The ability to sense androstenone was found to be genetic and the gene responsible was identified.

The sense of smell in the human female is intimately tied to the menstrual cycle. The height of olfactory sensitivity peaks at the time of ovulation. The androstenone and skatole scents are perceived to be less offensive or more attractive at the time of ovulation. The androstenone skatole connection also explains why the feces and flatus of males is considered more powerful or offensive than that of females.

Diet also plays a role in that the ingestion of more meat and fat also leads to more skatole production than a diet with higher fiber content. This is partly due to the diet containing more tryptophan, the amino acid precursor of skatole, as well as the diet induced change in the microbiome. Androstenone also occurs naturally in some plants, including celery, parsnip, and truffle. The celery has long had a reputation as an aphrodisiac dating from Greek and Roman times.

Thiol, Sulfhydryl, Mercaptans

The sulfur hydrogen functional group may also be referred to as a thiol group or a sulfhydryl group. Thiols are also referred to as mercaptans. The term mercaptan (Latin mercurium captans 'capturing mercury') is used because the thiolate group bonds so strongly with mercury compounds. Hydrogen sulfide is known for its characteristic odor of smelling like rotten eggs. Surprisingly women tend to produce more hydrogen sulfide then men. Diet certainly plays a role as cruciferous vegetables such as broccoli, cabbage, cauliflower, and Brussels sprouts are common offenders. Dried fruits such as apricots are often treated with sulfur products that create odiferous gasses. Red meat, beer, garlic, and aromatic spices are other significant contributors. The offensive smell of sulfur products led to religious authorities ascribing an association between the devil and sulfur.

Hydrogen sulfide is a toxic substance in high concentrations yet very valuable and beneficial on a cellular level when present in minute quantities. The human nose is exceptionally sensitive to this toxin and can identify it in minute concentrations, such as in a fart. When present in very high concentrations the olfactory cells are overwhelmed and can no longer sense it. This has led to a severe hazard for farmers and workers in animal waste manure pits and sewage treatment facilities. A worker collapses on exposure to the high concentration of hydrogen sulfide and fellow workers coming to their aid are likewise stricken because there was no olfactory warning. With a toxic potency equivalent to cyanide, workers in such hazardous occupations are urged to use self-contained breathing apparatus to avoid exposure.

Volatile thiols have distinctive and strong garlic like odor. The spray of skunks consists mainly of thiols and derivatives. These compounds are detected by the human nose at concentrations as low as ten parts per billion. Human sweat contains methyl-sulfanylhexan (MSH), found in higher concentrations in females, and has a fruity onion-like odor. Not all thiols have unpleasant odors. The aroma of roasted coffee is due to thiols as is the characteristic scent of grapefruit. Dimethyl sulfide has an aroma that is often described as sweet. Natural gas distributors were required by law to add odorants such as thiols to odorless natural gas after a tragic school explosion in New London, Texas, in 1937 due to an undetected gas leak.

Most natural odorant additives used today contain mixtures of mercaptans and sulfides. T-butyl mercaptan is often utilized as the main odorant constituent. The characteristic and pungently offensive odor of animal flesh decay is caused by the odorant additives putrescence and cadaverine. Putrescence and cadaverine are the breakdown products of the amino acids ornithine and lysine, respectively. Cadaverine and putrescence were also used as odorant additives for natural gas before improved odorants became commercially available.

Methanethiol

Methanethiol (methyl mercaptan) is a flammable, colorless compound with a powerful smell like rotten cabbage or decomposing vegetables. It is a natural substance found in certain foods such as some nuts and cheese, and is released from decaying organic matter. Methanethiol is also a byproduct produced by the metabolism of asparagus. The change in the odor of urine may be apparent within thirty minutes of eating asparagus. It is one of the main chemicals responsible for bad breath and the smell of feces and flatus.

Natural gas and propane are both colorless and odorless, and an undetected leak can lead to tragic consequences. To serve as an odorous marker that a gas leak is occurring small amount of methyl mercaptan or ethyl mercaptan may be added as an odorant. The addition of an odorant is often required by law to prevent the danger of natural gas leaks going undetected leading to death and injury.

Fatty Acids

A fatty acid is a saturated or unsaturated carboxylic acid with a long aliphatic tail or chain. Fatty acids with carbon–carbon double bonds are known as unsaturated, and those without such bonds are known as saturated. Fatty acids are derived from triglycerides or phospholipids, and when unattached to other molecules are described as "free". Fatty acids are an important cellular fuel and yield large quantities of the energy storing molecule adenosine triphosphate (ATP) when metabolized. Many cell types can use either glucose or fatty acids for this purpose. Heart and skeletal muscle prefer fatty acids, although most cells can use glucose interchangeably. The brain has the ability to use fatty acids, glucose, or ketone bodies as a fuel.

Fatty acids that must be obtained via the diet because humans cannot synthesize them are called essential fatty acids. Fatty acid chains are categorized by their length. Short-chain fatty acids (SCFA) have aliphatic tails of fewer than six carbons. Medium-chain fatty acids (MCFA) have tails of six to twelve carbons and can form medium-chain triglycerides. Long-chain fatty acids (LCFA) have tails of thirteen to twenty-one carbons, while very long chain fatty acids (VLCFA) are longer than twenty-two carbons.

Short- and medium-chain fatty acids are absorbed by the intestines directly into the blood stream. Long-chain fatty acids are absorbed into the cells of the intestinal villi and converted into a triglyceride cholesterol compound known as a chylomicron. These enter lymphatic capillaries called lacteals and are transported via the thoracic duct of the lymphatic system, eventually entering the circulatory system via the left subclavian vein. Fatty acids and chylomicrons in the blood circulation may be processed in the liver and subsequently circulate as very low-density lipoproteins (VLDL), low-density lipoproteins (LDL), and high-density lipoproteins.

Aromatic Amino Acids

Aromatic amino acids are amino acids that include an aromatic ring. Examples include phenylalanine, tryptophan, histidine, and tyrosine. Phenylalanine, histidine, and tryptophan are essential amino acids in that animals cannot synthesize them and they must be obtained from the diet. Tyrosine is semi-essential in that it can be synthesized but only if phenylalanine is ingested. The disorder phenylketonuria occurs when there is an absence of the enzyme phenylalanine hydroxylase, which is required for tyrosine synthesis.

All plants and microorganisms synthesize their aromatic amino acids, unlike animals, which obtain them through their diet. Animals have lost these energy intensive metabolic pathways, since they obtain aromatic amino acids through their diet. Herbicides and antibiotics inhibiting enzymes involved in aromatic acid synthesis, are toxic to plants and microorganisms dependent on this pathway, but not to animals which do not utilize these enzymes.

Volatile Organic Compounds

The term volatile refers to the ability of a substance to evaporate or readily vaporize at room temperature. Most instances of vaporization refer to evaporation where a liquid becomes a gas, such as liquid water boiling into gaseous steam and water vapor. Some solids vaporize from the solid state directly without entering an intermediate liquid phase, a process is known as sublimation. One example would be dry ice, frozen carbon dioxide, which leaves the solid state and is immediately transformed into a gas.

Vaporization also has another form that is not evaporation, but is the scattering or diffusing of molecules or particles through the air. The particles have so little mass that they can remain airborne for extended periods of time, and become airborne again upon being disturbed or moved even by a gentle gust of air. This is frequently noticed when a bright beam of light enters a darkened room and the dust particles circulating in the air become visible.

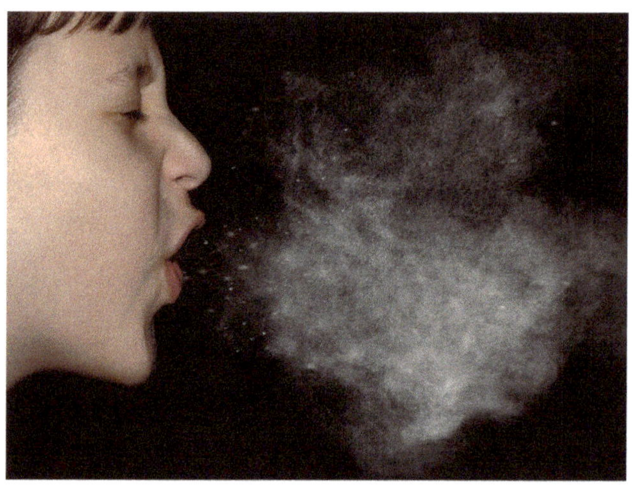

Mold, spores, pollens, viruses, bacteria, fecal matter of mites, volatile organic compounds and others can circulate and spread through large open spaces. Allergies, acquiring viral or bacterial infections from the sneeze or cough of others even hours earlier, occur because of this aerosolization. The ability to detect the aroma of certain compounds, and volatile organic compounds are the result of this form of vaporization, as well as their ability to enter the gaseous state by vaporizing at room temperatures.

A list of the volatile organic compounds found in strawberries includes approximately two dozen chemicals including methyl butyrate, octyl acetate, hexanol, and others. Since these compounds are volatile they may vaporize and if they reach your olfactory receptors you may detect them and identify them as coming from a strawberry.

Fart, Social Standards (see Fart Survey)

The Ontario Ministry of Health embarked on a public education campaign to curb tobacco usage. A common theme used by smokers to avoid the stigma of nicotine addiction was to describe their habit as that of being a social smoker. The public education campaign focused on that denial as being analogous to describing oneself as a social farter that enjoyed farting while in the company of others.

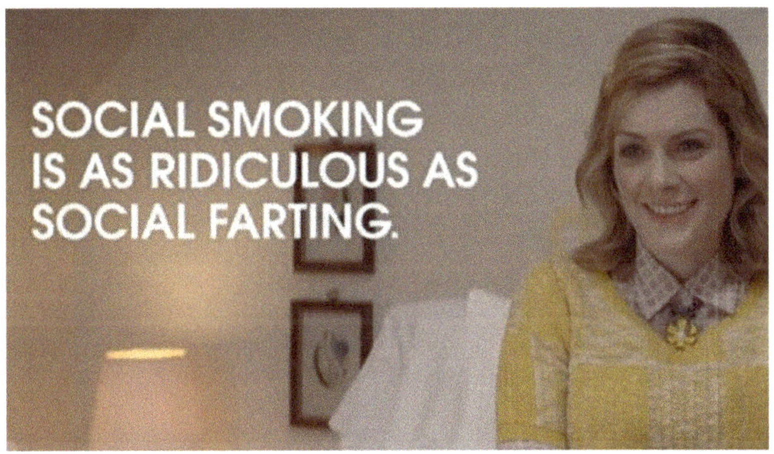
SOCIAL SMOKING
IS AS RIDICULOUS AS
SOCIAL FARTING.

Creative Commons License

Fart, Sound (Acoustics, Auditory)

The physics involved in the generation of the sound of a fart is very complex. Variables of the colonic and anal components, as well as the surrounding environment when it is released are multiple. Within the colon and rectum this includes the pressure, volume, temperature, moisture content, chemical nature of the gasses within the colon, and whether it is being released concomitantly with any liquid, semisolid, or solid material.

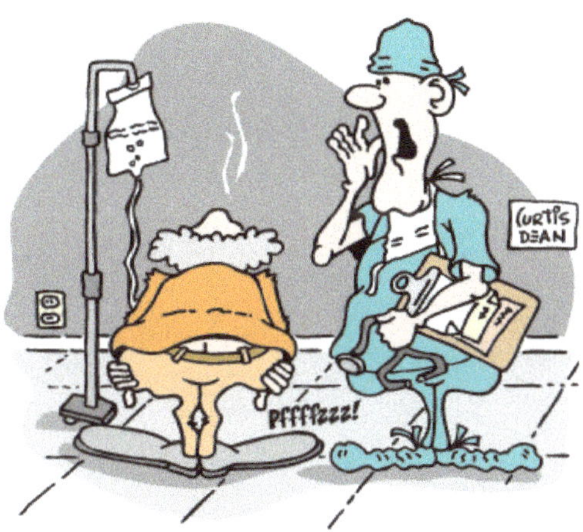
Pffffzzz!
CURTIS
DEAN

"Yes, that was very loud, but I said I wanted to hear your HEART!"

sciblogs.co.nz Creative Commons License

Within the anal canal it includes the anatomy of the sphincter including whether it is symmetrical or irregular such as with fissures, hemorrhoids, anal tags, etc., sphincter tone and pressure, elasticity and degree of relaxation, and the velocity and physical nature of the expelled material. In the immediate post expulsion state, factors include the atmospheric pressure, temperature, and volumetric constraints such as whether by clothing, sitting on a cushion, under a blanket, or voluntary social considerations.

The physics of gas and fluid dynamics allow calculations with the understanding and application of natural laws. If you have taken a course in physics you may recall with great fondness Laplace's Law, Boyle's Law, Charles' Law, Avogadro's Law, Gay-Lussac's Law that were integrated into what is called the Ideal Gas Law. This summarizes the close interrelationship between the pressure, volume, and temperature of gasses. To understand the physics of farts you need to incorporate the additional principles of physics and engineering called the "choked" compressible flow effect. The character that becomes choked or limited is the velocity, although after release the term choked may take on an entirely different meaning.

The velocity of the material increases as it is passed through a constriction. You may have experienced this if you have used a garden hose and notice that as the opening at the nozzle tip becomes smaller the velocity increases. You may also have noticed that the frequency of the sound generated also changes both by constricting the nozzle orifice or rotating the faucet leading to the garden hose. This involves recognition that the Venturi effect causes the static pressure, and therefore the density of the gasses, to decrease once released from the anus.

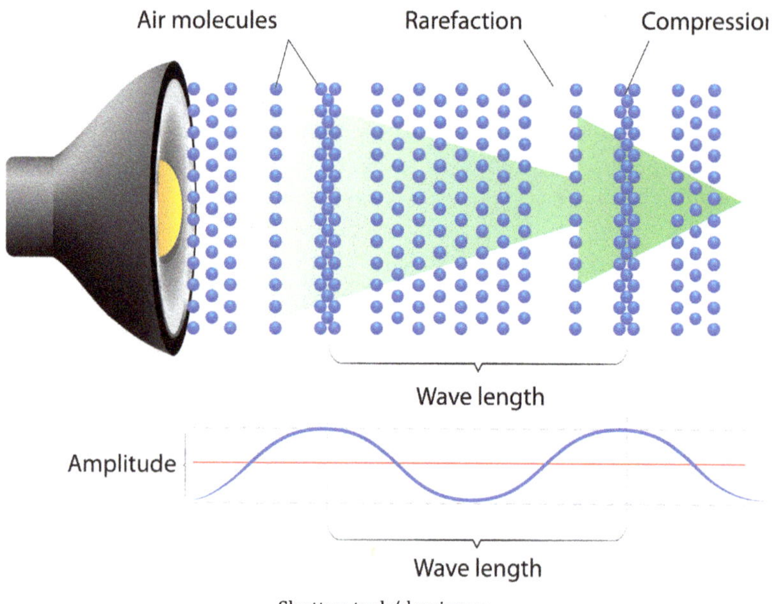

Shutterstock/dersignua

If the material passed includes a liquid component, a different type of choked flow can occur. In unusual circumstances dependent on the vapor pressure and temperature of the liquid, the liquid may partially flash into bubbles of vapor that collapse in a process called cavitation. When this occurs in a closed system of pipes such as plumbing fixtures the effect can be very noisy and sufficiently violent as to cause physical damage to valves, pipes, and associated equipment. Thankfully, humans are not a closed system but the noise and reverberations they generate may be comparable.

In general, the more tone the anal sphincter has the tighter it can hold on to the gasses to create a greater pressure gradient. The greater the pressure gradient the louder the potential sound will be. If the opposite occurs, then less noise is generated. As an example, it is said that if you blow air slowly into a trumpet without puckering your lips to generate an air pressure gradient the air will just flow through the instrument without "trumpeting".

The anal sphincter tone changes with age becoming more lax. This is also the case after childbirth, and any activities that stretch the anal opening on a regular basis, such as passing large stools with constipation, or engaging in anal receptive intercourse. With the loss of sphincter tone farts may escape involuntarily, but they also tend to be quitter as the larger the opening of the orifice the slower the velocity.

With so many variables it should come as no surprise that the sounds generated are equally variable. As the famous Greek philosopher Heraclitus (c 535 BCE- 475 BCE) said, "You could not step twice into the same river; for other waters are ever flowing on to you." It would be fair to say that no two farts are identical, much like snowflakes, although somehow pure white innocent snowflakes do not seem to be the right analogy.

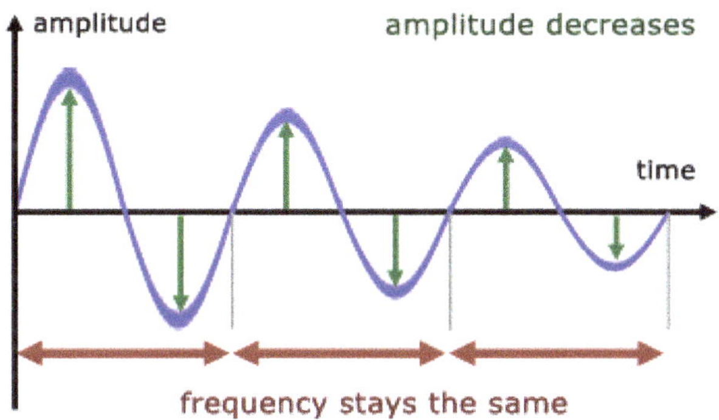

www.a-levelphysicstutor.com Creative Commons License

At the time that a fart is about to be released the variables under the control of a talented and experienced professional farter include the velocity of its release, the tension and symmetry of the sphincter, and the selection of the environmental nature of the location of its liberation. Yes, there is a significant amount of science behind the fart, but there is also an 'art to the fart'. As to the teleological question, is there an advantage to audible fart sounds, there are several theories. One is that the fart sounds are an auditory warning that noxious gasses are being released and to seek shelter or at least distance to protect oneself. A second theory suggests that these are actually primitive mating calls, especially an attempt of adolescent males to attract the female of the species. The third theory is so that people with anosmia, the loss of the sense of smell, can participate in the experience of a fart as well.

Using the principles of speed of travel of various phenomena, you may recall that you can calculate the distance of a lightning strike. The speed of light is 186,282 miles per second; the speed of sound is seven hundred and sixty-eight miles per hour in dry air at sixty-eight degrees Fahrenheit at sea level. Obviously the light will reach you first and you will see the flash, but no sound as it is lagging behind. The more distant you are from where the lightning struck, the greater the time lag. If you see the flash of lightening count the number of seconds before you hear the thunder. Now simply divide the number of seconds of lag time by the number five to adjust for the differences in speed of light and sound, and voila, you have a good approximation of the distance in miles that you are from where the lightning struck.

The lightning flash of a fart is a very special event discussed in greater detail in the section on combustible farts containing hydrogen and methane in the presence of oxygen, and the section on spontaneous human combustion. Can one use science to compare the speeds of sound and smell transmission? The answer is an unequivocal yes, but circumstances are rarely optimal. The speed of sound of a fart is the same as the speed of sound of a lightning strike, seven hundred and sixty-eight miles per hour in dry air at sixty-eight degrees Fahrenheit at sea level. The speed of smell diffusion has been measured at ten feet per second (nearly seven miles per hour) in an unventilated room with no circulating airflow.

Using the sound of the fart as a shotgun start for the stopwatch, count how many seconds it is until you smell the fart. To simplify calculations, the fart sound is about one hundred times faster than the fart smell. For a crude approximation simply take the number of seconds from the fart sound until the smell arrives as the number of feet you are distant to its source. Any circulation of air in the room, clothing that the fart has to pass through, and direction of the jet exhaust blast with which it is released can either accelerate or delay its arrival at your nose. This formula is at its most accurate in identifying the source of the fart if there are no more than two people in the room. The adage he who smelt it dealt it, is usually accurate unless the other party was in a compromised position with his own nose closer to the anus of the emanation.

The pressure generated by the abdominal muscles can be infinitely adjusted by the individual (the Valsalva maneuver generates this pressure with a bearing down motion with the breath held) and will affect the velocity and sound of a fart. Leaning to one side to deform the anal canal into an irregular shape to allow the fart to escape with less velocity is a technique learned by experience even if one does not recognize the principles of physics underlying its utility. Sitting on a cushion to muffle the sound and absorb the aroma is a common technique. With practice, some individuals have developed the remarkable musical ability to play their own human wind instrument. They have performed in public to great acclaim like Joseph Pool, known as Le Ptomaine on the Moulin Rouge of Paris. The sound of farts can be a source of entertainment and humor or offense and embarrassment, but it is a natural phenomenon that follows the laws of nature.

Scientific papers entitled "Sounds produced by herring (*Clupeid harangues*) bubble release" by Magnus Wahlberg and Haman Westerberg in the journal *Aquatic Living Resources* (2003, 16.271-275), and "Pacific and Atlantic Herring Produce Burst Pulse Sounds" by Ben Wilson, Robert S. Batty and Lawrence M. Dill in *Biology Letters* (2003, 271.S95-S97) confirm that herring communicate distress signals to the rest of the school of fish by farting. The papers are demonstrations of scholarly research and have spectrographic confirmation of the high frequency sound bursts at up to twenty-two kilohertz with visual confirmation of a stream of bubbles from the anus.

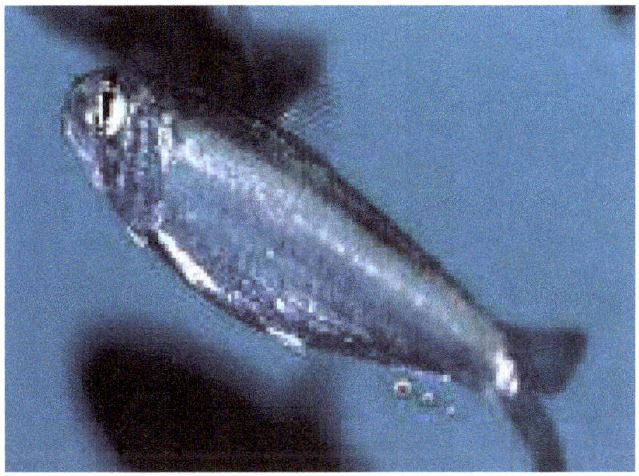

Herring communicate danger by high frequency sounds generated from bubbles escaping their anus described as F.R.T. fast repetitive ticks in published scientific papers first reported in 2003. Creative Commons License

Herring travel in enormous schools of fish that number in the billions. During the height of the cold war during the 1980's U.S. and NATO forces believed they had detected by sonar a unique sound pattern that was the signature of a new secret Soviet nuclear submarine. The new submarine appeared to be making provocative incursions into the territorial waters of Sweden and Norway, which protested vigorously through diplomatic channels. When the sound pattern was detected deep in the territorial waters of a Norwegian fjord NATO forces decided to trap the submarine and blockaded the entrance to the fjord. After days of waiting for the submarine to surrender they finally realized that the sonar sounds they were hearing were not a Soviet submarine but the sounds of a school of herring farting their way through the fjord.

During interviews with the National Geographic Society research team leader Ben Wilson a marine biologist studying pacific herring at the Bamfield Marine Science Centre, British Columbia, Canada was quoted saying "We know [herring] have excellent hearing but little about what they actually use it for. It turns out that herring make unusual farting sounds at night." Their collaborator Robert Batty, senior research scientist at the Scottish Association for Marine Science in Oban, Scotland added "In video pictures we can see the bubbles coming out of the anal duct at the same time. It sounds very much like someone blowing a high-pitched raspberry. "They labeled the sounds generated as F.R.T. for fast repetitive tick. They were awarded the 2004 IgNobel Prize in Biology.

There is a phrase called 'holding back the helium' which refers to farting by substituting the name of another gas, in this case helium. Is there another possible connection between helium and farting? Because gases have different densities, the speed of sound in helium is nearly three times the speed of sound in air. Inhaling a small volume of helium changes the sound of the human voice into a characteristic high resonant frequency sound. The sound generated is similar to the famous cartoon character Daffy Duck. Inhaling helium gas is actually very dangerous because the human body respiratory drive is not based on low levels of oxygen, but rather by high levels of carbon dioxide. When helium is inhaled the carbon dioxide levels remain normal even though oxygen may be so low that asphyxiation occurs without the expected warning of air hunger and suffocation.

The opposite effect, with low resonant frequencies more like the Star Wars character Darth Vader, can be obtained by inhaling a gas with higher density such as xenon, sulfur hexafluoride, or tungsten hexafluoride. Helium is by far the most readily available, typically associated with access through party favor stores to fill helium balloons for parties and entertainment. Helium actually plays a major role in industry and the biomedical sciences and is critical for scientific research in the fields of quantum mechanics, super fluidity, and superconductivity.

Now to the question that is undoubtedly keeping you up at night, what happens to the sound quality of a helium fart. First question is how does the helium get into the digestive tract. Inhaling pure helium will not lead to helium farts because you would die of asphyxiation within minutes. This is why even playing with the idea of helium to make your voice sound like a cartoon character is a very foolish and dangerous idea. Those who have done so and died from oxygen deprivation are considered candidates for what is called the Darwin Awards. This is offered, usually posthumously, to those who have improved the human gene pool for future evolution by removing themselves and their substandard intelligence genes from future procreation activities.

So let's say you know better than to breathe in helium, but undertake a swallowing effort to fill your digestive tract with helium to get it to pass as a fart. Not much of an improvement as the helium is such a small molecule that it easily diffuses through most membranes, as you can tell by how quickly the helium

escapes from a rubber balloon, and over a period of a few days, even from a metallic balloon.
Which leaves only one last logical way to fill the colon with helium, yes go to a party store and ask them to 'fill it up' for you. Now that you have a colon filled with helium you don't want to waste much time, as the helium will once again diffuse through the colonic epithelium. Will you fart like a duck? The answer is yes, but not because of a high frequency sound, but because a duck fart sounds like any old fart. What went wrong with the common expectation that it would sound like fingernails scratching a chalkboard? The problem is that the anal opening does not have a structure equivalent to the vocal cords of the human larynx also so appropriately called the voice box.

Phonation, the creation of sound and voice arises from the ability of the vocal cords to open and constrict to exceptionally nuanced degrees, allowing an infinite variety and modulation of frequencies. Humans are not the sole possessors of such a talent as songbirds and other animals can generate sounds in an even greater range of frequencies, often beyond the auditory abilities of our ears to hear the sounds. You are probably familiar to dog whistles that dogs respond to but are outside of our hearing range. It is the ability of the vocal cords to generate the range of frequencies that is impacted by the density of the gasses passed through that makes the voice reach higher frequencies with helium. It also can reach much lower frequencies sounding like Darth Vader from the *Star Wars* movie franchise if you use a much denser gas like xenon, sulfur hexafluoride, or tungsten hexafluoride.

The anal opening has hemorrhoid sinusoids, the internal anal sphincter, the external anal sphincter, and the occasional skin tag and in spite of the great control of some individuals like Joseph Pujol (Le Pétomane) it does not even come close to the resonance and sensitivity of sound creation of the vocal cords. Which is too bad, as a new *Star Wars* character a very short and squat Farth Vader could have become a cult hero. Another species creates sounds in a different fashion. Many fish have a swim bladder that is inflated or deflated as needed to maintain buoyancy. Usually expelled air bladder gas exits the mouth but the sand tiger shark, *Carcharias taurus*, discharges it out the anus. The carbon dioxide produced is eliminated via the gills. Methane, hydrogen, and other gasses would typically be released as a fart.

Fart, Speed (Velocity)

The word fart in northern European languages including German and the Scandinavian languages literally means speed. In you go by a school or hospital you may go by a no farting zone. Or you might receive a police citation for exceeding the fart limit! So a title of fart speed might seem redundant. A sneeze, or sternutation, is a powerful rapid expulsion of air from the lungs through the nose and mouth. The average velocity of a sneeze is forty-two meters/second) equivalent to approximately ninety-five miles per hour. A single sneeze can disperse up to forty thousand aerosol droplets, which can transmit pathogens and disease. The sneeze is a much more effective dispersant of infectious material than a cough or peaking. The average velocity of a cough was 15.3 meters per second and the average velocity of the breath of normal speech is 4.07 meters per second.

Although the mechanism of increasing intra-abdominal pressure is similar to generating intra-thoracic pressure for a sneeze the exit orifice is a major determinant of velocity. No one has voluntarily gotten close enough to a fart blast to measure its ejection velocity or count the vapor droplets. The brave soul who does so may not get a Nobel Prize, but would certainly be worthy of nomination for an IgNobel Prize.

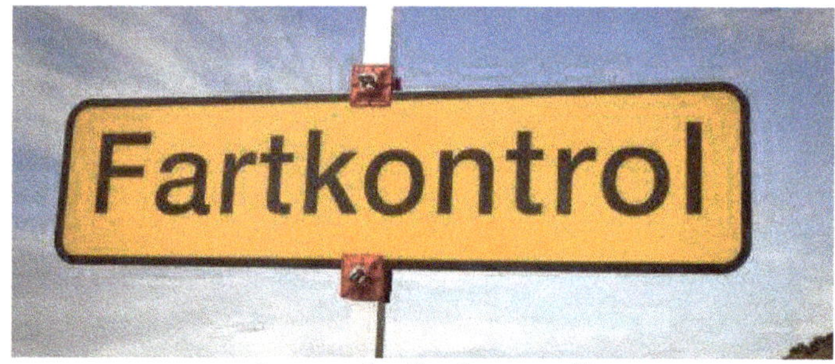

onpasture.com Creative Commons License

Coughing and sneezing release a large plume of aerosolized droplets impregnated with microbial pathogens. The sneeze and cough, which can easily reach a velocity of over one hundred miles per hour (one hundred and sixty kilometers per hour) and has been recorded at speeds up to five-hundred miles per hour (eight-hundred km/hour), will spread throughout a large size room. Even the flushing of a toilet will aerosolize fecal microbes that would cover a room in dimensions of twenty feet by twenty feet in a matter of seconds.

Farts have been recorded with the speed of aroma travelling at an extremely conservative ten miles per hour. It was not clear if this was from an individual wearing clothing at the time. A vigorous blast from a wet fart would probably look like the third photograph humorously labeled as Save the Whale. Perhaps science will one day answer the question about fart speed, or perhaps a watch company will sponsor a competition for the Guinness book of world records which has a number of fart categories already entered into the competitive arena. Another aspect that defines the extent of the reach of a fart besides its initial velocity and volume is the rate of diffusion. This is dependent on physical barriers such as layers of clothing or sitting on a cushion as well as air turbulence and ventilation. Please see entry on fart diffusion for more details.

Back in the 1946 a spoof recording of the International Crepitation Contest was created, and it is still commercially available today. It was apparently produced by some recording engineers for the Canadian Broadcasting Corporation and was held on February 31, 1946 as the World Championship Crepitation Contest at the

Maple Leaf Auditorium at Thunderblow, Canada between competitors Paul Boomer and Lord Windesmear.

Fart, Survey

The following Internet based survey of over one thousand three hundred male participants and an unspecified number of female participants does not qualify as scientifically or statistically valid. However for anecdotal and entertainment purposes it is as good as it gets when it comes to this subject matter.

Number of times women fart per day:

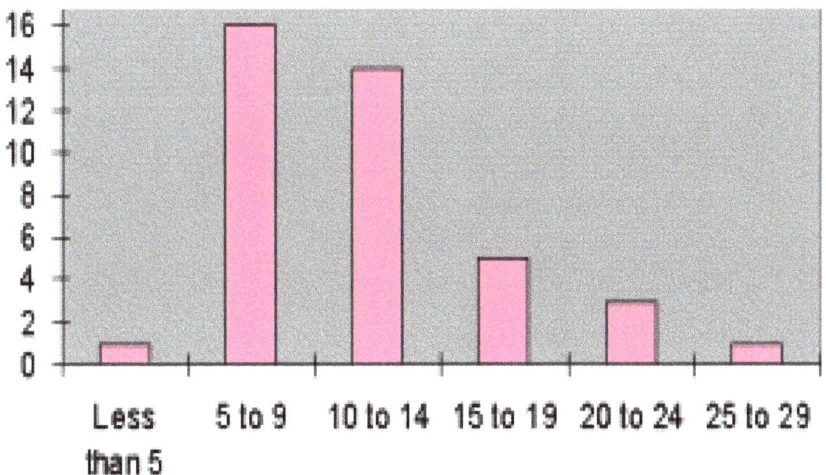

Women fart an average of eight times per day. Fifty percent of the women surveyed fart between five and ten times per day.

Women: Can you fart on command also called "Butt Breathe"?

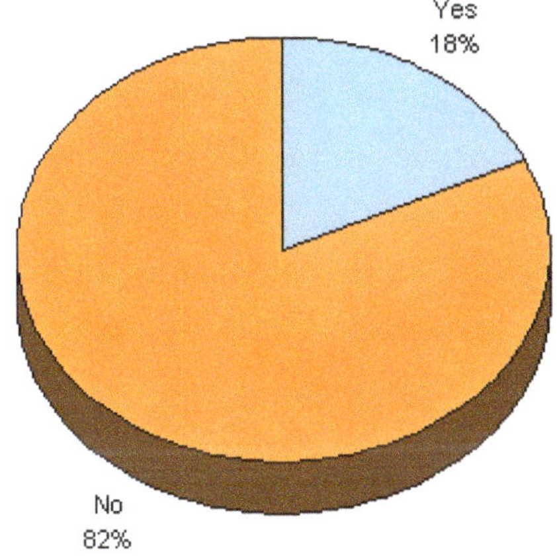

Eighteen percent of the women surveyed can fart on command by sucking air into the colon.

Women: Do you like to fart?

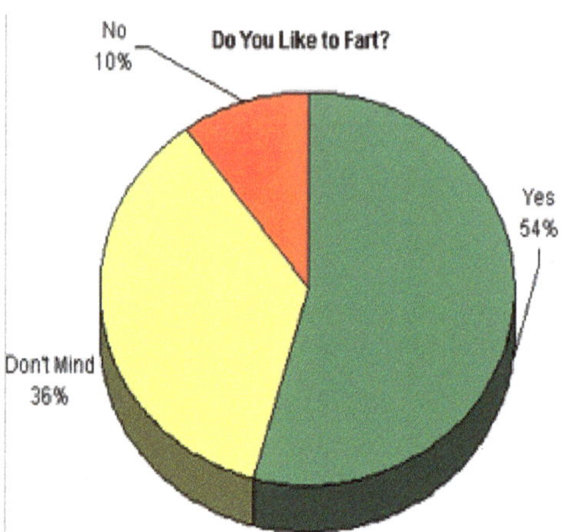

Only half of the women surveyed admit that they like to fart. About twenty percent don't mind farting, but don't necessarily like it. Only ten percent of women are absolutely insistent that they do not like to fart, but they would certainly change their mind if they experienced the results of being unable to fart!

Women: When you were younger did you like to fart in water to make bubbles?

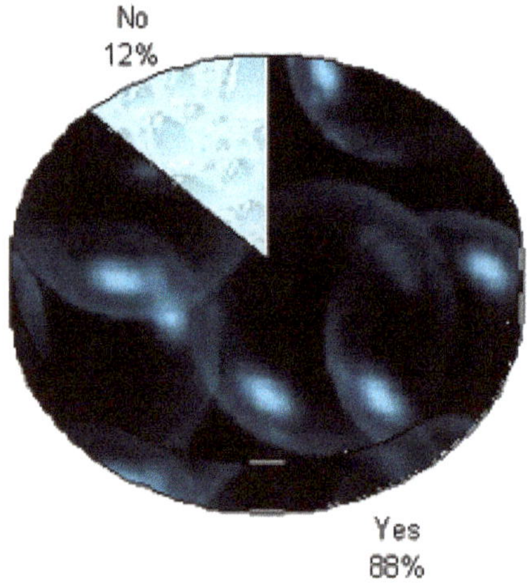

Most women liked to fart in the bathtub or pool to make bubbles.

Number of times men fart per day:

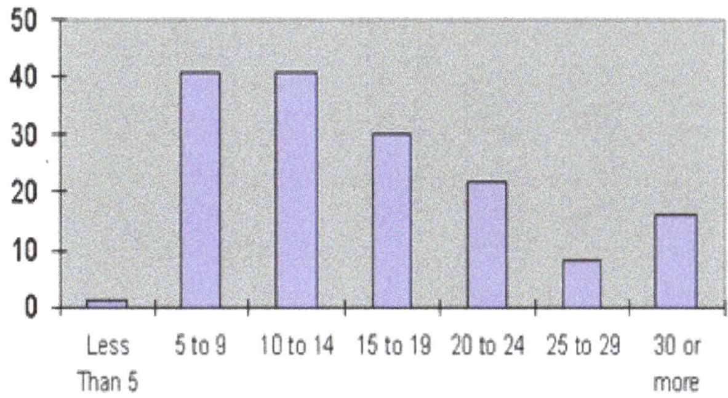

Men fart an average of fourteen times per day. Fifty percent of the men surveyed fart between five and fifteen times per day.

Men: Can you fart on command also called "Butt Breathe"?

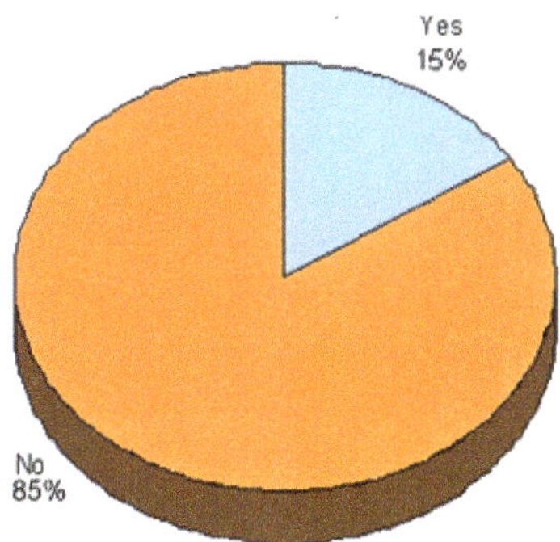

Only fifteen percent of the men surveyed can fart on command by sucking air into the colon. One third of all men did not even know that this is possible.

Men: When you were younger did you like to fart in water to make bubbles?

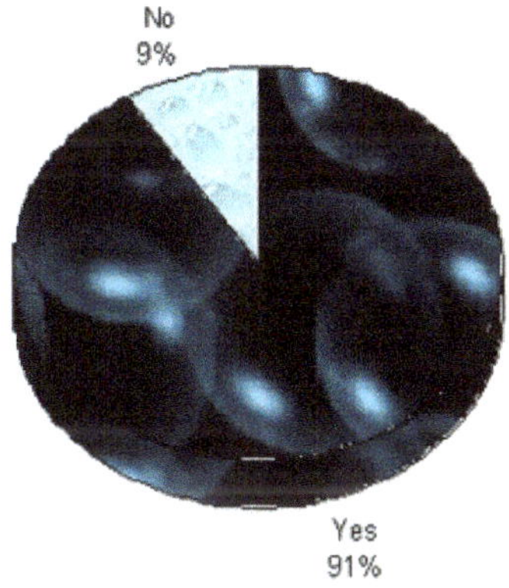

The vast majority of men liked to fart in the bathtub or pool to make bubbles.

Fart, Therapeutic Options

Many individuals have issues with unpleasant fecal odors, and unfortunately it is not as easily remedied as flushing or walking away. The fecal aroma generated by the gut microbiome that offers the characteristic smell of defecated feces is the identical aroma that may be discharged with intestinal gas, fecal incontinence, fistula, ostomies, diarrhea, inflammatory bowel disease, after gastric bypass surgery, and a host of other conditions. The numbers of individuals affected is in the millions in the United States alone. Unfortunately, the majority of the general public remains uninformed and impose a social stigma on a medical condition over which they have limited or no control.

Fortunately there are a number of effective therapeutic options available, but too many sufferers are not aware of or have access to them. They range from external appliances and clothing, to external and internal deodorants and suppressants. Of course there are also tongue-in-cheek suggestions, such as getting a dog to blame as the source of the fart odor. The Merck Manual a few years back suggested working on perfecting one's glare, just glare at someone else as if they were the source.

More direct references to farts has been employed in the advertising campaign of air-freshener company Poo-Pourri. Although the advertising campaign received a nomination as one of the worst ads by a national newspaper, it was a major hit on social media with over thirty million views. For a holiday themed advertisement Santa Claus is farting on the toilet, while an attractive model sings a parody of a seasonal tune.

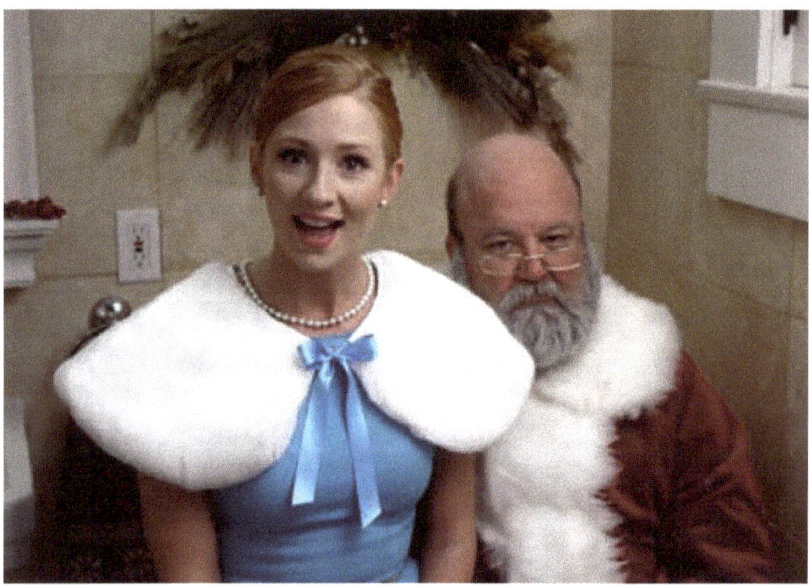

Poo-Pourri Advertising video www.ninjamarkweting.it

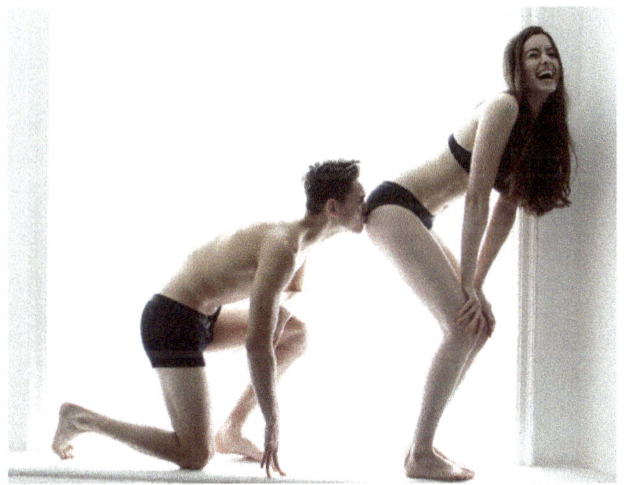

Shreddies advertising campaign for activated charcoal odor adsorbing underwear myshreddies.com

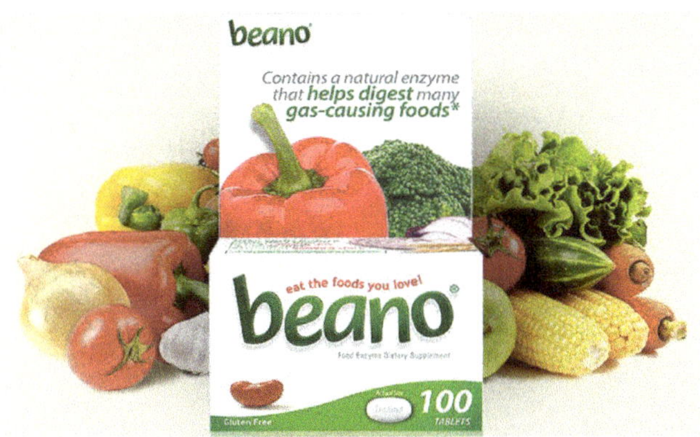

Beano was one of the first products to advertise a product designed to reduce intestinal gas.
Its ad first appeared in *Vegetarian Times*

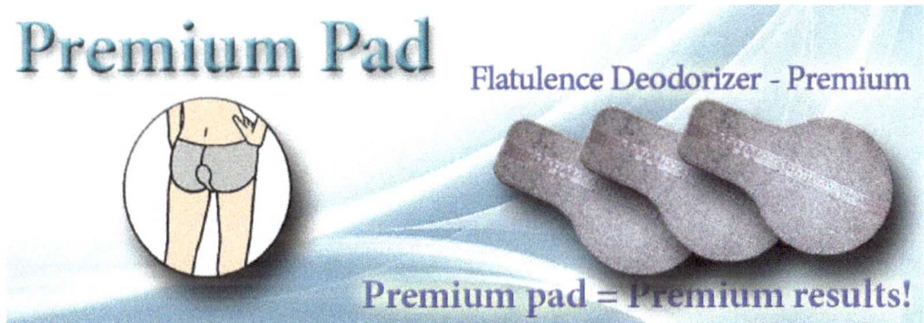

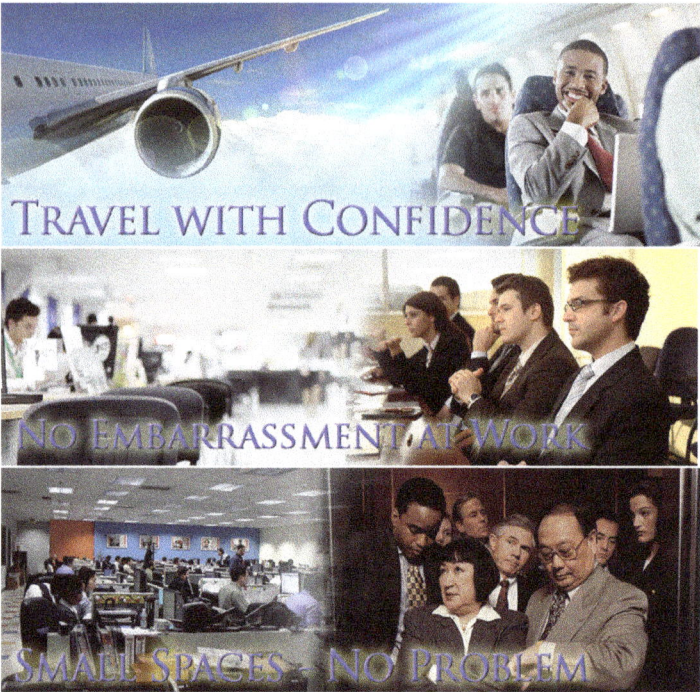

Flat-D advertises and markets a wide variety of activated charcoal products to adsorb the aroma of flatus and other body odors. www.flat-d.com

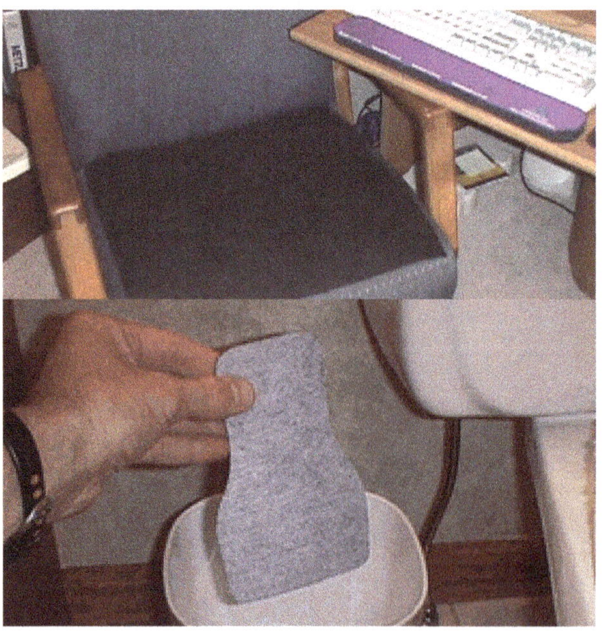

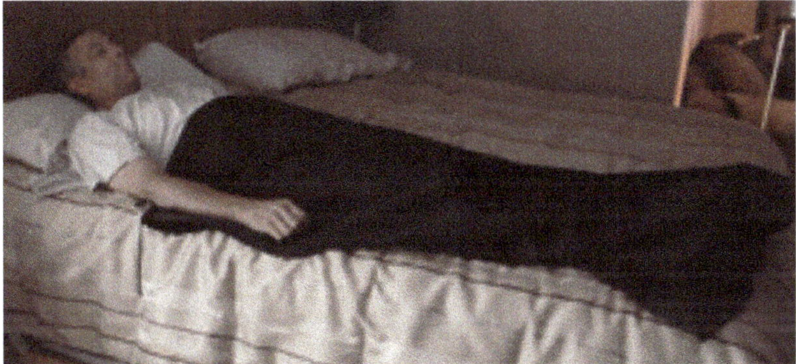

Flat-D advertises and markets a wide variety of activated charcoal products to adsorb the aroma of flatus and other body odors. Activated charcoal seat cushions, liners for underwear and clothing, and sleeping sack are amongst the numerous products they offer. www.flat-d.com

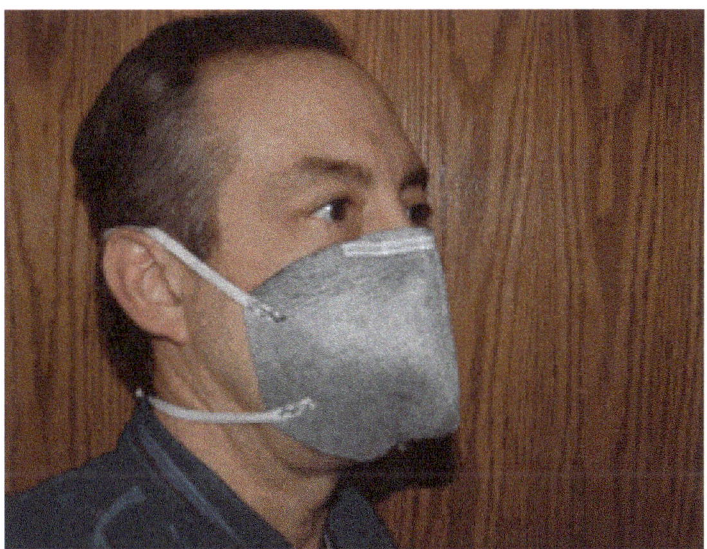

Flat-D offers another approach to protect the individual from offensive odors, by wearing an activated charcoal facemask covering the mouth and nose. www.flat-d.com

Surprisingly, while it can provide relief and comfort to many sufferers, some media outlets refuse to place advertisements for products dealing with flatulence and ostomy odors. Deodorants, feminine hygiene douches, tampons, sanitary napkins for menstruation, diapers for adults with incontinence, erectile dysfunction prescriptions, etcetera have been seen by the public without the downfall of social order. Devrom, an effective internal deodorant that suppresses fecal odor was not allowed to place their advertisement in *Reader's Digest* or *AARP Magazine* (Association for the Advancement of Retired People) because it contained the word stool and referred to smelling flatulence. Somehow the publications did not see the irony in that their policy did not pass the proverbial smell test of good judgment.

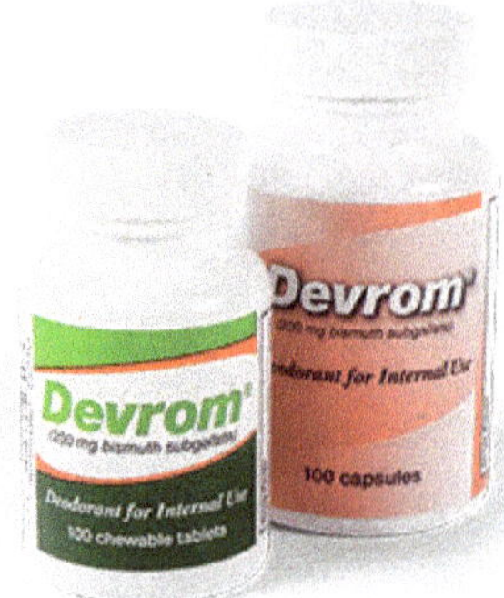

Devrom is an over the counter preparation of bismuth subgallate and has been marketed for over fifty years as an internal deodorant. Bismuth does have antibacterial properties it may change the microbiome by reducing the organisms that contribute to offensive flatulence. Another bismuth product that has been popular in the marketplace is Pepto-Bismol, which is a bismuth subsalicylate. Bismuth subsalicylate is related to aspirin (salicylic acid) and does not appear to provide as significant relief from the unpleasant odors as has been reported with Devrom.

It has been particularly popular for individuals who have undergone gastric bypass surgery, inflammatory bowel disease, as well as those with ostomies, and others. With advances in surgery, and the ability to preserve sphincters or create artificial sphincters, ostomies are seen less frequently. This is where the intestinal discharge exits the body through an artificial opening, the ostomy, created at surgery. Because the bowel is diverted from the colon less moisture is absorbed and the feces may be semi-formed or liquid.

The more liquid form allows for the more rapid vaporization of volatile organic compounds and gasses that give rise to the feculent odor. In spite of being in otherwise excellent health, many individuals with these issues find themselves socially restricted in their activities because of concern about embarrassment or offending others. Safe and effective products are available, but many individuals are unaware and suffer unnecessarily because of the lack of information and understanding.

Bismuth is a chemical element, number eighty-three on the periodic table, which has long history of being used in preparations designed to treat gastrointestinal complaints. It is a heavy metal with a low level of toxicity. Its various compounds have also been used historically to treat syphilis and the severe diarrhea from cholera. Bismuthinite is a mineral consisting of bismuth sulfide (Bi_2S_3) and is an important ore for bismuth.

The mechanism of action is unknown and may be related to its known antimicrobial activity, perhaps inhibiting the microbes that generate some of the more offensive gasses that usually contain sulfur as well as aromatic and volatile organic compounds. Bismuth also reacts directly with sulfur generating bismuth sulfide, a dark black insoluble compound. This can cause darkening or blackening of the tongue if sulfur is found in high concentrations in the saliva. It will also cause blackening of the stool as it binds with the sulfur that would otherwise give rise to hydrogen sulfide and other offensive sulfur gasses. The dark black color of the stool may be mistaken for melena, a sign of internal bleeding that results from the digestive process on blood cells and hemoglobin. The black coloration is not a health concern and is temporary, clearing with cessation of bismuth intake.

Activated carbon is used to treat oral poisonings by binding to and preventing the poison from being absorbed by the gastrointestinal tract. Charcoal biscuits were marketed in the early nineteenth century as an antidote to flatulence, and are still marketed today for diarrhea, indigestion, flatulence, and as a pet care product. Unfortunately orally ingested charcoal pills are not effective in appreciably reducing intestinal gas. This may be because the adsorptive capacity of the activated charcoal is fully utilized before it finally gets to the colon where its gas adsorbing properties are most needed. Fortunately, bismuth products do provide a significant advantage by binding to the sulfur compounds and eliminating them without producing offensive gas.

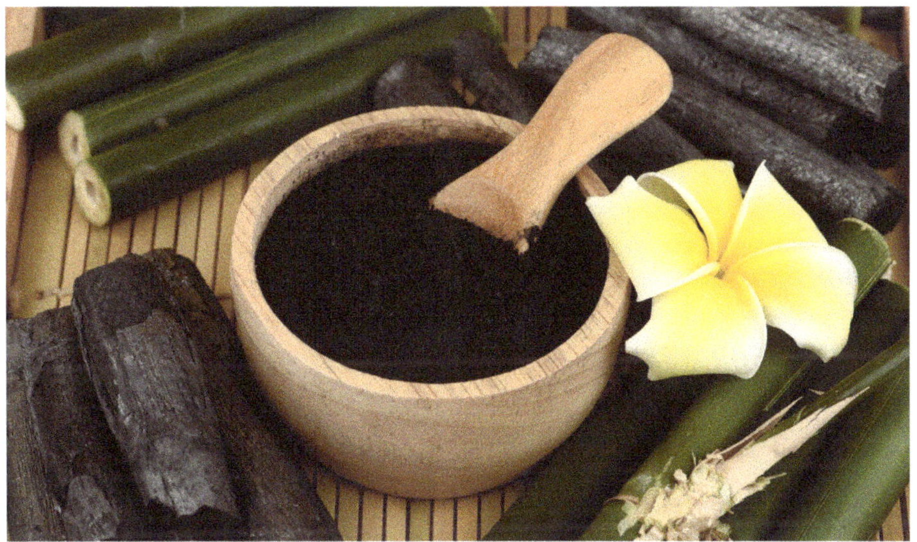

Activated charcoal used as a treatment of aerophagia. Shutterstock/wasanajai

Fart, Underwater

It is to be expected that all living creatures that pass gas on land and in the air will do so underwater as well. A large number of humans find this to be a particularly pleasurable activity as confirmed on a large Internet based survey. Of course other animals will release gas underwater as a matter of nature, although they may find it entertaining as well as humans. For more information about the sounds generated by underwater farts please see entry on fart, sound (Acoustic, auditory).

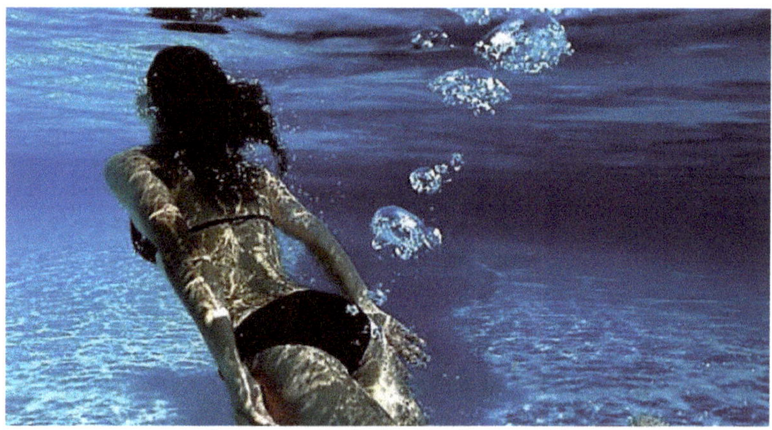

www.home-remedies.br Creative Commons License

The hippopotamus (Greek hippos-horse and potamus-river) is considered by many experts to be the most dangerous animal in Africa (excluding the malaria carrying mosquito) having killed many more people than lions have. The hippo is extremely aggressive with its huge canine teeth and sharp incisors, has unpredictable behavior, and is fearless of humans. Most deaths occur when the victim gets between the hippo and deep water or between a mother and her calf.

Hippos weigh up to eight thousand pounds, gallop at eighteen miles per hour (twenty-nine kilometers per hour), sleep or lounge around on riverbanks and in the water most of the day, and graze on the grasslands at night. Their skin secretes sticky pinkish oil that helps protect them from the sun. They defecate generous amounts of excrement into the rivers and ponds in which they wallow all day, punctuated by voluminous farts.

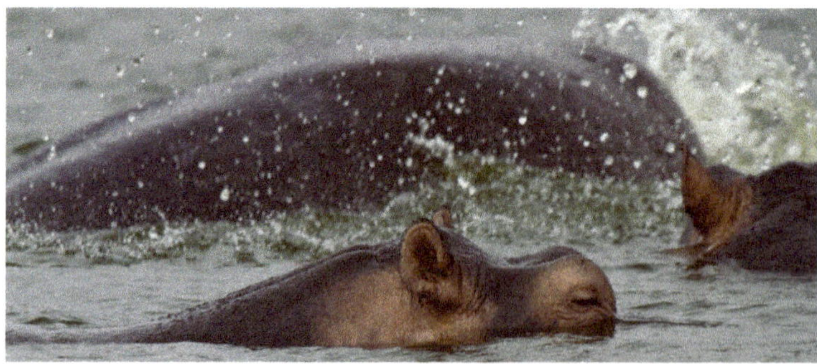

white-voodoo.deviantart.com Creative Commons License

They also participate in marking territory by what the hippo experts refer to as "dung showering." They blow feces mixed with urine over a large area around their watering hole, twirling their relatively short tails like fans to distribute the aromatic spray.

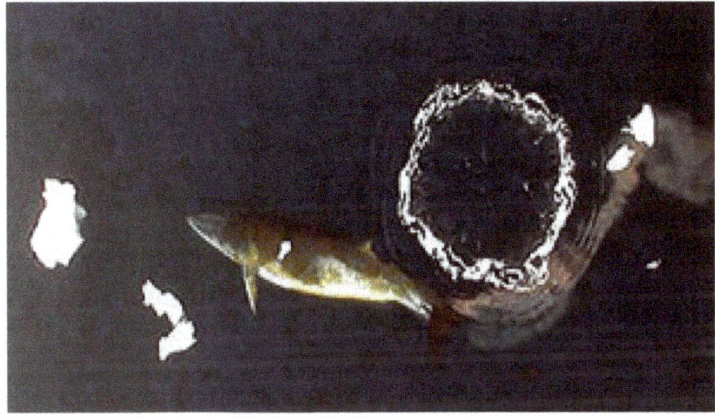

Marine research scientists studying the Minke whale population near Antarctica were able to capture a whale fart on film for the first time. The photograph was taken from the bow of the research vessel and the fart subsequently surfaced right under their noses. "We got away from the bow of the ship very quickly ... it does stink," said Nick Gales, a research scientist from the Australian Antarctic Division. However, the skunk like episode did not detract them from completing their mission of collecting DNA from whale dung and attaching satellite tracking devices to the whales to study their migration patterns.

Many fish have a swim air bladder that is inflated or deflated as needed to maintain buoyancy. Usually expelled swim air bladder gas exits the mouth but the sand tiger shark, *Carcharias taurus*, discharges it out the anus. The carbon dioxide produced is eliminated via the gills. Methane, hydrogen, and other gasses would typically be released as a fart. Fisherman knew about herring farts and they were even written about back in 1914 by Swedish author Ludvig Runebergwrote in his masterpiece Bottenhavsfiskare (Bothnian Bay Fishermen). The section below is freely translated from the Swedish.

"In the evening they were rowing away to the barren islands, pulled up the boats, lit a fire and made coffee, opened the dinner box and ate. While they were sitting there a group of fishermen were staring out towards the sea, the sun sinking, the sky turning red, and the waves smoothing, wind dying, moon sailing out, lonely and large, the ducks moving back and forth in trains, and in all this, which no longer looked like the earth but more seemed to be an advection into the sky, a distant boiling was seen on the blank water surface. Thousands and thousands of small blisters glaring into the sea, without it being possible to say wherefrom they came, and only in one small defined place: it was the herring which was approaching them on its migration."

Fart, Vagina

Fart is also a term used for an emission or expulsion of air from the vagina. It may occur during or after sexual intercourse or during other sexual acts, stretching, exercise, getting up from a chair, etcetera. Puffs or small amounts of air passed into the vaginal cavity during cunnilingus are normally not associated with vaginal fart. However, "forcing" or purposely blowing air at force into the vaginal canal can cause an air embolism which is dangerous for the woman, and if pregnant for the fetus.

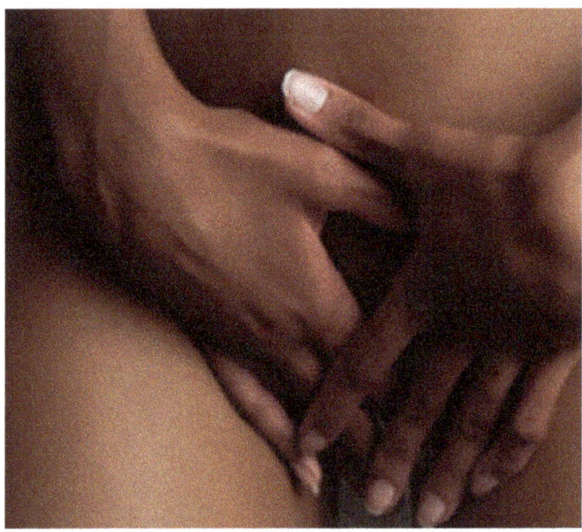

i9.photobucket.com Creative Commons License

The sound of flatus from the vagina is somewhat comparable to flatulence from the anus but does not have a feculent odor in the normal state. If a feculent odor is present it may be because of a colovaginal fistula, a serious condition involving a tear between the vagina and colon. A colovaginal fistula can result from surgery, childbirth, diseases such as the inflammatory bowel disease Crohn disease, trauma such as rape and sexual abuse, infections, and other causes. This condition can lead to urinary tract infection and other complications. Slang terms for vaginal flatulence include *vart, queef* and *fanny fart* (mostly British).

Fart, Visual

It may sound hard to visualize a fart, but it is actually fairly simple, it's that the circumstances have to be just right. Yes, in releasing an invisible gas into invisible air you would normally not expect to see it with the limited visual spectrum of the human eye. However if you had vision in the infrared portion of the electromagnetic spectrum it would be very visible. With the advent of infrared photography and thermographic imagery the invisible fart can be visualized.

You can also see the fart if the temperature and humidity are just right. If you were in the polar zones, at very high altitude, in frigid weather, or even in a walk-in freezer, dropping a fart from exposed buttocks would look much like the steamy cloud of warm breath on a cold winter day. One should be careful about trying this when it is dangerously frigid as frostbite of this sensitive part of the anatomy may result in a new medical malady, which I hereby name 'frostbutt'.

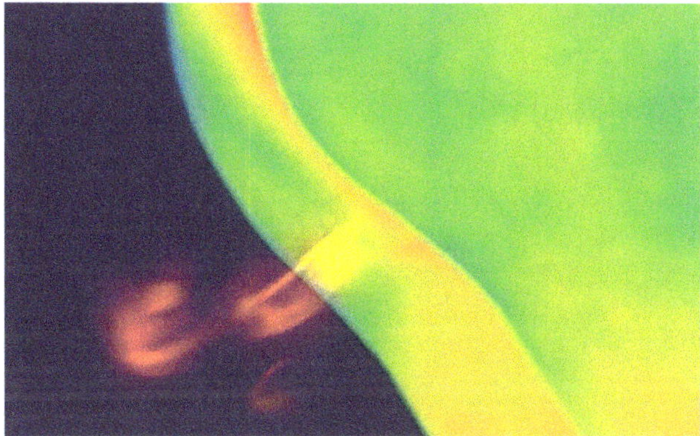

i.telegraph.co.uk

Frostbite is a real risk for mountaineers, and for Mount Everest climbers the comforts of base camp at an altitude of 17,590 feet may be the last chance they have for a protected bowel movement without exposing their behinds to the extreme winds and weather approaching the summit. Frozen poop stays permanently frozen and does not decompose at that altitude, so there is a growing collection from earlier expeditions that is of concern. Climbers are having a more challenging timed finding ice that has not been contaminated for melting into drinking water. Drinking contaminated water and developing diarrhea at that high altitude and hostile environment would increase the exposure to frostbite dramatically.

The most visible of the visual farts occur in the bathtub or when immersed in water, like a swimming pool or hot whirlpool tub. If you are sharing the water with someone else the innocent looking telltale bubbles underwater can deliver a powerful bouquet to the unsuspecting nose. The intensity of the olfactory message of the human sense of smell is modulated by the brain and limbic system. If you are in a bathroom having a bowel movement the fart odor is less noticeable and certainly less alarming then when you are in an elevator, theater, or restaurant, and you are aromatically assaulted without forewarning.

Fart, Volume (Quantity)

The fact is that all living creatures create gas from the cellular respiration, which is ubiquitous through various life forms. The bacteria in your intestinal flora generate microscopic nanofarts and microfarts, which collect into larger bubbles of gas in the bowel. They are intermixed with the atmospheric air swallowed throughout the day and particularly at meals, when chewing gum, or when chewing or smoking tobacco or other recreational products. Aerophagia is universal and we swallow on average three to five milliliters (one teaspoonful) of air with every swallow. Now add into the mixture the gasses produced during the enzymatic digestive processes as well as the neutralization of gastric hydrochloric acid and pancreatic and duodenal bicarbonate and you have a virtual windstorm of voluminous gasses transiting the bowel.

Fortunately, the vast majority of the gasses produced are absorbed by the gut, then dissolve into the bloodstream through diffusion and as a solution, finally being exhaled when they reach the alveoli of the lungs and can be exchanged with atmospheric air. The component gasses have very different properties of diffusion through the bowel wall and into the bloodstream. Carbon dioxide readily diffuses and enters solution and is exhaled, such that although it is the largest volume of gas generated by far, and temporarily is a major contributor to distension and postprandial (after meal) discomfort, it is the easiest to eliminate from the bowel and is only a minor contributor to flatulence.

Nitrogen is the largest volume component of atmospheric air, and as would be expected, represents an identically high proportion of the gasses swallowed through aerophagia. Once in the body the carbon dioxide of the air is absorbed and eliminated as discussed above. The nitrogen however is a very poorly absorbed gas, and in essence will either come back up as a burp, or will sooner or later, comes out the other end as a fart.

The oxygen in the air, representing nearly twenty-one percent of the air gasses swallowed during aerophagia, is absorbed slowly, as the gut is not nearly as efficient at absorbing oxygen as the lungs are for respiration. As the carbon dioxide and oxygen are absorbed the percent of the gastrointestinal tract air that is nitrogen increases. As soon as the digestive process begins, hydrochloric acid of the stomach is neutralized by sodium bicarbonate of the duodenum and pancreas. Large volumes of carbon dioxide gas are generated, as are smaller quantities of hydrogen, methane, and other aromatic gasses discussed later. The volume of gasses in the gastrointestinal tract is dependent on the quantity and nature of foods ingested, the body's ability to synthesize and utilize specific enzymes for the various food types, the nature and quantity of the bacteria in the gut flora, the speed of gastrointestinal transit which may be influenced by drugs, hormones, food product and illness, the absorptive capacity and health of the mucosal lining, and the physical length of the individual's gastrointestinal tract.

The question of what is the average number of farts per day is similar to the question if what is an average price for a normal used car. What year, make, model, condition, diesel or gas or electric or hybrid, mileage, etc. etc. The quoted figure of eleven and one-half farts per day is a reasonable approximation from a very small sample size of male medical students, but normal has a very wide range depending on the variables. The female medical students were too smart to participate in the study so as far as science is concerned, women do not fart. Later suggestions that they fart, but less than the guys, is just as suspect.
The differences in the physical attributes between male and female of a species represent their sexual dimorphism. The theory of sexual selection advanced by Charles Darwin in 1871 is closely related to sexual dimorphism. On average adult human males are four percent taller and eight percent heavier than females. In a number of other species it is the female that is larger, occasionally dramatically so.

The triple wart sea devil, an anglerfish, exhibits extreme sexual dimorphism, with the male becoming little more than a stunted sperm-producing body that lives a parasitic existence off of the females hard work and effort in providing livelihood and producing the next generation of offspring. Some human males appear to have evolved their behavioral patterns from the anglerfish modus operandi.
In most mammals, humans included, the males are larger in size, mass, and caloric intake. In most species it is the female that is diminutive in size, sometimes dramatically so. It would only make sense that males would generate more gas, but how do the two compare if the caloric intake and composition were identical? Since there are no identically comparable cases, the studies would have to compare averages of large populations of each gender to minimize the variables as much as possible.

As curious as we may be to know the answer to this question vital to gender politics and security, no studies are planned or anticipated. There have been reports of extreme flatulence in the medical literature of what may be considered the upper limits of the normal range, up to one hundred and fifty farts in a twenty-four hour period. There are probably more accurate reports of what is the upper limit of spousal tolerance in divorce court proceedings and depositions. So for general health we talk about achieving our target heart rate during exercise. Is there an equivalent for a target fart rate? For harmonious relationships ideal would be below the quoted figure of eleven and one-half farts per day, that way you could reasonably suggest that you fart less than average. You could also argue that the twenty-three farts you passed were each only a half-fart so you still are within the normal range.

As we age we produce less digestive enzymes and there is an argument to be made that there should be an adjustment and tolerance allowed for 'old farts'. The sheer number of variables allow 101+ explanations for why you fart much less than expected for your given circumstances. But perhaps the best excuse is that you did not do anything, it's the billions of nanofarting and microfarting bacteria that are to blame. If you are told to pick on someone closer to your own size you could blame the dog and claim it is a talented ventrilo-farter. Trying to arrive at a definition of what constitutes a discrete individual fart is a challenge worthy of drafting and approving a United Nations resolution. Is a staccato stutter of ten small farts completed in rapid succession to count as one or ten? Is one large long loud fart the equivalent of four small farts over thirty seconds. Should a loud tuba blast count the same as a faint toot?

Fart, Weight

As a fart is composed of atoms and molecules it has physical properties, including a mass and weight. Since it is composed of gasses and volatile molecules it is very light, yet the weight is measureable. In addition, each fart carries a sampling of the gut microbiome, aerosolized microbes the significance of which has never been evaluated in terms of potential for disease transmission. Each person's microbiome and thus fart is unique, much like fingerprints, although don't expect it to be used for personal identification on a television forensic science drama anytime soon. The total mass of the average fart is 0.0371 grams. For those wishing to lose weight every fart means you weigh just a little bit less. The constituent gasses and mass of the average fart is listed below:

Nitrogen: 0.0263 grams
Hydrogen: 0.0003 grams
Carbon Dioxide: 0.0063 grams
Methane: 0.0018 grams
Oxygen: 0.0016 grams
Odiferous Products: 0.0008 grams

Fecal Microbiota Transplant

A Fecal Microbiota Transplant (FMT) is also known as a stool transplant, fecal transplant, fecal bacteriotherapy, fecal transfusion, fecal enema, human probiotic infusion, and in its most ancient form of oral administration as coprophagia. One of the side effects of taking antibiotics is that they not only eliminate the harmful pathogenic microorganisms, but they also harm the normal commensal microbiome. When the balance of the microbiome is disrupted, an organism named *Clostridia difficile* may predominate the gut microbiome with horrific and life threatening consequences. This condition is known as antibiotic associated colitis, and is also known as pseudomembranous colitis. It results in severe and often intractable diarrhea. For many years, the treatment required multiple and prolonged course of ever stronger antibiotics, which all too often failed to eradicate the infection and led to relapses.

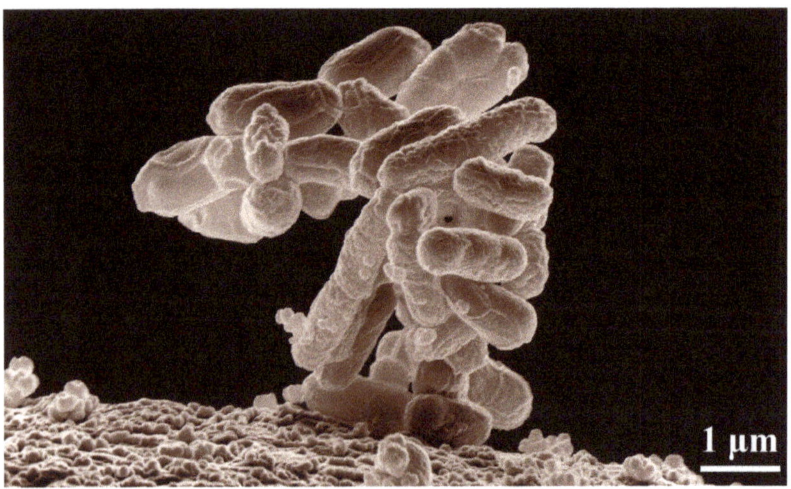

Low-temperature electron micrograph of a cluster of E. coli bacteria, magnified ten thousand times. Each individual bacterium is oblong shaped. 2005 Photo by Eric Erbe Public Domain

The alternative approach of transplanting feces from a healthy donor into the bowel of the patient with antibiotic associated colitis courses was initially perceived as counterintuitive, if not offensive to the sensibilities of modern medicine and the Western ethic of hygiene. The fact that the treatment is remarkably effective, and much safer and less expensive that intensive antibiotic therapy, surprisingly did not result in its rapid adoption. A lack of understanding on both the part of the public, as well as the medical industrial complex, brought fecal transplantation into the crosshairs of regulators and industry. Instead of recognition and accolades of the heroic status of fecal donors and establishment of national Brown Cross donation centers and stool banks, the Food and Drug Administration attempted to regulate the procedure into the realm of multi-year and multi-billion dollar research studies within academia and industry.

Fecal transplantation is becoming more established, not only as the treatment of choice for antibiotic associated colitis from *Clostridia difficile,* but is being investigated for its reported benefits in a whole host of digestive disorders such as inflammatory bowel disease (ulcerative colitis, Crohn Disease), irritable bowel syndrome, leaky gut, constipation, and other non-digestive conditions such as arthritis, cancer, heart disease, multiple sclerosis, Parkinson Disease, autism, metabolic syndrome, diabetes, autoimmune disorders, obesity, etc. The role of the gut microbiome is an area of intense research interest, and preliminary research data suggests it will revolutionize our understanding of disease and treatment.

With further progress in understanding the optimal gut microbiome for an individual, the future of repopulating the gut with a healthy microbiome to treat and prevent disease will advance. Rather than the relatively crude approach of transplanting the feces of a healthy donor, the gut microbiome will be repopulated (repoopulated is a popular pun in the fecal transplant world) with a scientifically designed and formulated culture with the proper mixture and proportion of desired microbes. With the nature of the biomedical industry, one can envision specific patents and branding of gut microbiome cocktails for specific diseases, conditions, and desired outcomes.

The administration of fecal transplants will also expand beyond colonics, enemas, nasogastric tubes, and high tech and expensive administration via colonoscopy or endoscopy. Freeze dried, purified, healthy microbiome probiotics in sealed odorless tasteless sterile time released capsules with reduce the less than appealing stigma of a fecal transplant. Undoubtedly, even the terminology will be adapted to appeal to modern sensibilities. Perhaps Super Microbiome Supplementation will reach the level of popularity of protein supplements in nutritious organic fruit and vegetable juice blends!

Interestingly enough, fecal transplants were part of the armamentarium of ancient medicine from the days of Ayurveda, Chinese Medicine, and beyond. Bedouins have used consumption of fresh, warm camel feces as a remedy for bacterial dysentery for ages. Its efficacy may attributable to the antibiotic subtilisin from *Bacillus subtilis* or the wholesale substitution of the gut flora. German soldiers in Africa confirmed the effectiveness of the camel feces during World War II to whom it was administered when they had dysentery. Another possibility is that a number of the 'cured' did not get better but refused to admit it in order to avoid another dose of a 'medicine' that literally tasted like shit.

Fecal Oral Contamination Route (see Pathogen)

Fecal oral route (fecal oral contamination) is the transmission of a disease pathogen via feces particles that are ingested by the now infected host. The process of transmission may be by gross contamination as described by the term coprophagia, but much more often the transmission is less visible or microscopic (although it technically remains coprophagia). Examples may include a scenario where a fly that had been feeding on feces lands and feeds on open food at a picnic, which it contaminates by the feces residue on its feet. Swimming in a pool that had an undisclosed recent toddler 'accident'. Poor hand washing after a bowel movement with less than perfect toilet paper wiping, then eating finger foods such as potato chips or popcorn from a common bowl.

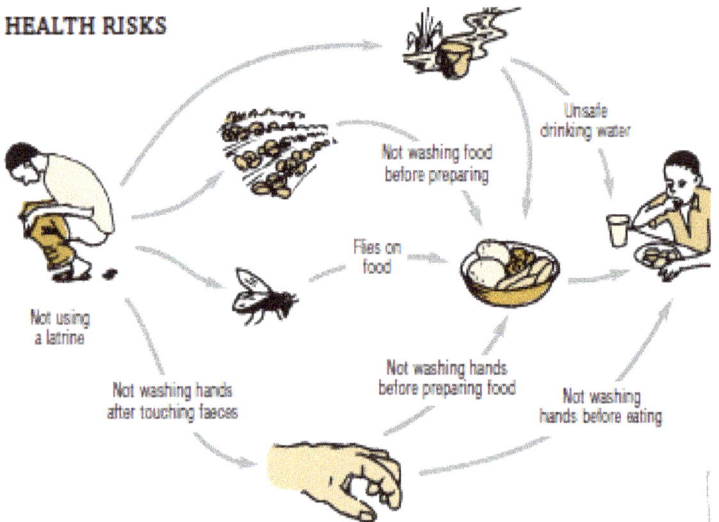

The degree of fecal oral contamination that takes place on a daily basis in even the most sophisticated and highest levels of socioeconomic achievement are sobering. An illness that is easily transmitted by purely fecal oral contamination will infect nearly all members of any closely living household within a matter of days. The number of infectious particles we are exposed to each and every day is astronomical. Rotavirus is transmitted by the fecal oral route and is the most common cause of severe diarrhea among infants and young children. Nearly every child in the world has been infected with rotavirus at least once by the age of five. If is estimated to cause about forty per cent of all hospital admissions due to diarrhea among children under five years of age worldwide, leading to one hundred million episodes of acute diarrhea that result in three hundred and fifty thousand to six hundred thousand child deaths each year.

The number of infectious viral particles in one gram (less than one thirtieth of an ounce) of feces from a child with rotavirus is more than ten trillion (10,000,000,000,000). One child in a household has more than enough viral particles in a thimble of stool to infect every human on the planet Earth and another ten thousand planets with the same population. Some of the diseases that can be passed via the fecal-oral route include poliomyelitis, norovirus acute gastroenteritis, giardiasis, hepatitis A, hepatitis E, rotavirus, shigellosis (bacillary dysentery), typhoid fever, *Vibrio parahaemolyticus* infections, enteroviruses, cholera, clostridium difficile, cryptosporidiosis, ascariasis, and many others.

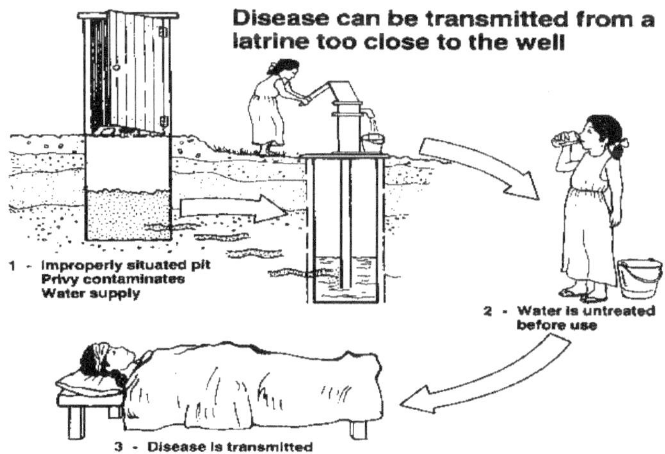
Disease can be transmitted from a latrine too close to the well
1 - Improperly situated pit Privy contaminates Water supply
2 - Water is untreated before use
3 - Disease is transmitted

Feces

Feces (Latin fæx "dregs") (excrement, shit, turd, and dozens of other euphemisms) are the excreted waste product from the digestive tract expelled through the anus during defecation. Although the digestive tract has extracted nutrients the fecal matter often has fifty percent of its energy value remaining. This is a vital resource for organisms such as bacteria, fungi, and insects such as the fly and dung beetle. Human fecal matter varies significantly in appearance, depending on diet and health. A sticky gummy texture is often noted with substantial internal bleeding, which also often presents as black tarry stool called melena.

Brown Stool - Human feces ordinarily has a light to dark brown coloration, which results from a combination of bile and bilirubin that is derived from the breakdown products of dead red blood cells.

Yellow Stool - Stool that is yellow may suggest presence of undigested fat in the stool. The stool containing the undigested fat may appear yellowish in color, greasy, and also may smell foul. Yellowing of feces may also be caused by an infection that may also cause diarrhea, such as from *Giardia lamblia* a protozoan parasite.

Black Stool (Melena) - Feces can be black due to the presence of red blood cells that have been broken down by digestive enzymes. This is known as melena, and is typically due to bleeding in the upper digestive tract, such as from a bleeding peptic ulcer. The same color change can be observed after consuming foods that contain a substantial proportion of animal blood, such as black pudding or tiết canh.

Black feces can also be caused by a number of medications containing bismuth products (such as Pepto-Bismol and the newer formulation of Kaopectate in the United States), iron supplements, or foods such as beetroot, black liquorice (also spelled as licorice), or blueberries.

Red Stool - Hematochezia is similarly the passage of feces that are bright red due to the presence of undigested blood, either from lower in the digestive tract, or from a more active source in the upper digestive tract. Ingestion of red beets will also color the stool and can be easily misinterpreted as a sign of internal bleeding. Besides the dramatic blood red color of beets, a similar red color may also come from natural or artificial coloring such as red gelatin, popsicles, Kool-Aid, and dragon fruit.

Blue Stool - Prussian blue, used in the treatment of radiation, cesium, and thallium poisoning, can turn the feces blue. Substantial consumption of products containing blue food dye, such as blue curaçao or grape soda, can have a similar effect.

White (Acholic) Stool - Acholic stools, which are pasty white in color, are characteristic of complete biliary obstruction.

Silver Stool - Silver or aluminum feces color results when biliary obstruction of any type (acholic or white stool) combines with gastrointestinal bleeding from any source that would normally present as black stools or melena

Green Stool - Feces can be green due to having large amounts of unprocessed bile in the digestive tract. When stool passes through the intestines rapidly (diarrhea) there may be little time for bilirubin to undergo its usual chemical changes. Green feces may occasionally be the result from eating liquorice (also spelled as licorice) candy, as it is typically made with anise oil rather than liquorice herb and is predominantly sugar. Excessive sugar consumption or a sensitivity to anise oil may cause loose, green stools.

When a pediatric colleague was in medical school a professor was quizzing the medical students about the significance of different colored stools. The group was asked what question they would ask if a young lady patient told them she was passing golden stools. My friend Dick Buchta told me this story in the presence of his wife Diane so he assured us it was a different medical student, not him, who quickly responded with the question that should be asked: Will you marry me?

Feces are often used as fertilizer, both manure and guano becoming large commercial enterprises. Historically, human waste euphemistically called night soil was used as a major source of fertilizer. Animal feces, especially those of camel, bison, oxen, yak, water buffalo, and cattle can be used as fuel or building material when dried. Terms such as dung, scat, spoor, manure, castings, spraint, fewmets, guano, and droppings are used to refer to specific animal feces.

Common animal dropping (scat) names are:

cattle - tath
otter -spraints
cow - bodewash, cowpies, buffalo chips, dung, cow pats
seafowl - guano,
earthworm - wormcast
dinosaur - coprolite
Hart and deer - fewmets
hare - crotiles, crotisings
boar, bear, and wolf - lesses
fox - billitting
vermin - fuants;
hawk – mutes
dog - scumber
caterpillars and leaf beetles – frass
horse – manure, roadapple
wild carnivores - scat

Feces Waste Management

Feces waste management has been a concern from pre-Biblical times:
"And thou shalt have a paddle upon thy weapon; and it shall be, when thou wilt ease thyself abroad, thou shalt dig therewith, and shalt turn back and cover that which cometh from thee: For the LORD thy God walketh in the midst of thy camp, to deliver thee, and to give up thine enemies before thee; therefore shall they camp be holy: that he see no unclean thing in thee, and turn away from thee." (Deuteronomy 23:13-14).

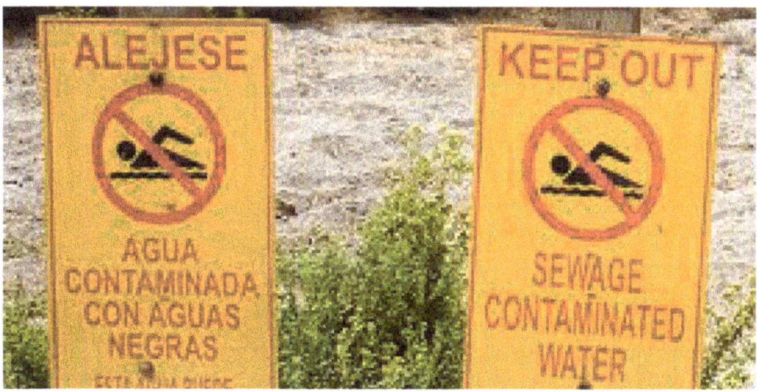

Composting Toilet

A composting toilet is a dry toilet that uses managed aerobic decomposition to treat human waste. They are an alternative to flush toilets where there is a limited water supply or no waste treatment facility is available. The human excrement is normally mixed with sawdust, coconut coir, or peat moss to support aerobic processing, absorb liquids, and to reduce odor. The decomposition process is typically faster than the anaerobic decomposition used in wet sewage systems such as septic tanks.

Urine can contain ninety percent percent of the nitrogen, fifty percent of the phosphorus, and seventy percent of the potassium present in human excreta. In healthy individuals the urine is sterile and thus pathogen free. Undiluted urine may contain inorganic salts and organic compounds toxic to plants. The requirement critical for aerobic microbial action is sufficient oxygen. Some units require manual methods for periodic aeration of the solid mass. Significant reductions in the volume of waste occurs through the process with only ten percent of the inputs coming out as a humus-like material which can be used as a soil amendment.

Pit Toilet

A pit toilet is a dry toilet system which collects human excrement in a large container and can range from a simple slit trench to a more elaborate outhouse with a ventilation pipe. They are used in rural and wilderness areas as well as in much of the developing world. When the pit is improved with a small enclosed structure with a roof for shelter and a seat with a hole in it it is commonly known as an outhouse.

The ventilated improved pit latrine, or VIP, is a pit toilet outhouse with a ventilation pipe and a screen at the top outlet. VIP latrines are an improvement over simple pit latrines by reducing odors, flies, and mosquito nuisance and unpleasant odors. The ventilation pipe also removes the explosive danger of accumulated methane gas from the decomposition of the human waste in the pit.

Sewers

A sewage system may convey the wastewater by gravity, pumping, or vacuum to a sewage treatment plant. Pipelines range in size from six inches (one hundred and fifty millimeters) to tunnels of up to thirty feet (ten meters) in diameter. Although sewer systems are intended to transport only sewage and not storm runoff all sewer systems have some degree of infiltration of groundwater which can lead to sewer overflows.

The first sanitation system has been identified in prehistoric ruins near Zabol, Iran. The ancient cities of Harappa and Mohenjo-daro of the Indus Valley civilization developed networks of brick-lined sewers around 2600 BC and also had outdoor toilets that were flushed with water from reservoirs. Ancient Minoan civilization also had stone sewers that were flushed with water. Roman towns and garrisons in the United Kingdom between 46 BC and 400 AD had sewer networks sometimes constructed out of hollowed-out logs.

In the developed world sewers are usually pipelines from buildings to larger underground trunk mains, which transport the sewage to sewage treatment facilities. Vertical pipes, called manholes, connect the mains to the surface and are used for maintenance and to vent sewer gases. Sewers are generally gravity powered although pumping stations may be necessary. For decades sanitary sewer cracks or other damage could be repaired only by the expensive operation of digging up the damaged pipe and replacing it. In the mid-1950's technology advanced where a special cement mixture coated the inside of the pipe sealing all cracks and breaks.

Many cities built sewer systems to control outbreaks of disease such as typhoid fever and cholera. Initially these systems discharged sewage directly to surface waters such as rivers and lakes without treatment. As pollution of water bodies grew cities added sewage treatment plants to their systems to chlorinate and filter the water and sewage discharged. The institution of sewerage systems was a great public health advance.

Dung Beetle

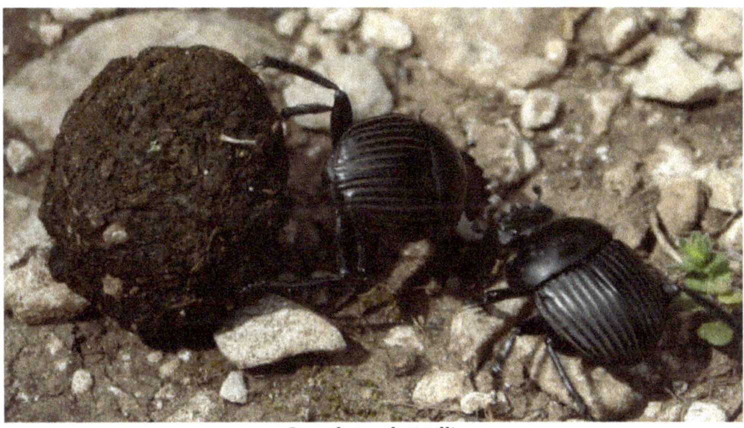

Scarabaeus laticollis

Dung beetles are beetles that feed partly or exclusively on feces. "Never did adventurers hurrying from the four corners of the earth display such eagerness," the French entomologist Jean-Henri Fabre once wrote. "They are there in the hundreds, large and small, of every sort, shape and size, hastening to carve themselves a slice of the common cake." Some grab what dung they can and cram it underground on the spot. Dung beetles have been known to steal treasured dung balls from each other. Others, the ball-rollers, embark on a journey that requires the heavens to navigate.

All the species belong to the superfamily Scarabaeoidea which alone comprises more than five thousand species. Many dung beetles, known as *rollers*, roll dung into round balls, which are used as a food source or brooding chambers. They can roll up to ten times their weight and some species can pull up to one thousand times their weight. Other dung beetles, known as *tunnelers*, bury the dung wherever they find it. A third group, the dwellers, neither roll nor burrow: they simply live in manure. Dung beetles are currently the only animal, other than humans, known to navigate and orient themselves using the Milky Way.

Dung beetles play an important role in agriculture by burying and consuming dung that improves nutrient recycling and soil structure. They also protect livestock, such as cattle, by removing the dung which, if left in the open could provide habitat for pests. Many countries have introduced the creatures for the benefit of animal husbandry and as an adjunct for improving standards of hygiene. Several species of the dung beetle, most notably the species *Scarabaeus sacer* often referred to as the sacred scarab, enjoyed a sacred status among the ancient Egyptians. The scarab was linked to Khepri ("he who has come into being") the god of the rising sun. The image of the scarab symbolizing transformation, renewal, and resurrection, is ubiquitous in ancient Egyptian religious and funerary art.

The ancients believed that the dung beetle was unique in that only the male gender existed, and that it reproduced by depositing semen into a dung ball. The supposed self-creation of the beetle resembles that of Khepri, who creates himself out of nothing. The dung ball rolled by a dung beetle resembles the sun. In ancient Greece Plutarch wrote: The race of beetles has no female, but all the males eject their sperm into a round pellet of material which they roll up by pushing it from the opposite side, just as the sun seems to turn the heavens in the direction opposite to its own course, which is from west to east.

The dung beetle has several appearances in the classical literature. In Aesop's fable *The Dung Beetle and the Eagle*, the eagle kills a hare despite the beetle's appeals. The beetle takes revenge by twice destroying the eagle's eggs. The eagle, in despair, flies up to Olympus and places her latest eggs in Zeus's lap, beseeching the god to protect them. When the beetle finds out what the eagle has done, it stuffs itself with dung, goes straight up to Zeus and flies right into his face. Zeus is startled at the sight of the unpleasant creature and jumps to his feet. The eggs are broken. Zeus then learns of the beetle's plea which the eagle had ignored. He scolds the eagle and urges the beetle to stay away from the bird. But his efforts to persuade the beetle fail; so he changes the breeding season of the eagles to take place at a time when the beetles are not above ground.

The ancient Greek playwright Aristophanes alluded to Aesop's fable several times in his plays. In *Peace*, the hero rides up to Olympus to free the goddess Peace from her prison. His steed is an enormous dung beetle which has been fed so much dung that it has grown to monstrous size. In Franz Kafka's *The Metamorphosis*, the transformed character of Gregor Samsa is called an "old dung beetle" (alter Mistkäfer) by the charwoman.

Chamber Pot

A chamber pot (French: pot de chambre) is a pit like receptacle for receiving human waste. It was usually kept in the same chambers and under the sleeping bed and since the sixteenth century often enclosed in a stool with a lid. Chamber pots were used in ancient Greece at least since the sixth century BC and remained in common use in any parts of the world until the mid-twentieth century. In rural areas lacking indoor plumbing they are still in use today. They have also been modified to serve as bedpans for the ill and disabled.

The affectionate term "potty" is often used with children especially during toilet (potty) training. The term potty is also used to describe child size chamber pot type toilets that are at the appropriate height and have a child size opening to sit on. Regular adult toilets have an opening that is too large and frightening for a child who could accidentally fall in if not assisted. The height of the adult toilet does not allow their feet to touch the ground to assist in the squatting maneuver that assists defecation. A foot stool to give their feet a place on which to rest can assist squatting which eases the initiation of a bowel movement and can accelerate toilet training.

Close (Night) Stool

A close stool, also called a necessary or night stool, was in popular use for nearly five hundred years from the sixteenth century until the advent of indoor plumbing. It was an enclosed cabinet at chair height with an opening in the top often covered by a lid. It contained a pewter or earthenware chamber pot. In the nineteenth century it was referred to as a night commode, and in the twentieth century the commode euphemism was extended to the flush toilet.

Gong Farmer

Gong farmer was a term used in Tudor England for the worker who removed human excrement from outhouses, privies, cesspools, and cesspits. "Gong" is derived from the Old English gang, which means "to go", and since the eleventh century has been used to refer to a toilet facility, or privy, and its contents. They were only allowed to work at night and later became known as "night soil men" or "night men". The human feces they collected was known as night soil and was used as fertilizer. The emptying of cesspits today is usually accomplished with mechanical suction, by specialized tankers or trucks referred to by the euphemism Honey Truck.

Towns usually provided public latrines, known as houses of easement. Cesspits were often placed under cellar floors some of which had wooden chutes to convey the excrement. Cesspits allowed the liquid waste to drain leaving only the solids.

Besides the offensive odor cesspits were a continual problem as the accumulation of solid waste required the services of gong farmers to dig out and remove the excrement. Perhaps to avoid overfilling their cesspit it was not uncommon for the contents of chamber pots to be thrown into the streets from upstairs windows.

Despite being well paid being a gong farmer's job was not considered an enviable occupation. They were only allowed to work between nine in the morning and five in the evening and were permitted to live only in certain areas. Besides the occupational hazard of infectious diseases, the concentrations of noxious and toxic gasses sometimes led to asphyxiation. Gong farmers often employed young boys to fill and lift buckets of excrement out of the pit because of the confined spaces. The excavated solid waste was removed in large barrels which were loaded onto a horse-drawn cart called the honey cart or wagon. It was not an infrequent event to discover the corpse of an unwanted infant during the clearing of cesspits.

The job is still commonplace in India where it has estimated that up to one million and three hundred thousand Indians work with the collection of human waste. These workers are considered the lowest of the untouchable caste. They confine marriage to within its members leading to a waste collecting caste passing the profession and caste burden on to the next generation. The recent film *Slumdog Millionaire* showed a brief glimpse of their existence.

Honey Bucket & Honey Wagon

A honey bucket is a bucket that is used as a toilet in locations that do not have more advanced facilities available. It often has a frame with a toilet seat lid and may be lined with a plastic bag for ease and convenience of disposal. A cover material such as sawdust may be used to reduce the odors from collected waste. Honey buckets are common in the far northern Arctic type climates especially where permafrost makes the installation of septic systems or outhouses impractical. They are seen throughout the world, especially in rural and undeveloped areas.

A honey wagon is a cart, wagon or truck for collecting and carrying excrement or manure. The term is often applied to the trucks that service septic tank systems as well as the bathroom on commercial aircraft. A recent news incident of a motor home bungled burglary of the siphoning of gasoline was reminiscent of a honeywagon. The police were called to investigate what was presumed to be an attempt to steal the gasoline from a parked vacation motor home. They found several empty gasoline transport containers, a length of rubber tubing, a pool of fecal material and vomited food.

The nighttime would be fuel thieves opened the flap door, removed the cap, and put the siphon hose in an applied oral suction to start the flow of what they assumes would be gasoline. The thieves opened the cap and valve to the septic system by mistake, got a mouthful of sewage which they vomited up and fled the scene leaving their paraphernalia behind.

Night Soil

Night soil is the common name used for human fecal waste collected at night from cesspools and outhouses. It is often used as a fertilizer in developing countries where it contributes to risk of acquiring parasites because the feces may contain eggs, such as is commonly seen in the roundworm *Ascaris lumbricoides*. Rarely, diseases have been transmitted into developed countries by the importation of vegetables with contaminated soil.

The use of night soil as fertilizer was common in Japan. The feces of rich people were sold at higher prices because their diet was better and it was thought that there would be more nutrients remaining in their waste. It brings a new level of understanding to the common phrases "filthy rich" and the "rich get richer". It could also serve as a learning and teaching model for salespeople in a competitive business to recognize that the salesperson who sold the shit of the rich at a higher price was the ultimate salesperson and marketer who could sell anything and would be a valuable addition to any company's sales force.

Selling night soil as fertilizers became less common after World War II for sanitary reasons as well as the increased availability of chemical fertilizers. Modern Japan still has some areas with ongoing traditional night soil collection and disposal. The Japanese name for the 'outhouse within the house' style toilet, with the night soil collected, is Kumitori Benjo (汲み取り便所). China, Singapore, and Hong Kong also had extensive use of night soil collection, especially from urbanized areas where open honey buckets were carried through the streets. Hong Kong has a euphemism called 倒夜香, which literally means "pour night fragrant".

Septage

The partially treated waste in a septic tank that does not drain into the soil or is decomposed by the bacteria in the tank is called septage. This term should not be confused by a septuagenarian who in their seventies may occasionally feel like a septagegenarian. It can be transported to local waste water treatment centers or stored to be used as fertilizer.

The septage in a septic tank is usually considered in one of three categories. Scum which floats to the top generally harbors the greatest concentration of bacteria. The layer below is called the effluent and is a semi-treated liquid. The layer of solids at the bottom of the tank is called sludge, or more descriptively as fecal sludge. The sludge accumulates over time and dependent on the number and volume of deposits and usage as well as the septic tank capacity, may function for many years of use before requiring emptying or service. An overflowing or backed up septage system is not a pleasant experience. A septage pump truck removes the septage material from septic tanks, portable toilets, recreational vehicles such as motor homes, and boats. In commercial aviation and other industries, this type of vehicle may also be called a honey wagon.

Outhouse

Many outhouses are simply holes in the ground, once the capacity is reached a new site selected and the outhouse structure moved. Keeping the waste site away from the source of drinking water important from a disease prevention and hygiene perspective. Many of the deaths attributed to military campaigns were actually caused by poor sanitation and waste management. The lack of hygiene and contaminated drinking water frequently led to more death and incapacitation of soldiers than those injured or killed in battles.

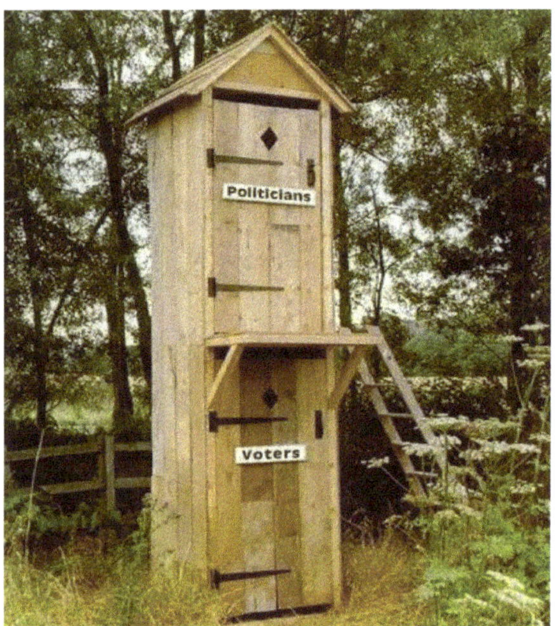

A two story outhouse with a political satire message.

I have been in locations with primitive toilet facilities, but had the most unusual experience in a very old three story building in Egypt. Much like in modern times the bathrooms were stacked directly over each other for ease of plumbing and drains. When this building was built the bathroom was a simple room with a hole in the ground, with lined up holes in the floors of the levels above. If you were using the ground floor hole as bathroom you had to make sure that you could see skylight through the holes above. If any of the floor holes above was eclipsed by a human moon, better get out of the way because sewage is about to be deposited!

Deities associated with defecation and elimination have an ancient history preceding Babylonian times. They were worshipped in Roman times and still have a role in folk beliefs of indigenous peoples of Japan, China, New Zealand and other parts of the world. Such deities have been associated with bowel health, general well-being, and fertility because of the use of human waste as a fertilizer for agriculture.

Ancient Rome had three gods involved in the passage of human waste. The sewer goddess Cloacina (Latin sewer) had her origins in Etruscan beliefs and was the protectors of the Cloaca Maxima, Rome's sewage system. Titus Tatius, who ruled early Rome with Romulus, built a shrine to her in his toilet and she was appealed to if sewers backed up. She was also the Goddess protector of sexual intercourse in marriage and her worship was later combined with that of Venus. Her image was placed on Roman coins.

Crepitus was described as the Roman god of flatulence but probably was a fiction created to denigrate Roman theology. He appears as a god in several works of French literature by Voltaire, Baudelaire, and Flaubert as well as material promoting Roman Catholicism as the true faith. Stercutius (Latin stercus 'excrement') was the god of dung who was particularly important to farmers when fertilizing their fields with manure. Worshipping the porcelain god, or ceramic throne, is a jocular reference to past toilet worship when heaving into the toilet bowl during vomiting.

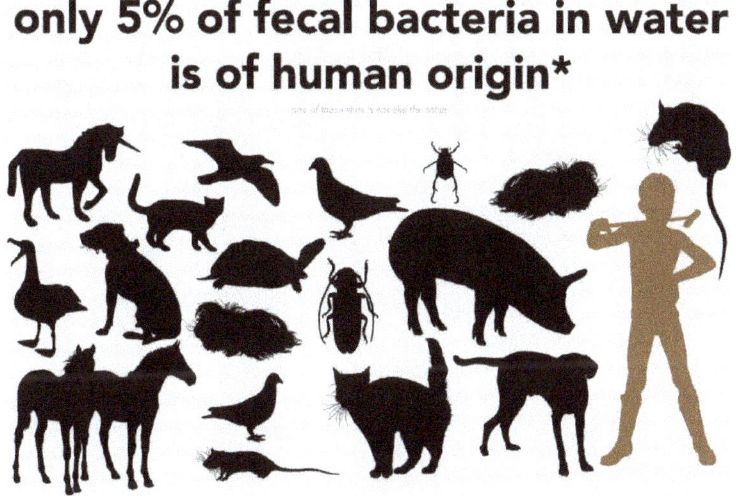

only 5% of fecal bacteria in water
is of human origin*

Continued in Volume Two

Afterword

Medicine and the life sciences are undergoing dramatic advances in knowledge and understanding. We are at the threshold of a revolutionary understanding of genomics and the microbiome, with the analogy being made that this is the equivalent of the discovery of an enormous unexplored continent. Actually this analogy is inadequate, it is more as if an entire parallel universe has been identified. This discovery is partly due to advances in technology which allow deeper exploration of the universe around us, including peering more deeply into the previously invisible microscopic and molecular worlds. Another contributing advance is the enhanced ability to communicate, a critical aspect of the collaboration that most often results in scientific breakthroughs. It is ironic and tragic that many of the lifesaving advances in science and medicine such as immunization, antibiotics, and effective therapeutics were delayed for hundreds of years, resulting in the deaths of millions, because of lapses in communication, usually because of language barriers.

Humans on Earth use six thousand five hundred different languages and 46 different alphabets. Approximately four hundred of these languages belong to the Indo-European family, which includes Greek, Latin, English, Sanskrit and many languages spoken in Europe, Iran, and the Indian subcontinent. Although they only account for seven percent of all languages, they are spoken by three billion people, nearly half the world's population. In spite of the rich tapestry of world culture, the communication challenges have contributed to a fragmented world community, hostilities, and a barrier to societal, scientific, and human achievements. The English language is the richest language on the planet with over one million words using its twenty-six character alphabet. Although English has become the dominant language in medicine and science, computers have advanced translation capabilities to become virtually universal and instantaneous. Imagine the world with one universal language and only one alphabet. Now imagine that the alphabet consists of only four main characters or letters. Welcome to the universal world of genomics, where all life forms on the planet communicate and understand this single language.

Although, for better or for worse, we consider ourselves closer relatives to the other humans on the planet than all other life forms, we actually share a deeper level of a common communication language with all living creatures on the planet. This is the language of the universal genetic code, consisting of a limited alphabet of characters that can be counted on one hand. The sequence of the acid bases, adenine, guanine, cytosine, and thymine, encodes the genetic information within genes on the double helix of deoxyribonucleic acid. The single helix of ribonucleic acid uses the nucleic acid uracil in place of thymine. The Swiss scientist Friedrich Miescher (1844-1895) discovered nucleic acids in 1869, and later proposed their possible role in heredity. Nobel Laureate Erwin Schrödinger (1887-1961) further developed the theory that heredity must be transmitted by a chemical structure found in the nucleus with a provocative publication entitled *What is Life?* Francis

Crick (1916-2004) and James Watson (1928-) identified the double helix structure of DNA based on the groundbreaking work of Rosalyn Franklin who tragically died at a young age before the Nobel Prize was awarded for the discovery.

The theory of evolution posits that all life on earth originated with a single organism, and mutations that proved beneficial for survival and reproduction eventually led to further advancement of life forms. Mutations that were not beneficial and that did not contribute to survival of the fittest were removed from the gene pool with the demise and eventual extinction of the disadvantaged species. As expected with this theory, one can trace the progress of evolution over eons and the course of present day and extinct life forms that inhabited the planet. The oldest evolutionary life forms have a genetic fingerprint of genes that have remained vital for enhanced survival, and are virtually universal in spite of otherwise significant genetic diversity. If we accept our anthropomorphic notion that humans are the highest evolutionary life form, it can be humbling that we share approximately one third of our entire genome with the most primitive of microscopic life, bacteria and Archaea. Perhaps just as humbling is that our nearest genetic relative the chimpanzee shares just under ninety-nine percent of the human genome.

One of the most startling of the scientific advances of the last generation is actually a reassessment of the consensus one hundred years ago that Charles Darwin (1809-1882) was correct in genetic inheritance, and his contemporary Jean-Baptiste Lamarck (1744-1829) was wrong in proposing that genetics can be influenced by the environment. It appears that actually they were both right dependent on different circumstances. The original belief that mapping the human genome would unlock the secrets of human health and disease was disproven with the discovery of a new field called epigenetics. This rapidly evolving science has demonstrated that the environment and external factors can determine the activity or restriction of genes. Not only the environment, but also other genes can have potent and consequential epigenetic properties. It is no longer just the human genome that is key to human health and disease, but it is also the environment and the genes and epigenetic activity of all of the nonhuman genes we are constantly exposed to.

Humans have approximately twenty-three thousand genes of which between thirty percent to ninety-eight point five percent are already shared with and interchangeable with other organisms on the planet. The trillions of organisms representing thousands of different species that live within the human microbiome, the majority within the gut microbiome, represent an exposure pool of over one million nonhuman genes. Because all genes, no matter the origin, speak a universally understood language, the instructions from a nonhuman source are not necessarily recognized by the host as being of alien origin. Of particular importance is that the universal communication has distinct advantages for the human host, and indeed its survival is dependent on these gene supplements from the microbiome.

Although pathogenic organism occurs, and can contribute to disease and mortality, the vast majority of the microbiome are commensal organisms which enhance human health and longevity. There is growing evidence that most human disease is related to a disruption of the normal healthy microbiome. Ironically, the lifesaving development of antibiotics appears to be a contributor to the disruption of the healthy microbiome, a condition called dysbiosis. Not only has antibiotic usage become profligate, but its common incorporation into the animal food supply as a growth enhancer has led to its widespread dissemination into the environment, food, water supply.

It is clear that the human microbiome, especially the gut microbiome, is dependent on the host diet. The presence of fiber in the diet is critical for microbiome health, as it is a main source of microbial nutrition, and is thus referred to as a prebiotic. Dietary changes, above and beyond prebiotics and probiotics, can lead to major changes in the microbiome, and thus human health and disease. A previously underappreciated implication of the universal communication of nonhuman genes and the human host is that humans are exposed to additional millions of genes in the diet. All food sources have their own genomes and whether plant or animal, Archaea or bacteria, virus or prion, parasite or protist, a gene of any origin can be understood by the human host, and if acted upon can change the host. The diet can play a critical, and direct role in human health and disease, both through manipulation of the microbiome as well as directly from food based genomic information.

The gut-brain axis has been known for a long time with its origins in the concept of gut instincts and gut feelings. The discovery of the extremely well developed enteric nervous system gave rise to the concept that the gut is actually a secondary or primitive brain. Surprisingly the major neurotransmitter serotonin, most often thought of in association with depression, is found to be unevenly distributed in the human body, only five percent is in the brain, ninety-five percent is in the gut. The neurotransmitter dopamine is found in equal fifty percent proportions in both the brain and the gut. The condition of Parkinson disease associated with dopamine deficiency is now believed to originate in the gut, and after many years or decades eventually affect the brain. The ability of microbes to affect the brain has been known since their discovery, especially with the recognition that infections of the brain can lead to severe symptoms, such as seen with syphilis, rabies, encephalitis, etc. The role of parasites, such as the extremely common cat protist parasite *Toxoplasma gondii* is just becoming more recognized. With the enormous domesticated cat population around the world, it is not surprising that humans may become infected directly by contact with cats and their droppings, or by ingesting undercooked foods that contain the cysts. The number of people infected because of their proximity to cats is numbered in the billions.

Although many people are impressed with cats use of a litter box and their reputation for cleanliness, the feral outdoor cat population more than compensates by leaving contaminated droppings everywhere. As far as an outdoor cat is concerned, a children's playground sandbox is just an oversized kitty litter box. When a pregnant human is exposed to Toxoplasma catastrophic and tragic infection of the fetus is all too common. It had previously been believed that only a minority of infections with Toxoplasma led to symptoms of the disease state known as toxoplasmosis. Growing evidence highlights the importance of the parasite in modulating the brain and behavior. There is growing evidence that *Toxoplasma gondii* may contribute, or perhaps even be the single causative agent in specific individuals, of mental health disorders such as depression, schizophrenia, mood disorders, hostility, psychosis, risk taking behavior and other conditions.

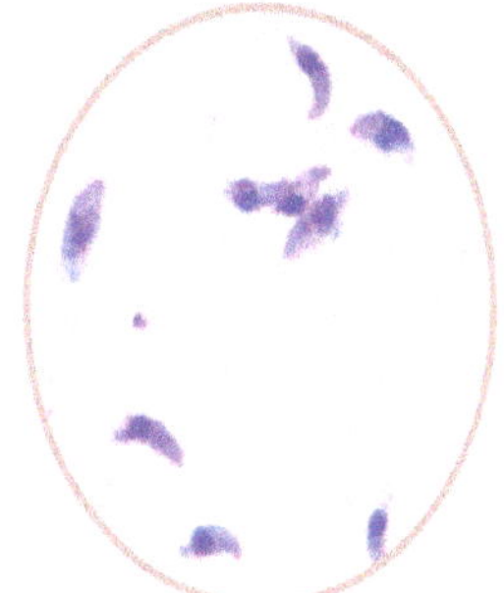

NEGLECTED PARASITIC INFECTION:
Toxoplasmosis
Toxoplasmosis is the 2nd leading cause of death from foodborne illness in the United States.

The effect of hormones on mood and mental function has likewise been long recognized. The ability of food, drink, tobacco, alcohol, psychoactive mushrooms and seafood, herbs, etc. to effect human mood and behavior has long been apparent. The concept of psychopharmacology was originally based on plant isolated and derived pharmaceuticals and chemicals. The most recent scientific advances suggest that depression, anxiety, Parkinson, Alzheimer, and perhaps even autism and multiple sclerosis may have gut origins related to the microbiome. Probiotics that may be beneficial in therapy for these conditions are now being classified as potential pscychobiotics. Manipulation of the microbiome is a potential approach to managing obesity and diabetes mellitus. Fecal microbiota transplants in animal models shows a reversal of obesity and mood disorders. Investigation of its utility in humans is ongoing for these conditions, after already been proven effective in managing dysbiosis due to the life threatening colitis caused by the antibiotic resistant organism *Clostridia difficile.*

The gut-brain-microbiome-diet axis is just beginning to be fully explored and holds great promise for major advances in human health and longevity. The golden age of discovery is not in the past, but hopefully in the present and the near future. Unfortunately, medicine and the life sciences have a long history of missteps and false hopes, especially when commerce has an opportunity for financial gain. The burgeoning industry of probiotics has already exceeded forty billion dollars of revenue each year, in spite of the lack of the lack of knowledge about the optional microbiome. It is more than likely that the optimal microbiome will have to be tailored and individualized for each person based on genomics, environmental exposure, diet, and other yet to be identified variables.

The other important message to remember about the microbiome is that it is not one organism, but a community of hundreds if not thousands of distinct species that together create the optimal microbial environment. The probiotics offered in the marketplace today offer only a single or several species. The results of supplements of a single or a few species of microbes may be beneficial to a limited number of individuals who may offer well-meaning testimonials. It is just as likely that a limited number of others will have adverse reactions, and the majority will probably not notice a change one way or the other. When it comes to the probiotic marketplace it is not regulated by the Food and Drug Administration (FDA), and even if it were, that would not be a meaningful assurance of either safety or benefit. Until there is scientific validation, hopefully that will be generated over the next few years, it would be prudent to use probiotics that occur naturally in foods that have been consumed for generations. Yogurt, kefir, sauerkraut, pickles, kimchi, etc. are safer and much less expensive.

The personalized and precision medicine that is on the horizon will be a major advance. The previous concept of population based medicine based on the statistical average patient has been a poor substitute for recognizing the unique needs and requirements of the individual. Everything from selection of therapy, dosage, risks of side effects, diet, exercise, probiotics, etc. will be based on the genomics and physiology of the individual. Further advances will undoubtedly make even this most current concept outdated and obsolete. The greater the knowledge base, the more we can define effective and beneficial approaches. Although the books in this series will with time be superseded by future writings, the knowledge contained provides our current understanding and wisdom. It is the author's hope that they have provided practical and useful information in an enlightening and entertaining manner, yet encouraged an open mind that future advances may either validate or disprove and replace current concepts. With future advances all but certain, it is important to seek competent professional advice on health matters, and not rely on books and readings. It is also prudent to remember a witticism from Mark Twain (1835-1910): "Be careful about reading health books. You may die of a misprint!" With that caveat, the reader is encouraged to peruse the author's other offerings that will hopefully likewise be found to be intriguing, informative, and entertaining.

To 'Air' is Human: Everything You Ever Wanted to Know About Intestinal Gas cover everything you ever wanted to know about the burp, belch, bloat, fart, and digestive topics but were either too afraid or too embarrassed to ask. Intestinal gas has been produced and released by virtually every human who has ever lived, yet very few people have been provided with the knowledge that can offer comfort and relief. These volumes are overflowing with practical information, fascinating facts, surprising trivia, and tasteful humorous insight about this universal phenomenon. The following companion volumes may also be of interest.

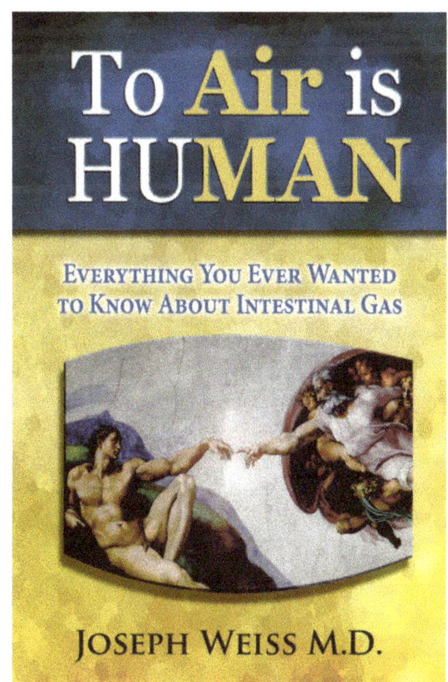

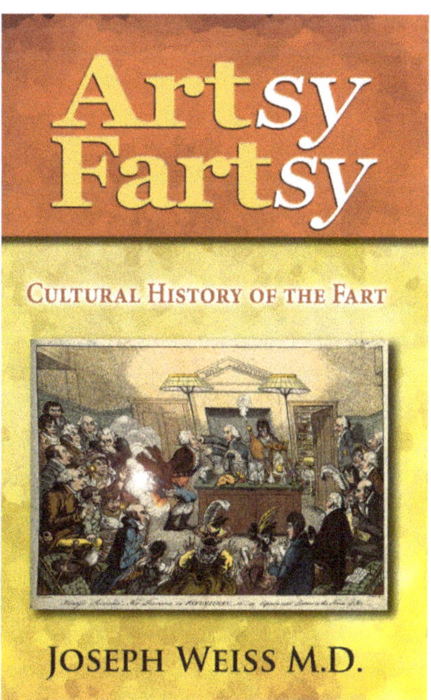

Artsy Fartsy, Cultural History of the Fart is a fascinating and factually correct review of the common fart through human culture and history. The cough, sneeze, hiccup, stomach rumble, burp, belch, and other bodily sounds simply cannot compete with the notoriety of the fart. Whether encountered live and in person or through the medium of literature, television, film, art, or music it may leave a powerful and lingering memory. The intent of the book is to demonstrate that the ubiquitous fart has a more illustrious story to share than just lowbrow humor. The societal standards and cultural acceptance of this normal physiologic event have evolved over the years, and it is currently popular as a point of humor even in sophisticated circles.

The history of the fart in culture and society is a seldom told but fascinating tale. The very same fart that has triggered wars and the deaths of thousands of innocents (see entry on Josephus Flavius) has also led to the laughter and entertainment of millions worldwide (see entry on Joseph Pujol and Cinematic Arts). Even today the response to a fart can reach from the extremes of triggering violence to inducing spasms of uncontrollable laughter. This volume is a chronological survey of some of the high and low points in the cultural history of this ubiquitous but inherently controversial activity. Rather than an exhaustive and long-winded discourse, this volume is meant to introduce the reader to the colorful and extremely varied response to the fart over the course of human history.

The Scoop on Poop, Flush with Knowledge is the equally unique volume that continues the series in a scatological vein. Digestion, genomics, gut-brain-microbiome-diet axis, and poop are just some of the important topics covered that profoundly impact human health and wellness. It provides a wealth of knowledge on the rarely told but engrossing subject of the digestive residue of the gastrointestinal tract. From potentially life-saving information to the bizarre and obscure, the book completely covers a subject many people mistakenly consider a simple waste. It is much more complex than that, and this book uncovers and airs its mysteries! The wealth of valuable information and trivia in these volumes can sustain a long social conversation, or cut it short abruptly!

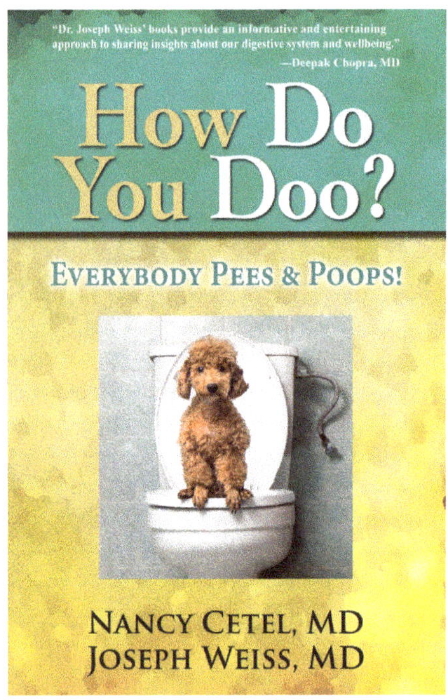

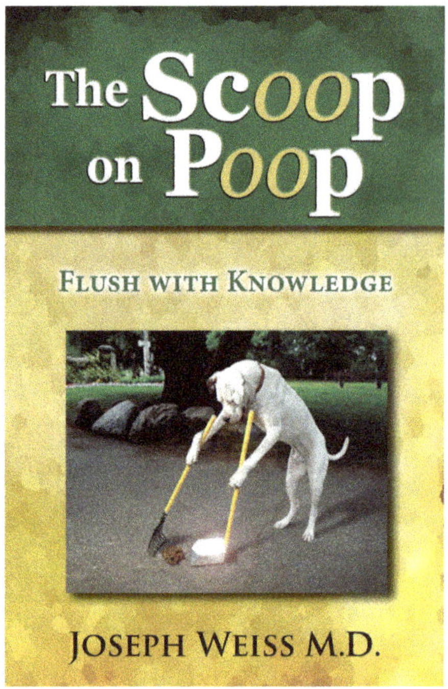

How Do You Doo? Everybody Pees & Poops! A delightfully informative, entertaining, and colorfully illustrated volume with valuable practical insights on toilet training. Tasteful color photographs of animals answering the call of nature allows the child to understand that everybody does it! Additional informative relevant content to entertain the adult while the child is 'on the potty' is included.

The Quest for Immortality, Advances in Vitality & Longevity provides an informative and enlightening overview of the remarkable advances in science and medicine that are dramatically enhancing human health and lifespan. The volume is written in clear, understandable, and engaging language with striking colorful illustrations. From groundbreaking nanotechnology to genomics and stem cells, the secrets of vitality and longevity are being uncovered along with more traditional advances and practical insights into disease prevention and health enhancement.

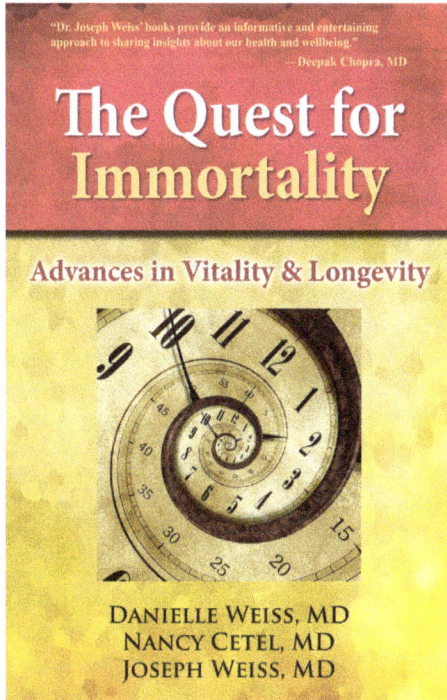

An even more comprehensive yet entertaining series are the extensive volumes of ***Digestive Health & Disease, an Illustrated Encyclopedia of Everything You Ever Wanted to Know About Digestion & Nutrition***. These volumes are a uniquely informative, entertaining, and lavishly illustrated compendium of alimentary knowledge and eccentricities. It covers everything you ever wanted to know about digestion and nutrition in health and disease. Volumes One through Five are available on Amazon.com. Organized as a reader friendly encyclopedia, the volumes cover over two thousand five hundred subject topics. Each volume may be utilized as an independent fully contained resource for the subjects it covers. The extensive size and scope of the series allows topics to be included that are rarely discussed in other books in the field and may be of great interest to the curious mind. The website www.smartaskbooks.com has a complete list of books and programs.

Index

www.ingramcontent.com/pod-product-compliance
Lightning Source LLC
Chambersburg PA
CBHW051243020426
42333CB00025B/3034

9781943760183